CLINICAL FOCUS SERIES

DISORDERS OF
THYROID

CLINICAL FOCUS SERIES

DISORDERS OF
THYROID

Series Editor
Romesh Khardori MD PhD
Professor
Division of Endocrinology and Metabolism
Eastern Virginia Medical School
Consultant
EVMS Strelitz Center for Diabetes
Endocrine and Metabolic Disorders
Norfolk, Virginia, USA

Editor
KM Prasanna Kumar MD DM
Consultant Endocrinologist
Centre for Diabetes and Endocrine Care
Former Senior Professor and Head
Department of Endocrinology
MS Ramaiah Medical College
Bengaluru, Karnataka, India

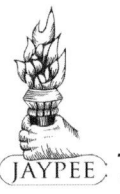

JAYPEE The Health Sciences Publisher
New Delhi | London | Panama

Jaypee Brothers Medical Publishers (P) Ltd

Headquarters
Jaypee Brothers Medical Publishers (P) Ltd
4838/24, Ansari Road, Daryaganj
New Delhi 110 002, India
Phone: +91-11-43574357
Fax: +91-11-43574314
Email: jaypee@jaypeebrothers.com

Overseas Offices

J.P. Medical Ltd
83 Victoria Street, London
SW1H 0HW (UK)
Phone: +44 20 3170 8910
Fax: +44 (0)20 3008 6180
Email: info@jpmedpub.com

Jaypee-Highlights Medical Publishers Inc
City of Knowledge, Bld. 237, Clayton
Panama City, Panama
Phone: +1 507-301-0496
Fax: +1 507-301-0499
Email: cservice@jphmedical.com

Jaypee Brothers Medical Publishers (P) Ltd
17/1-B Babar Road, Block-B, Shaymali
Mohammadpur, Dhaka-1207
Bangladesh
Mobile: +08801912003485
Email: jaypeedhaka@gmail.com

Jaypee Brothers Medical Publishers (P) Ltd
Bhotahity, Kathmandu, Nepal
Phone: +977-9741283608
Email: kathmandu@jaypeebrothers.com

Website: www.jaypeebrothers.com
Website: www.jaypeedigital.com

© 2017, Jaypee Brothers Medical Publishers

The views and opinions expressed in this book are solely those of the original contributor(s)/author(s) and do not necessarily represent those of editor(s) of the book.

All rights reserved. No part of this publication may be reproduced, stored or transmitted in any form or by any means, electronic, mechanical, photocopying, recording or otherwise, without the prior permission in writing of the publishers.

All brand names and product names used in this book are trade names, service marks, trademarks or registered trademarks of their respective owners. The publisher is not associated with any product or vendor mentioned in this book.

Medical knowledge and practice change constantly. This book is designed to provide accurate, authoritative information about the subject matter in question. However, readers are advised to check the most current information available on procedures included and check information from the manufacturer of each product to be administered, to verify the recommended dose, formula, method and duration of administration, adverse effects and contraindications. It is the responsibility of the practitioner to take all appropriate safety precautions. Neither the publisher nor the author(s)/editor(s) assume any liability for any injury and/or damage to persons or property arising from or related to use of material in this book.

This book is sold on the understanding that the publisher is not engaged in providing professional medical services. If such advice or services are required, the services of a competent medical professional should be sought.

Every effort has been made where necessary to contact holders of copyright to obtain permission to reproduce copyright material. If any have been inadvertently overlooked, the publisher will be pleased to make the necessary arrangements at the first opportunity.

Inquiries for bulk sales may be solicited at: jaypee@jaypeebrothers.com

Clinical Focus Series
Disorders of Thyroid / Romesh Khardori, KM Prasanna Kumar

First Edition: **2017**

ISBN: 978-93-5270-027-1

Printed at: Paras Offset Pvt. Ltd., New Delhi

CONTRIBUTORS

SERIES EDITOR

Romesh Khardori MD PhD
Professor
Division of Endocrinology and Metabolism
Eastern Virginia Medical School
Consultant
EVMS Strelitz Center for Diabetes
Endocrine and Metabolic Disorders
Norfolk, Virginia, USA

EDITOR

KM Prasanna Kumar MD DM
Consultant Endocrinologist
Centre for Diabetes and Endocrine Care
Former Senior Professor and Head
Department of Endocrinology
MS Ramaiah Medical College
Bengaluru, Karnataka, India

CONTRIBUTING AUTHORS

Unnikrishnan AG MD DM DNB MNAMS
CEO and Endocrinologist
Chellaram Diabetes Institute
Pune, Maharashtra, India

Rana Bhattacharjee MD DM MRCP FICP
Faculty
Department of Endocrinology
Institute of Post Graduate Medical
Education and Research
Kolkata, West Bengal, India

Subhankar Chowdhury MD DTM&H DM MRCP
Professor and Head
Department of Endocrinology and Metabolism
The Institute of Post-Graduate Medical
Education and Research and Seth Sukhlal
Karnani Memorial Hospital
Kolkata, West Bengal, India

Partha P Chakraborty MD DNB DM
Assistant Professor
Department of Medicine
Midnapore Medical College and Hospital
Midnapore, West Bengal, India

Vaibhav V Dukle MD
Senior Resident
Department of Endocrinology
CARE Hospital
Hyderabad, Telangana, India

Sujoy Ghosh DM FRCP FACE
Associate Professor
Department of Endocrinology
Institute of Post Graduate Medical
Education and Research
Kolkata, West Bengal, India

Smita Gupta MD
Consultant Endocrinologist
Diabetes, Thyroid, and Endocrine Clinic
San Jose, California, USA

Anjana Hulse MRCPCH MSc
Consultant
Department of Pediatrics
Apollo Hospitals
Bengaluru, Karnataka, India

Pramila Kalra MD DM MAMS
Professor
Department of Endocrinology
MS Ramaiah Medical College
Bengaluru, Karnataka, India

Jayant V Kelwade MD
Senior Resident
Department of Endocrinology
CARE Hospital
Hyderabad, Telangana, India

Gumpeny Lakshmi MD
Registrar
Department of Internal Medicine
MS Ramaiah Medical College
Bengaluru, Karnataka, India

Vivek Mathew MD DM
Associate Professor
Department of Endocrinology
St John's Medical College and Hospital
Bengaluru, Karnataka, India

Puthezhath SN Menon MD MNAMS FIAP FIMSA
Consultant and Head
Department of Pediatrics
Jaber Al-Ahmed Armed Forces Hospital
Kuwait

Shrivalli Nandikoor DMRD DNB
Senior Consultant
Department of Radiology
Apollo Hospitals
Bengaluru, Karnataka, India

Kaushik Pandit MD DNB DM FACE
Chief Endocrinologist
Department of Endocrinology
Belle Vue Clinic
Kolkata, West Bengal, India

Harsh Y Parekh MD
Senior Resident
Department of Endocrinology
CARE Hospital
Hyderabad, Telangana, India

Vedavati B Purandare MD
Consultant
Diabetes Clinic
Chellaram Diabetes Institute
Pune, Maharashtra, India

Rajesh Rajput MD DM FACE FICP FIACM FIMSA
Senior Professor and Head
Department of Endocrinology
Post Graduate Institute of Medical Sciences
Rohtak, Haryana, India

PS Venkatesh Rao MS DNB FRCS FACS
Consultant Endocrine Surgeon
Kadri Clinic
Bengaluru, Karnataka, India

Krishna G Seshadri AB
Visiting Professor
Sri Balaji Vidyapeeth
Pondicherry, India

Bipin K Sethi MD DM
Consultant and Head
Department of Endocrinology
CARE Hospital
Hyderabad, Telangana, India

Vageesh Ayyar S MD DM DNB
Professor and Head
Department of Endocrinology
St John's Medical College and Hospital
Bengaluru, Karnataka, India

Chitra Selvan MD DM MRCP
Assistant Professor
Department of Endocrinology
MS Ramaiah Medical College
Bengaluru, Karnataka, India

Mythri Shankar MD
Senior Consultant
Nuclear Medicine
Cytecare Cancer Hospital
Bengaluru, Karnataka, India

Gumpeny R Sridhar MD DM FACE FRCP
Director
Department of Endocrinology
Endocrine and Diabetes Centre
Visakhapatnam, Andhra Pradesh, India

Jagdeesh Ullal MD MS CCD ECNU FACE FACP
Associate Professor
Center for Endocrine and Metabolic Disorders
Eastern Virginia Medical School
Norfolk, Virginia, USA

Madhava Vijayakumar MD DCH DNB
Additional Professor
Department of Pediatrics
Institute of Maternal and Child Health
Government Medical College
Kozhikode, Kerala, India

Preface

This book "Disorders of Thyroid" is the combined effort and collected wisdom of senior thyroidologists, radiologists, and endocrine surgeons in India. It is essential for young endocrinologists and physicians to get latest information and practical aspects of management of thyroid disorders. We have made an earnest attempt to include clinically relevant topics which help clinicians understand the intricacies of managing thyroid disorders in every day practice.

It is also a review of latest clinical practice in India. We have incorporated a few cases in each chapter to sustain the interest of the reader in the topic and to help them take a pragmatic approach to a thyroid disorder. We have included a few novel chapters like interpreting thyroid tests, depression, and thyroid, as it will help a young endocrinologists and physicians to interpret the laboratory results, and any underlying depression which may alter the therapy for thyroid disorders.

I would like to thank Professor Romesh Khardori for inviting me to be the guest editor for this book; he has been my mentor in endocrinology for the last three decades. I wish to thank all the contributors to the book who have spent their precious time and energy in preparing the chapters assigned to them. I wish to thank the publishers Jaypee Brothers Medical Publishers (P) Ltd. for their efforts in bringing out this book. Special thanks to Dr Neeraj Choudhary and Barkha Arora for their continuous efforts to get this book published within time. I hope that this book meets the expectation of our readers and assists physicians in the management of thyroid disorders.

KM Prasanna Kumar

Contents

1. **Hypothyroidism** — 1
   Subhankar Chowdhury, Partha P Chakraborty

2. **Graves' Thyrotoxicosis** — 10
   Chitra Selvan, KM Prasanna Kumar

3. **Thyroid Disorders During Pregnancy** — 19
   Vivek Mathew, Vageesh Ayyar S

4. **Approach to the Solitary Thyroid Nodule and Cancer** — 27
   Krishna G Seshadri

5. **Thyroiditis** — 51
   Pramila Kalra

6. **Depression and Hypothyroidism** — 65
   Gumpeny R Sridhar, Gumpeny Lakshmi

7. **Subclinical Hyperthyroidism** — 71
   Rana Bhattacharjee, Sujoy Ghosh

8. **Subclinical Hypothyroidism** — 77
   Vedavati B Purandare, Unnikrishnan AG

9. **Thyroid Imaging: From an Endocrinologist's Point of View** — 87
   Mythri Shankar, Shrivalli Nandikoor

10. **Surgery in Thyroid Disorders** — 104
    PS Venkatesh Rao

11. **Thyroid Hormone Resistance Syndrome/Resistance to Thyroid Hormone** — 115
    Romesh Khardori, Jagdeesh Ullal, Smita Gupta

12. **Interpreting Thyroid Hormone Results** — 124
    Kaushik Pandit

13. **Thyroid-associated Orbitopathy** — 134
    Rajesh Rajput

14. **Juvenile Hypothyroidism** — 147
    Puthezhath SN Menon, Madhava Vijayakumar

15.	**Neonatal Hypothyroidism** *Anjana Hulse*	172
16.	**Sick Euthyroid Syndrome** *Bipin K Sethi, Jayant V Kelwade, Harsh Y Parekh, Vaibhav V Dukle*	182
	Index	*191*

PLATE 1

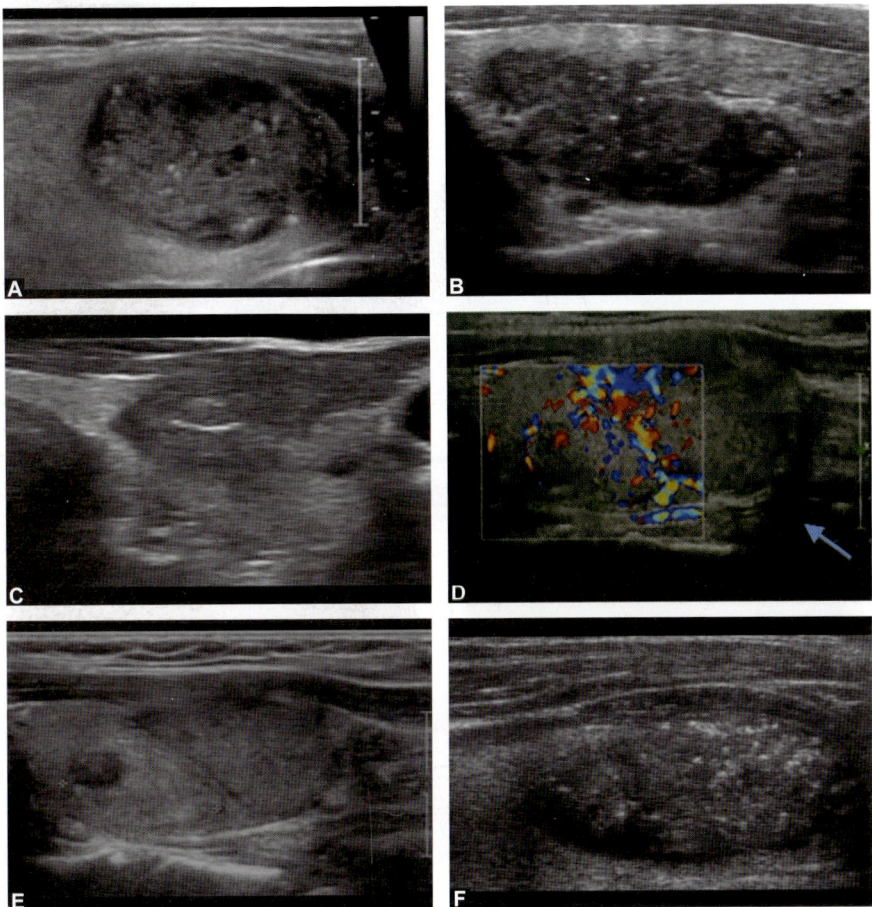

FIG. 4: Ultrasonographic features suggestive of malignancy. **A,** Microcalcifications; **B,** ill defined margins; **C,** extension beyond thyroid margin; **D,** increased central vascularity + reverberation halo; **E,** absent peripheral halo; **F,** cervical lymph node metastsis *(Chapter 9)*

PLATE 2

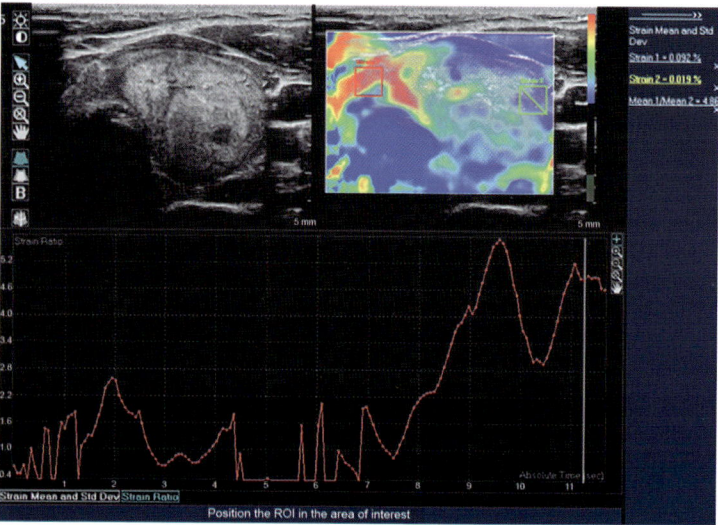

FIG. 5: Strain tissue elastography image showing varying grades of tissue stiffness *(Chapter 9)*

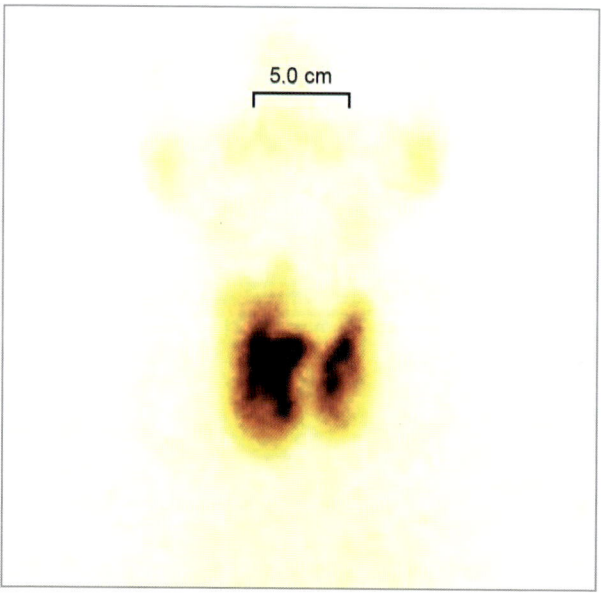

FIG. 7: Multiple nodules with heterogeneous uptake (multinodular goiter) *(Chapter 9)*

PLATE 3

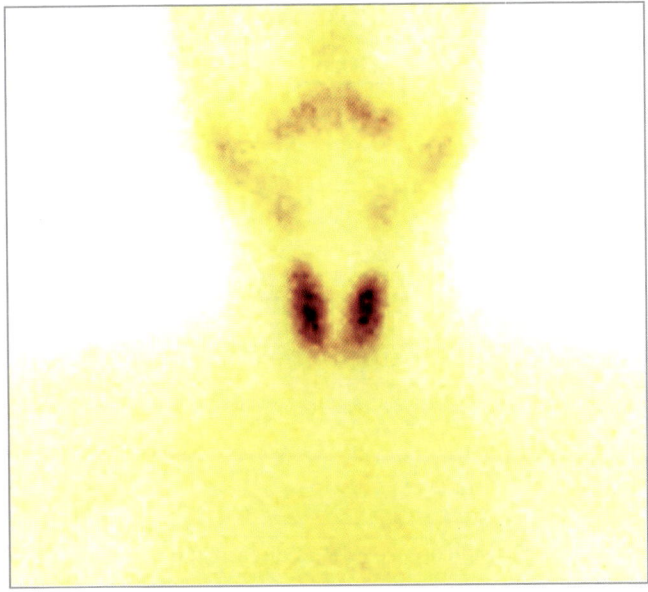

FIG. 8: Normal thyroid gland with normal uptake values *(Chapter 9)*

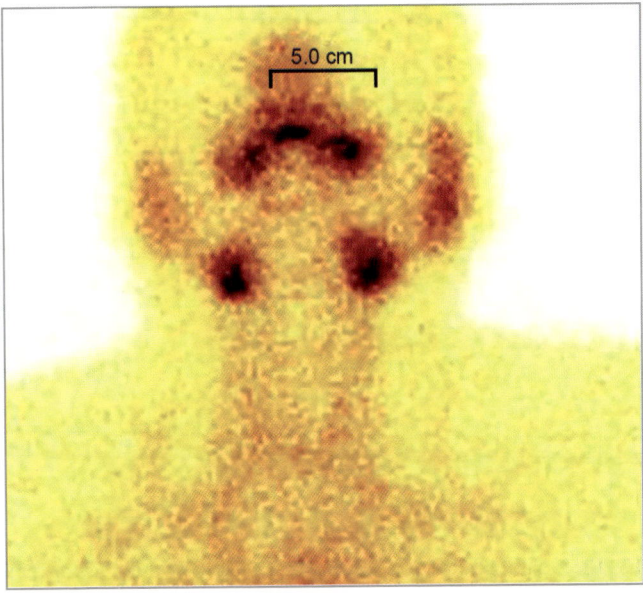

FIG. 9: Low uptake or decreased trapping function (thyroiditis) *(Chapter 9)*

PLATE 4

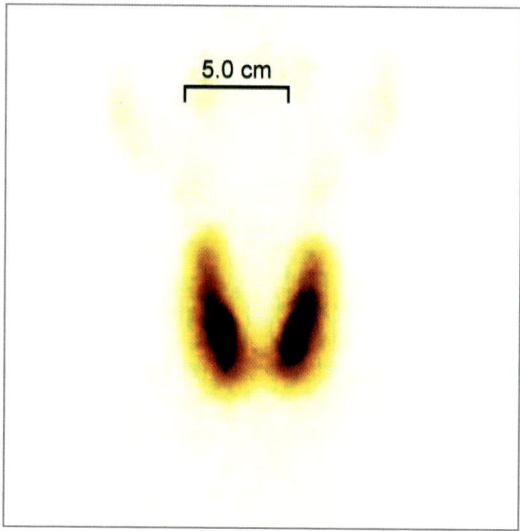

FIG. 10: High uptake (Graves' disease) *(Chapter 9)*

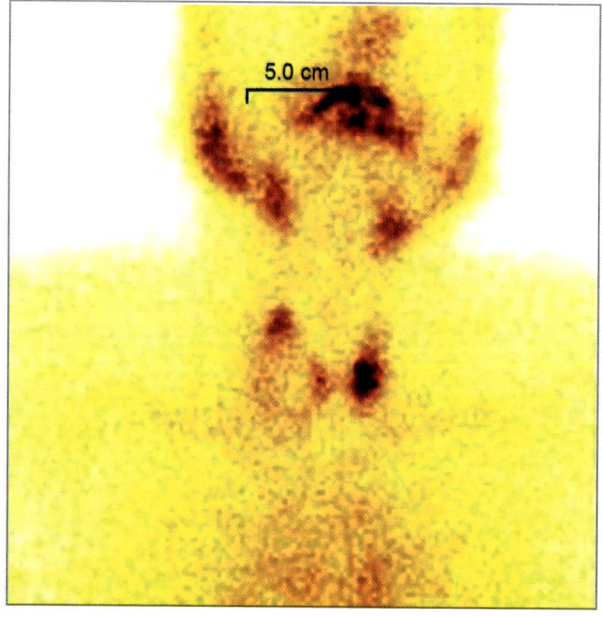

FIG. 11: Solitary nodule with low uptake (Cold nodule) *(Chapter 9)*

PLATE 5

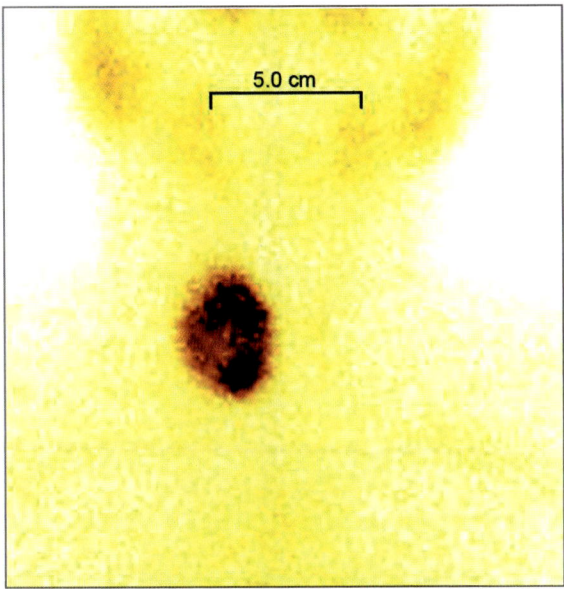

FIG. 12: Solitary nodule with high uptake and suppression of contralateral gland (toxic or autonomous nodule) *(Chapter 9)*

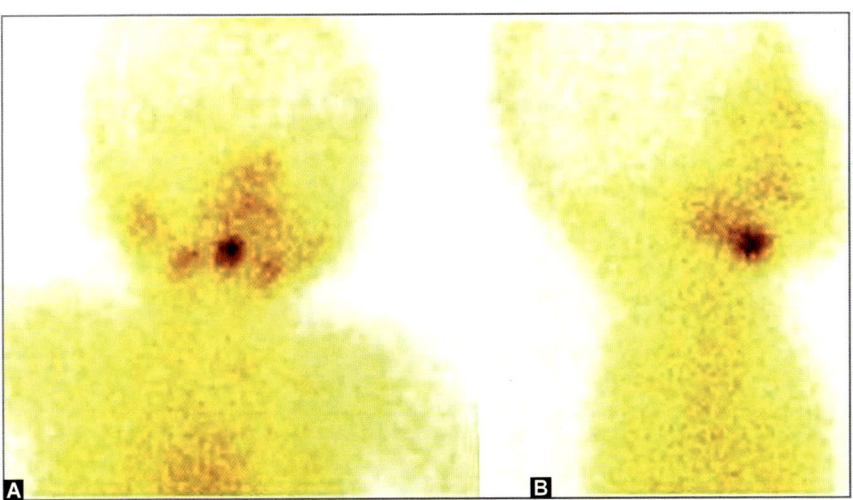

FIG. 13: Lingual thyroid in a pediatric patient (Better appreciated in lateral views). **A,** Anterior; **B,** right lateral *(Chapter 9)*

PLATE 6

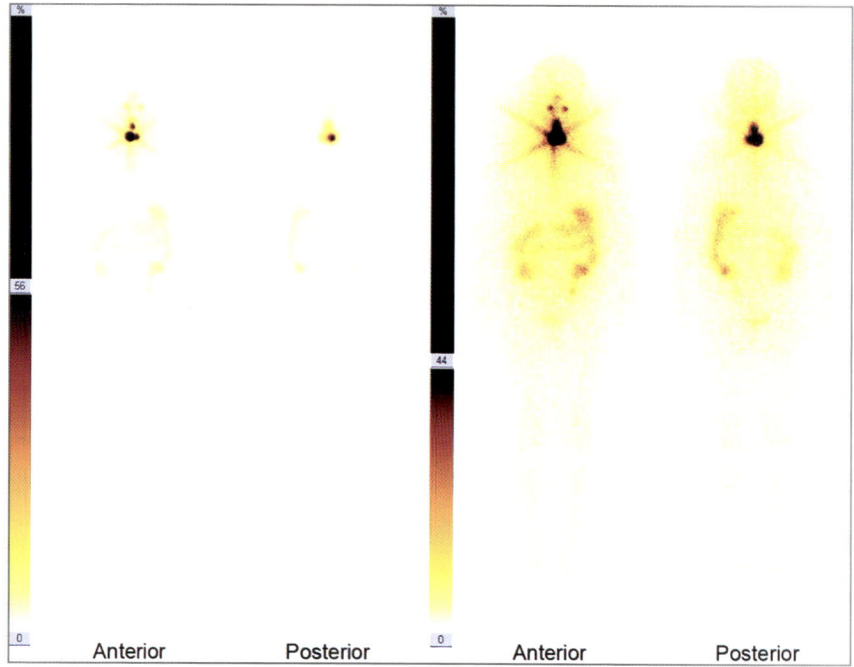

FIG. 14: Positive whole body iodine scan showing iodine avid tissue in the thyroid bed suggestive of residual thyroid tissue *(Chapter 9)*

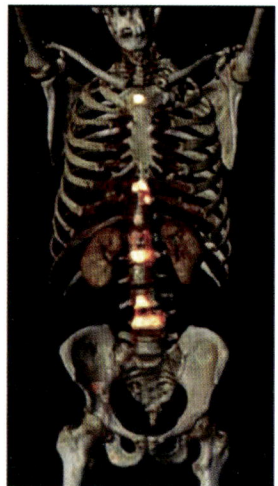

FIG. 15: Fluorodeoxyglucose positron emission tomography computed tomography showing multiple skeletal metastasis *(Chapter 9)*

PLATE 7

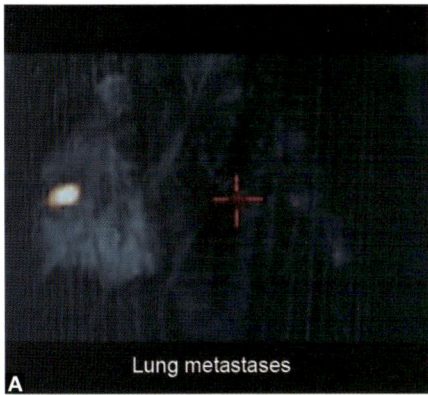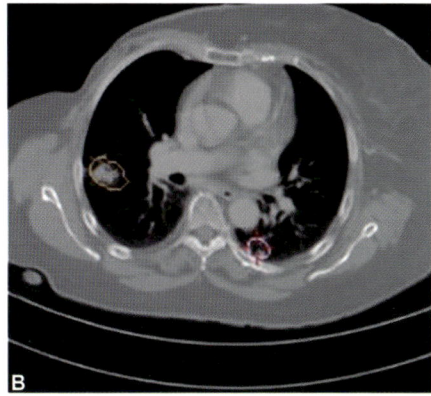

FIG. 16: Fluorodeoxyglucose positron emission tomography computed tomography showing pulmonary metastasis *(Chapter 9)*

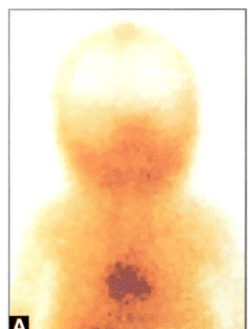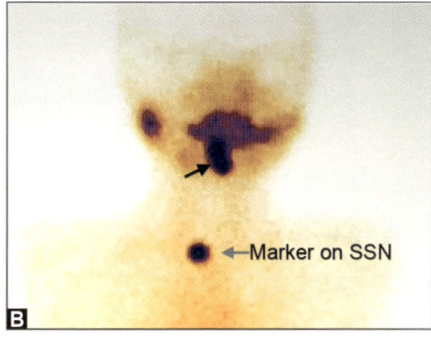

FIG. 2: A, Technetium scan showing agenesis of thyroid gland (note absence of concentration of the isotope in the neck); **B,** technetium scan showing ectopic thyroid (sublingual; note the arrows for location of suprasternal node and sublingual locations) *(Chapter 14)*

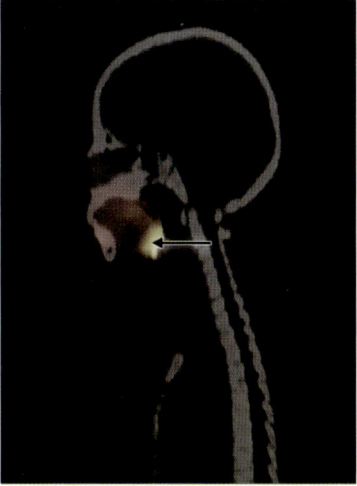

FIG. 6: Single-photon emission computed tomography image (after administration of technitium) showing a focal nodular area in the posteroinferior aspect of the tongue with intense uptake of tracer (arrow) *(Chapter 14)*

CHAPTER 1

Hypothyroidism

Subhankar Chowdhury, Partha P Chakraborty

CASE 1 (FIG. 1)

A 24-year-old female presented with short stature, mental retardation, primary amenorrhea, and absence of secondary sexual characters. Her growth and developmental milestones were satisfactory till 5 years of age when her school performances started deteriorating gradually and she left school at the age of 10 years. On examination, she had a typical puffy face, alopecia, madarosis, and dry and coarse skin. She had severe short stature with a height standard deviation score of −5.6. Ankle jerks were grossly delayed. She had breast buds only (Tanner stage 2) and no pubic or axillary hair.

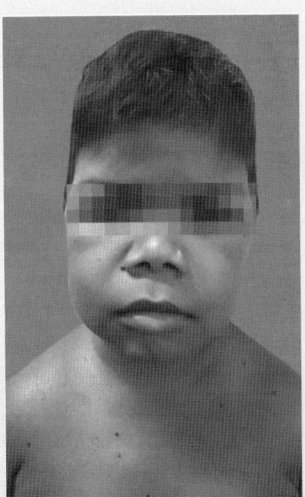

FIG. 1: A 24-year-old lady with primary hypothyroidism due to chronic Hashimoto's thyroiditis

Relevant investigations revealed the following:
- Free thyroxine (FT4): 0.2 ng/dL
- Thyroid-stimulating hormone (TSH): >150 mIU/L
- Total cholesterol (TC): 330 mg/dL
- Low-density lipoprotein cholesterol (LDL-C): 178 mg/dL
- Triglycerides (TG): 224 mg/dL

- Antithyroid peroxidase (anti-TPO) antibody: Positive
- Antithyroglobulin (anti-Tg) antibody: Negative
- Bone age: 10 years
- Neck ultrasonogram revealed a hypoplastic thyroid gland.

Diagnosis: Primary hypothyroidism due to chronic Hashimoto's thyroiditis.

CASE 2 (FIG. 2)

A 48-year-old lady got admitted to emergency ward with sudden onset disorientation following recurrent episodes of vomiting for 3 days. She was amenorrhoeic since her last child birth 27 years back and she could not breastfeed her youngest child. There were similar episodes of disorientation for several times in the past. The Glasgow Coma Scale score was 6 out of 15 with supine blood pressure of 76/42 mmHg. She had a typical pale-looking face with loss of lateral eyebrows. Pubic and axillary hairs were absent.

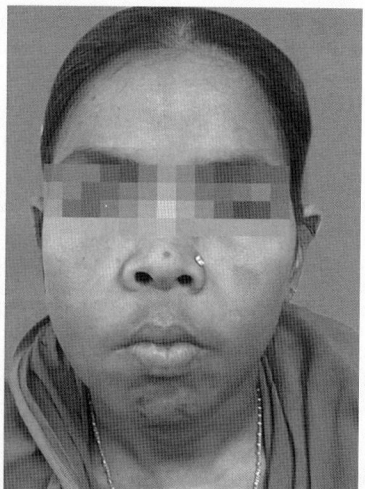

FIG. 2: A 48-year-old lady with secondary hypothyroidism due to Sheehan's syndrome

A detailed workup revealed the following:
- Random plasma glucose: 64 mg/dL
- Serum sodium level: 119.7 meq/L
- Potassium: 3.7 meq/L
- Morning cortisol: 2.2 µg/dL
- Triiodothyronine (T3): 55 ng/dL
- Free T4: 0.4 ng/dL
- Thyroid-stimulating hormone 0.25 mIU/L
- Follicle-stimulating hormone: 2.4 mIU/mL
- Urine spot sodium: 122 meq/L.

Magnetic resonance imaging of brain showed partial empty sella with flattened pituitary gland as a thin rim lining the sella. Patient was put on hypertonic saline, systemic steroid, and levothyroxine (LT4), following which she recovered remarkably within 48 hours.

Diagnosis: Secondary hypothyroidism due to Sheehan's syndrome.

INTRODUCTION

Hypothyroidism, one of the common endocrine diseases across the globe, has multiple etiologies and varied clinical manifestations. It is broadly classified into overt hypothyroidism (OH) and subclinical hypothyroidism (SCH) based on the thyroid function tests (TFTs). Subclinical hypothyroidism, essentially a biochemical diagnosis, is strictly defined as elevated serum TSH with a normal serum free thyroxine (FT4) level in absence of ongoing or recent severe illness and abnormal functioning of the hypothalamic-pituitary-thyroid axis. It, probably, represents a compensated early state of primary thyroid disease where an elevated level of TSH is required to maintain serum thyroid hormones (TH) within the normal range. Though, it is called subclinical, many patients are symptomatic and significant clinical improvement is noticed after LT4 supplementation. Low FT4 combined with elevated TSH constitutes OH. Appropriate and successful treatment requires an accurate diagnosis which is also influenced by coexisting medical ailments.

ETIOLOGY

Hypothyroidism can be primary, when the disease involves the thyroid gland itself with abnormal TH synthesis and/or release; or secondary when the defect lies in the hypothalamus and/or pituitary with inappropriate thyrotropin-releasing hormone (TRH) or TSH signaling; or peripheral/consumptive which results from accelerated conversion of thyroxine (T4) to reverse T3 and T3 to diiodothyronine (T2) by excessive production of type 3 deiodinase usually from a tumor.

The commonest type of hypothyroidism is primary hypothyroidism; its usual causes are:
- Autoimmune thyroiditis
- Iodine deficiency
- Surgical removal or radioiodine ablation of the thyroid gland
- Medications.

Usual causes of secondary hypothyroidism are:
- Sellar or suprasellar space-occupying lesions
- Vascular insult to the pituitary
- Inflammatory disorders of the hypothalamic-pituitary region.

PRESENTATION

The signs and symptoms of hypothyroidism have poor sensitivity and specificity and vary according to the degree of thyroid dysfunction. They are subjective and commonly include fatigue, somnolence, aches and pains, menstrual irregularities, cold intolerance, dry skin, constipation, vocal changes, and non-pitting edema.

Hypothyroidism, at times, may have monosymptomatic presentation like short stature in children, infertility, galactorrhea, polyserositis, and hypoosmolar euvolemic hyponatremia (secondary hypothyroidism).

Atypical presentations, like Van Wyk-Grumbach syndrome (combination of primary hypothyroidism, peripheral isosexual precocity, delayed bone age, feedback pituitary adenoma, and ovarian cysts), Kocher-Debre-Semelaigne syndrome (primary hypothyroidism with pseudomuscular hypertrophy in children), Hoffman's syndrome (primary hypothyroidism with pseudomuscular hypertrophy in adults), and delayed ejaculation, are not uncommonly encountered in clinical practice.[1,2]

HYPOTHYROIDISM AND COMORBIDITIES

A number of comorbidities are commonly associated with hypothyroidism of which dyslipidemia, cardiovascular morbidities, menstrual irregularities, infertility, depression, and diabetes are of significant clinical importance.

Thyroid hormones play an important role in different steps of cholesterol metabolism. It stimulates hepatic cholesterol synthesis by inducing 3-hydroxy-3-methyl-glutaryl-coenzyme A reductase. On the other hand, TH increases hepatic low-density lipoprotein receptor expression and decreases intestinal cholesterol absorption, and thereby, decreases serum TC and LDL-C concentration. Thyroid hormones can potentially decrease high-density lipoprotein cholesterol (HDL-C) concentration by stimulating cholesteryl ester transfer protein and hepatic lipase activity. However, effects on cholesterol clearance predominates over cholesterol synthesis; so, hypothyroidism, both overt and subclinical, are associated with increased TC, TG, very-low-density lipoprotein cholesterol, LDL-C, HDL-C, and lipoprotein(a) [Lp(a)] levels. There are suggestions of qualitative abnormalities of LDL-C particles in hypothyroidism as well. What is of interest is that even in patients with TSH level within the so-called reference range, lipid levels are more deranged as the TSH rises.

Patients of hypothyroidism have more cardiovascular risks due to underlying atherogenic lipid profile, abnormal hemodynamics, endothelial dysfunction, hypercoagulability, and abnormal nontraditional risk factors [elevated Lp(a), homocysteine, and C-reactive protein]. The trend is same for both OH and SCH; SCH with TSH more than 10 µIU/mL is considered as definite cardiovascular risk factor.

Hypothyroidism has long been associated with depression. Thyroid hormones has an established role in central nervous system (CNS) function and the prevalence of depression has been shown to be significantly high even in patients with SCH. Interestingly, patients with autoimmune hypothyroidism are more prone to mental disturbances compared to patients with hypothyroidism secondary to other etiologies as evidenced by a positive correlation of depression scores with elevated anti-thyroid peroxidase (anti TPO) antibody even in patients with normal TFT. Levothyroxine, though alone is ineffective in inducing complete remission, can enhance the effect of concurrent antidepressant medications. Conversely, patients with endogenous depression may manifest abnormal TFTs characterized by higher T4 and reverse T3 (rT3) with lower T3 and TSH. Absent nocturnal surge of TSH and blunted TSH response to TRH explain the suppressed value in those patients. Elevated circulatory glucocorticoids and resultant reduced activity of peripheral deiodinases alter the TH metabolism and the TFT resembles a state seen in sick euthyroid syndrome.

Diabetes and hypothyroidism are the two most frequently encountered endocrinological disorders and thyroid dysfunction is more common in diabetes, in particular type 1 diabetes. About 20% of children with type 1 diabetes may have antithyroid antibodies and 3–8% suffer from hypothyroidism. Thyroid hormones has its role in glucose homeostasis. It increases hepatic glucose output and stimulates intestinal glucose absorption, and thereby tends to increase blood glucose levels. It also stimulates peripheral utilization of glucose minimally. A particular polymorphism of type 2 deiodinase is associated with insulin resistance. The effect of hypothyroidism on blood glucose level, thus, varies but hypothyroidism is known to adversely affect the cardiovascular and nephropathy risks in patients with diabetes. Glycolsylated hemoglobin is a commonly used biochemical marker of long-term glycemic control; it could be spuriously high in patients with OH, making it unreliable as a glycemic marker.

Menstrual irregularities and infertility are common in hypothyroidism and the prevalence of infertility is estimated to be around 10–15% due to abnormal function of the hypothalamic-pituitary-gonadal axis. Abnormal pulsatility of the gonadotropins, hyperprolactinemia, and structural abnormalities of the ovaries are the important underlying mechanisms. Levothyroxine administration normalizes these abnormalities, reverses menstrual abnormalities, and improves chances of spontaneous fertility.

Obesity and Hypothyroidism

About a quarter of overweight or obese patients have abnormal TFTs which mimic SCH. In individuals with normal body mass index (BMI), T4 produces equal amount of T3 and rT3. There is increased T3 production and decreased rT3 production in obesity. The high leptin level in obesity is perhaps the main underlying mechanism for elevated TSH. Leptin stimulates TRH, proopiomelanocortin/cocaine- and amphetamine-regulated transcript (POMC/CART) neurons and inhibits neuropeptide Y/agouti-related protein (NPY/AGRP) neurons and pituitary conversion of T4 to T3, and thus, elevates serum TSH. The other postulations for elevated TSH in obesity are injury of thyroid cells and sodium-iodide symporter due to chronic systemic inflammation, low levels of TH receptors in hypothalamus/pituitary with resultant TH resistance, derangement of hypothalamic-pituitary axis with secretion of immunoreactive but bioinactive TSH, TSH receptor mutation, and impaired mitochondrial function and coexisting thyroid disease.

These patients usually have a TSH value of less than 10 μIU/mL and usually do not require LT4 therapy. Thyroid-stimulating hormone and BMI have a positive correlation, and with reduction of weight, the TSH value falls within the reference range.

DIAGNOSIS

Diagnosis of hypothyroidism is confirmed by simple laboratory test. It is suggested that when the clinical suspicion of hypothyroidism is high, a combination of FT4 and TSH should be ordered; however, as a routine screen for thyroid dysfunction, serum TSH alone is sufficient. A combination of elevated TSH and low FT4 fulfils the diagnostic criteria of overt primary hypothyroidism. Subclinical hypothyroidism is said to be present when TSH is elevated but the FT4 is within the laboratory reference range. Low FT4 with low or inappropriately normal or mildly elevated TSH constitutes secondary (pituitary) or tertiary (hypothalamic) hypothyroidism and should ask for imaging of the hypothalamus and pituitary gland, and ensuring normal serum cortisol level before starting on levothyroxine therapy. Though at present, TSH is commonly measured using a third-generation chemiluminescence assay, older generation assays are sufficient enough to diagnose primary hypothyroidism. There is much controversy worldwide as far as normal reference range of TSH is concerned and a value between 0.3 and 5.0 mIU/L is commonly used as the normal reference range. A monograph by the National Academy of Clinical Biochemistry suggested that 95% of euthyroid volunteers had a serum TSH between 0.4 and 2.5 mIU/L on routine screening.[3] Alterations in TFTs in different clinical situations mimicking primary or secondary hypothyroidism have been summarized in table 1.

Measuring thyroid autoantibodies (anti-TPO and anti-Tg) in hypothyroid patients not only helps to determine the underlying etiology of primary hypothyroidism, it can assess the risk of progression of SCH to OH. Though anti-TPO antibodies are commonly present in patients of chronic autoimmune thyroiditis, a subset of patients who are

Disorders of Thyroid

TABLE 1: Alteration in thyroid function tests in disorders of hypothalamo-pituitary-thyroid axis and non-thyroidal illnesses mimicking primary or secondary hypothyroidism

Free thyroxine	Free triiodo-thyronine	Thyroid-stimulating hormone	Possibilities
Low	Low/normal	High	Primary hypothyroidism
Normal	Normal	High	SCH/recovery from sick euthyroid syndrome/recovery from thyroiditis/heterophile antibody against TSH/macro-TSH/partial TSH resistance
Low	Low	Low/normal	Secondary hypothyroidism/sick euthyroid syndrome/drug effect like dopamine, steroid/patients of hyperthyroidism treated with antithyroid drugs or radioiodine in recent past
Low	Low	Mildly elevated (Usually <20 mIU/L)	Rule out secondary hypothyroidism/sick euthyroid syndrome

TSH, thyroid-stimulating hormone; SCH, subclinical hypothyroidism.

negative for anti-TPO antibody are tested positive for anti-Tg antibody. It has to be kept in mind that a minority of patients with histologically confirmed autoimmune hypothyroidism are negative for both antibodies. Thyroid scintigraphy and ultrasound do not provide any extra information in patients of hypothyroidism; the latter has a role to characterize any associated thyroid nodule.

It would be relevant to rule out hypothyroidism before embarking on statin treatment for dyslipidemia (especially, if any clinical suspicion). It is because if frankly hypothyroid, thyroxine treatment may be enough to correct or at least to improve the dyslipidemia, and the risk of statin-induced myopathy is significantly higher in untreated hypothyroidism.

TREATMENT

The initiating dose of LT4 replacement varies depending on etiology of hypothyroidism, age, body weight, and associated comorbidities. Neonates and infants with hypothyroidism should be initiated with a higher dose whereas children with long-standing severe hypothyroidism and elderly individuals should be put on a significantly lower dose of LT4 at the beginning. Caution should also be exercised when initiating and titrating LT4 therapy in individuals with known or suspected coronary artery disease to avoid development of new onset angina or worsening of preexisting ischemic heart disease. A typical starting dosage of 25–50 µg per day followed by a slow up-titration every 4–6 weeks is recommended in patients with underlying heart disease. Patients with complete absence of functional thyroid tissues typically require a replacement dose of 1.6–1.8 µg/kg/day and the calculation should be made using the ideal body weight.[4,5]

Thyroxine has a plasma half-life of about 6.7 days and provided that there is an intact hypothalamic-pituitary-thyroid axis, the dose adjustment is usually done every 8–12 weeks to allow achievement of a new steady state which requires 5–6 half-lives. However, in special circumstances like in pregnancy or in infants and children, dose titration every 4–6 weeks is recommended.

Many a time, patients on a stable dose of LT4 present with elevated TSH with normal FT4. A detailed history to ensure compliance is of importance before increasing the dose of LT4.

In nonpregnant, non-elderly individuals, the dose of LT4 is adjusted to maintain the TSH level within the normal reference range for the performing laboratory. Though, there are some suggestions for aiming a TSH within the lower half of the reference range (0.4–2.0 mIU/L), this level of TSH has not been consistently associated with symptomatic improvement, better quality-of-life scores or clinical outcomes.[6,7] However, a minority of patients prefer LT4 dosages that result in low-normal or even sub-normal serum TSH values.[8,9]

A recent reanalysis of the third National Health and Nutrition Examination Survey data, using age, sex, and ethnicity specific TSH reference limits, the 97.5 percentile for TSH values in whites between 70 and 79 years old was 5.6 mIU/L, and for those over age 80, it was 6.6 mIU/L. This age-dependent increase in serum TSH and the fact that longevity has been reported to be associated with high serum TSH should make the target TSH level in elderly individuals somewhat higher than the general population.

The current American Thyroid Association (ATA) guidelines for pregnancy and postpartum management of thyroid disease recommend that if trimester-specific TSH reference ranges are not available, the following target TSH ranges may be used: first trimester 0.1–2.5 mIU/L; second trimester 0.2–3.0 mIU/L; third trimester 0.3–3.0 mIU/L.

Many factors including food, medications, and disease processes are known to adversely affect the absorption of LT4. A number of commonly used drugs, like gastric antisecretory agents, antacids, calcium carbonate, and iron preparations, interfere with absorption of LT4. It is commonly advised that LT4 should be taken on an empty stomach, without other medications, supplements, or food for 1 hour to allow consistent absorption and to maintain serum TSH within a narrow target range.[10] Levothyroxine may also be taken in a similar fashion 4 hours after the last meal or at bed time with identical clinical and biochemical outcomes. In fact, it has been seen that the nocturnal absorption of LT4 is better because of higher basal secretion of gastric acid and slower intestinal motility overnight combined with the fasting state.[11]

However, considering the food habits of the majority of Indian population, patients should be instructed to take LT4 tablets at empty stomach in the morning, and bed time administration of LT4 should not be entertained. Poor compliance and difficulty with adherence to a daily regimen is common in clinical practice. Study with randomized crossover design has shown that euthyroidism can be achieved with once-weekly dosing of LT4, at a dose slightly higher than 7 times the usual daily dose, without systemic side effects,[12] and once-weekly LT4 administration may be tried only in exceptional cases to counteract noncompliance.

Different brands of LT4 are available in the market with different bioequivalence, and changes in LT4 brands are strongly discouraged as such a wide difference in bioequivalence may put patients at risk for incorrect dosing, if different brands are used interchangeably.

Animal studies have demonstrated that LT4 therapy in post-thyroidectomy subjects may not achieve euthyroidism in all tissues simultaneously and required the combination of LT4 and liothyronine.[13,14] However, randomized clinical trials comparing LT4 monotherapy with LT4 plus liothyronine combination therapy were unable to support the superiority of the combination therapy in general.[15] The positive outcome of combination therapy in some of the studies may be explained by favorable effects of combination therapy in a subset of patients harboring genetic polymorphism in relevant TH transporters or deiodinase enzymes resulting in low levels of T3 in the tissues.

In some of the studies, weight loss was somewhat higher in patients receiving combination therapy or desiccated thyroid compared to LT4 monotherapy[16,17] and was thought to be the explanation for patients' preference for combination therapy or desiccated thyroid which contains significant amount of T3. Though the determinants of patients' preferences for combination therapy still remain unknown, it has been speculated that higher serum and tissue T3 levels might be associated with improvement in T3-dependent functions of the CNS, including regulation of body weight. Despite all these evidences, only the European Thyroid Association have offered specific guidance for the use of LT4 and liothyronine combination therapy, but still consider it experimental.[18] On a futuristic note, based on a landmark study published in 2012 that has described the generation of functional thyroid tissue from embryonic stem cells, we can speculate that hypothyroid patients can also be treated with thyroid-generating stem cells in the coming years.[19]

CONCLUSION

Hypothyroidism may be primary, secondary, or peripheral. Biochemically, it can also be classified into overt or subclinical. Primary hypothyroidism is the most commonly encountered form of the disease while peripheral type is rare. Signs and symptoms of hypothyroidism are nonspecific and a high degree of clinical suspicion is required for diagnosis. Monosymptomatic presentations or atypical presentations are not uncommon. A number of comorbidities like dyslipidemia, cardiovascular disease, menstrual irregularities and infertility, depression, and diabetes are commonly associated with hypothyroidism, both overt and subclinical. One-fourth of overweight or obese patients have altered thyroid function, manifesting biochemically as SCH. Excess weight itself alters the hypothalamic-pituitary-thyroid axis by a number of mechanisms. There are significant controversies regarding management of SCH which requires individualization of therapy. The usual indications of treatment are pregnancy, infertility, cosmetically unaccepted goiter, TSH more than 10 µIU/mL, elevated antithyroid antibodies and dyslipidemia. Therapy with LT4 may also be tried in symptomatic patients of SCH if those are suggestive of hypothyroidism. Levothyroxine is the mainstay of therapy, which should preferably be taken at empty stomach in the morning. Changing of brands is discouraged. The target TSH in LT4-treated, nonpregnant patients depends on age, presence of comorbidities, and clinical scenarios. Trimester-specific TSH ranges provided by ATA may be used in pregnant patients.

REFERENCES

1. Van Wyk JJ, Grumbach MM. Syndrome of precocious menstruation and galactorrhea in juvenile hypothyroidism: An example of hormonal overwrap in pituitary feed-back. J Pediatr. 1960;57:416-35.
2. Werner SC, Ingbar SH, Braverman LE, Utiger RD. In: Werner and Ingbar's The Thyroid: A Fundamental and Clinical Text, 9th edition. Philadelphia: Lippincott Williams and Wilkins; 2005. pp. 894-5.
3. Baloch Z, Carayon P, Conte-Devolx B, Demers LM, Feldt-Rasmussen U, Henry JF, et al. Laboratory medicine practice guidelines. Laboratory support for the diagnosis and monitoring of thyroid disease. Thyroid. 2003;13(1):3-126.
4. Fish LH, Schwartz HL, Cavanaugh J, Steffes MW, Bantle JP, Oppenheimer JH. Replacement dose, metabolism, and bioavailability of levothyroxine in the treatment of hypothyroidism. Role of triiodothyronine in pituitary feedback in humans. N Engl J Med. 1987;316(13):764-70.
5. Santini F, Pinchera A, Marsili A, Ceccarini G, Castagna MG, Valeriano R, et al. Lean body mass is a major determinant of levothyroxine dosage in the treatment of thyroid diseases. J Clin Endocrinol Metab. 2005;90(1):124-7.
6. Boeving A, Paz-Filho G, Radominski RB, Graf H, Amaral de Carvalho G. Low-normal or high-normal thyrotropin target levels during treatment of hypothyroidism: a prospective, comparative study. Thyroid 2011;21(4):355-60.

7. Walsh JP, Ward LC, Burke V, Bhagat CI, Shiels L, Henley D, et al. Small changes in thyroxine dosage do not produce measurable changes in hypothyroid symptoms, well-being, or quality of life: results of a double-blind, randomized cliniical trial. J Clin Endocrinol Metab. 2006;91(7):2624-30.
8. Carr D, McLeod DT, Parry G, Thornes HM. Fine adjustment of thyroxine replacement dosage: comparison of the thyrotrophin releasing hormone test using a sensitive thyrotrophin assay with measurement of free thyroid hormones and clinical assessment. Clin Endocrinol (Oxf). 1988;28(3):325-33.
9. Toft AD, Beckett GJ. Thyroid function tests and hypothyroidism. Measurement of serum TSH alone may not always reflect thyroid status. BMJ. 2003;326:295-6.
10. Bach-Huynh TG, Nayak B, Loh J, Soldin S, Jonklaas J. Timing of levothyroxine administration affects serum thyrotropin concentration. J Clin Endocrinol Metab. 2009;94(10):3905-12.
11. Vanderpump M. Pharmacotherapy: hypothyroidism-should levothyroxine be taken at bedtime? Nat Rev Endocrinol. 2011;7(4):195-6.
12. Grebe SK, Cooke RR, Ford HC, Fagerström JN, Cordwell DP, Lever NA, et al. Treatment of hypothyroidism with once weekly thyroxine. J Clin Endocrinol Metab. 1997;82(3):870-5.
13. Escobar-Morreale HF, Obregón, MJ, Escobar del Rey F, Morreale de Escobar G. Replacement therapy for hypothyroidism with thyroxine alone does not ensure euthyroidism in all tissues, as studied in thyroidectomized rats. J Clin Invest. 1995;96(6):2828-38.
14. Escobar-Morreale HF, del Rey FE, Obregón, MJ, de Escobar GM. Only the combined treatment with thyroxine and triiodothyronine ensures euthyroidism in all tissues of thyroidectomized rat. Endocrinology. 1996;137(6):2490-502.
15. Grozinsky-Glasberg, S, Fraser A, Nahshoni E, Weizman A, Leibovici L. Thyroxine-triiodothyronine combination therapy versus thyroxine monotherapy for clinical hypothyroidism: meta-analysis of randomized controlled trials. J Clin Endocrinol Metab. 2006;91(7):2592-9.
16. Nygaard B., Jensen EW, Kvetny J, Jarløv A, Faber J. Effect of combination therapy with thyroxine (T4) and 3,5,3›-triiodothyronine versus T4 monotherapy in patients with hypothyroidism, a double-blind, randomised cross-over study. Eur J Endocrinol. 2009;161(6):895-902.
17. Hoang TD, Olsen CH, Mai VQ, Clyde PW, Shakir MK. Desiccated thyroid extract compared with levothyroxine in the treatment of hypothyroidism: a randomized, double-blind, crossover study. J Clin Endocrinol Metab. 2013;98(5):1982-90.
18. Wiersinga WM, Duntas L, Fadeyev V, Nygaard B, Vanderpump MP. 2012 ETA guidelines: the use of L-T4 + L-T3 in the treatment of hypothyroidism. Eur Thyroid J. 2012;1:55-71.
19. Antonica F, Kasprzyk DF, Opitz R, Iacovino M, Liao XH, Dumitrescu AM, et al. Generation of functional thyroid from embryonic stem cells. Nature. 2012;491:66-71.

CHAPTER 2

Graves' Thyrotoxicosis

Chitra Selvan, KM Prasanna Kumar

CASE 1

A 38-year-old woman presented with complaints of palpitations, tremulousness, and weight loss of around 8 kg (despite a good appetite) over the last 2 months. On examination, she was anxious, had a pulse rate of 100/min, warm and moist peripheries, fine tremors of the outstretched hands, and a visible goiter. She has mild proptosis of both eyes with ocular movements complete and visual acuity normal. Her younger sister has been diagnosed with primary hypothyroidism and is on treatment for the same.

Her laboratory examination revealed normal hemogram with an erythrocyte sedimentation rate of 25 mm in the first hour. Thyroid-stimulating hormone (TSH) less than 0.001 µIU/L and total thyroxine (TT4) 28 µg/dL (5–12 µg/dL). A technetium scan showed uniform diffuse uptake over the whole thyroid gland.

A diagnosis of Graves' disease with mild inactive ophthalmopathy was made and she was offered a choice of antithyroid drug, and radioiodine. Patient chose ATD. She was started on propranolol 30 mg/day and 20 mg of carbimazole with instructions to stop treatment in case of a pruritus, jaundice, acholic stools, fever, or pharyngitis. She was asked to review after 2 months with TT4 and TSH. At follow-up visit, she was feeling better, and had gained 4 kg weight. On examination, pulse rate was 78/min and no tremors. Laboratory investigations showed TT4 in the normal range with TSH less than 0.001 µIU/L. The β-blocker was stopped and the dose of carbimazole reduced to 5 mg/day with instructions to stop if any of the adverse features occurred. At review after 3 months, she had complaints of further weight gain of 5 kg and bodyache especially both shoulder regions and calves. Laboratory investigations revealed T4 in the lower quartile of normal with TSH 12 µIU/L. The patient was asked to stop ATD and asked to review in 3 months or earlier if symptoms of thyrotoxicosis recurred. At third visit, she was asymptomatic and her thyroid profile was normal. She was advised to repeat her thyroid function tests every 3–6 months for the next 1–2 years or if symptoms recurred.

CASE 2

A 30-year-old man presented with complaints of heightened anxiety, inability to concentrate at work, and insomnia since 4–6 months. On examination, he appears anxious, his pulse rate is 98/min, blood pressure normal, and minimal tremors of the outstretched hand with an palpable diffuse goiter. He has no eye signs. There is no family history of thyroid disease. He smokes 4–5 cigarettes per day.

> His laboratory examination revealed a suppressed TSH (<0.001 μIU/L), total T4 18 μg/dL (5–12) and free T4 2.8 ng/dL (0.8–1.9). A technetium scan revealed a diffuse uptake suggestive of Grave's disease.
>
> He was asked to stop smoking, started on propranolol, and offered radioablation as first-line treatment with 12 milicuries of iodine 131 (^{131}I). Following ablation, at follow-up visit, he had stopped smoking and was found to be feeling better and sleeping well, with weight gain of 4 kg in two months. On laboratory examination, he was found to have suppressed TSH and TT4 and free T4 in the normal range. He was taken off the β-blockers and asked to review after two months. At the second follow-up visit, he complained of generalized body ache and further weight gain. His thyroid profile showed TSH of 15 μIU/L with low levels of TT4 and free T4. A diagnosis of post-ablative hypothyroidism was made and he was started on levothyroxine 75 μg per day.
>
> In patients with mild to moderate thyrotoxicosis, radioablation can be offered without pretreatment with ATDs to achieve hypothyroid state.

INTRODUCTION

Thyrotoxicosis is a common condition and Graves' disease is the most common cause of persistent thyrotoxicosis. In this chapter, we review the diagnosis of Graves' disease based on clinical, biochemical, and imaging characteristics. We also review the pros and cons of modalities of management for this condition—antithyroid drugs, radioablation, and surgery.

EPIDEMIOLOGY: INDIAN DATA

Thyrotoxicosis is a common condition worldwide. In a community survey from Cochin, subclinical and overt hyperthyroidism was present in 1.6 and 1.3% of subjects.[1] In a hospital-based study in women in Puducherry, prevalence of thyrotoxicosis was 1.8% (overt 1.2% and subclinical 0.6%) of the total subjects, when the cutoff value for TSH was less than 0.1 μIU/ml.[2] In the latest survey of thyroid dysfunction in young females of South India, a low TSH was seen in 1.3% of the population.[3] The prevalence rates reported in India are similar to worldwide reported prevalence.[4] There is no pan India data of prevalence of thyrotoxicosis in India, as we do not have a national registry for thyroid disorders.

Thyrotoxicosis refers to the clinical state or manifestations seen due to excessive circulating thyroid hormones. The common clinical symptoms of thyrotoxicosis are nervousness, weakness, increased perspiration, heat intolerance, tremor, hyperactivity, palpitations, weight loss, and menstrual irregularities. The common signs of thyrotoxicosis are tachycardia, systolic hypertension, warm moist skin, tremors, hyperreflexia, staring look, and muscle weakness. Among the features that determine the manifestations of thyrotoxicosis are the age of the patient and the presence of concomitant disturbance in any organ system. Older patients are less likely to have signs and symptoms of sympathetic activation, such as anxiety and tremor, and more likely to have symptoms and signs of cardiovascular dysfunction such as congestive failure and atrial fibrillation.[5]

Thyrotoxicosis has multiple etiologies and thereby different treatment options. Hyperthyroidism, probably the most common cause of thyrotoxicosis, is the sustained increase in thyroid hormone biosynthesis by a hyperfunctioning thyroid gland. There can be thyrotoxicosis without a hyperfunctioning thyroid gland, e.g., release of stored thyroid hormones as in thyroiditis or ingestion of excess thyroid hormones.

Disorders of Thyroid

The causes of thyrotoxicosis are:[6]
- Primary hyperthyroidism
  - Graves' disease
  - Toxic multinodular goiter
  - Toxic adenoma
  - Functioning thyroid carcinoma metastases
  - Activating mutation of TSH receptor
  - Activating mutation of Gs alpha subunit (McCune-Albright syndrome)
  - Struma ovarii
  - Drugs and iodine excess
- Thyrotoxicosis without hyperthyroidism:
  - Subacute thyroiditis
  - Silent thyroiditis
  - Other causes of thyroid destruction (radiation)
  - Ingestion of excess thyroid hormone
- Secondary hyperthyroidism:
  - Thyroid-stimulating hormone secreting pituitary adenoma
  - Human chorionic gonadotropin secreting tumors
  - Gestational thyrotoxicosis
  - Resistance to thyroid hormone.

Of the various causes of thyrotoxicosis, Graves' disease, toxic multinodular goiter, and thyroiditis are probably the most common causes. The following points on history and examination will help in ascertaining the cause of thyrotoxicosis:
- Duration of symptoms
- Size, shape of thyroid gland
- Presence or absence of tenderness over thyroid
- Extrathyroidal manifestations of Graves' disease.

Graves' disease is usually the cause of thyrotoxicosis in patients with a family history, who have been symptomatic for several weeks to months, have a diffuse goiter, and has symptoms related to extrathyroidal manifestations of Graves', most commonly ophthalmopathy, e.g., feeling of grittiness in the eyes, increasing prominence of eyes. In severe instances, a thyroid bruit can be appreciated over the thyroid.

Patients with toxic multinodular goiter are generally older, have had the swelling in front of the neck for many years, have been symptomatic for months, and have a nodular goiter with no extrathyroidal features like in Graves'.

Subacute thyroiditis mostly have symptoms lasting from few days to weeks, is generally painful, the gland is firm to hard on palpation, and the erythrocyte sedimentation rate is almost always greater than 50 and sometimes over 100 mm/h.

It is prudent to remind oneself there are caveats to these pointers, e.g., not all patients with Graves' have extrathyroidal features, and about 10% of them might not have a palpable goiter. Not all nodular goiters are multinodular goiters.

UPTAKE STUDY

When the cause of thyrotoxicosis is not obvious on clinical examination, an uptake study should be asked. An uptake scan is added when thyroid nodularity is noted and when toxic multinodular goiter or toxic adenoma is suspected. If the cause of thyrotoxicosis is hyperthyroidism, then the uptake of radioiodine is increased [like in Graves' and toxic multinodular goiter (MNG)]. Whereas in conditions like thyroiditis, the uptake is close to zero.[7] It is important to make this distinction as ATDs and radioablation can be used for treatment only in patients with hyperthyroidism.

Amongst conditions with increased uptake, the pattern of uptake (in a scan study) will help with the definite diagnosis. The pattern of uptake is diffuse (unless there are coexistent nodules or fibrosis) in Graves' disease. Toxic adenoma generally shows focal uptake in the adenoma with suppressed uptake in the surrounding and contralateral thyroid tissue. The image in toxic MNG demonstrates multiple areas of focal increased and suppressed uptake.

Technetium is a molecule that is also rapidly taken up by the sodium iodine symporter in the thyroid gland, very much like radioiodine. Technetium scintigraphy offers the advantage of imaging in 20 minutes, lesser radiation exposure, and easier accessibility as compared to ^{123}I. Thus, in the differential diagnosis of thyrotoxicosis, more centers are using technetium than radioiodine. In centers where scintigraphy is unavailable, Doppler flow in the thyroid gland may be helpful in documenting increased blood flow in Graves' disease.[8] Serum levels of antibodies against the TSH-receptor antibody (TSHrAb) can also be used to diagnose Graves' disease.[9]

MANAGEMENT

Symptomatic management in the form of β-adrenergic blockade should be offered to all symptomatic patients with thyrotoxicosis, especially the elderly, and tachycardia.[10] Treatment with β-blockers leads to a decrease in heart rate, systolic blood pressure, muscle weakness, and tremor, as well as improvement in the degree of irritability, emotional lability, and exercise intolerance. Propranolol is a non-selective β-blocker most used in thyrotoxicosis, usually in the doses of 10–40 mg three times daily or four times daily. Other β-blockers used are atenolol and metoprolol. Caution should be exercised in patients with airway hyper-reactive disease before starting β-blockers. Calcium channel blockers like verapamil and diltiazem can be used in patients in whom β-blockers are contraindicated.

Once diagnosis is made, one of the following three modalities of management can be offered to a patient with Graves' disease such as antithyroid drugs, radioiodine ablation, or thyroidectomy. The modality best suited for each patient is a decision made after carefully considering the features pertaining to the disease, relative contraindications of a particular modality of treatment, availability, cost, logistics, and patient preferences.

Antithyroid Drugs

This class of drugs reduces the production of thyroid hormones by inhibiting iodine oxidation and organification of tyrosine residues in thyroglobulin.

In India, methimazole, its precursor carbimazole and propylthiouracil are available. Dose of 10 mg of carbimazole is equivalent to 6 mg of methimazole. Carbimazole or methimazole (MMI) is the preferred agent while propylthiouracil (PTU), due to concerns about hepatotoxicity is reserved for special situations like first trimester of pregnancy or thyroid storm.[11]

It is prudent to get a baseline complete blood count, including white count with differential, and a liver function profile including bilirubin and transaminases. A baseline absolute neutrophil count less than 500/mm^3 or liver transaminases enzyme levels elevated more than fivefold the upper limit of normal are contraindications to initiating ATD therapy.[10] Carbimazole and methimazole are started at a dose of 10–20 mg/day and has the advantage of being administered once daily. Propylthiouracil has a shorter duration of action and is usually administered two or three times daily, starting with 50-150 mg three times daily. The minor side effects include urticaria, arthralgia, arthritis, fever, transient granulocytopenia, gastrointestinal upset, and alterations in taste and smell.

The major side effects include agranulocytosis, and very rarely aplastic anemia, thrombocytopenia, toxic hepatitis (PTU), cholestatic hepatitis (MMI), vasculitis, hypoprothrombinemia (PTU), hypoglycemia due to anti-insulin antibodies (MMI), and pancreatitis (MMI).

Patients need to be educated at the initiation of therapy and at subsequent visits to stop the drug immediately and report back if they notice pruritic rash, jaundice, acholic stools or dark urine, arthralgias, abdominal pain, nausea, fatigue, fever, or pharyngitis (suggestive of agranulocytosis or hepatic injury).

Serum T4 levels should be obtained 4-6 weeks after initiation of therapy. In patients with triiodothyronine (T3) toxicosis, serum T3 levels should be used for monitoring. The dose of ATDs adjusted accordingly. Once the patient is rendered euthyroid, the dose of antithyroid drugs can be tapered down. Carbimazole in doses of 5-15 mg/day is the usual maintenance dose of ATD in most of the Indians with Grave's thyrotoxicosis. Thyroid-stimulating hormone can remain suppressed even after normalization of T4 and T3 levels, hence is not the ideal parameter for monitoring.

Most patients who develop agranulocytosis are symptomatic, hence a differential white blood cell count should be obtained during febrile illness and at the onset of pharyngitis in all patients taking antithyroid medication.[10] Similarly, liver function should be assessed in patients who experience pruritic rash, jaundice, light-colored stool or dark urine, joint pain, abdominal pain or bloating, anorexia, nausea, or fatigue. Routine monitoring of complete blood count and liver function tests are not recommended.

Minor cutaneous reactions may be managed with concurrent antihistamine therapy without stopping the ATD. Any patient who develops agranulocytosis or other serious side effects while taking either MMI or PTU, use of the other medication is absolutely contraindicated owing to risk of cross-reactivity between the two medications.

Once the patient is rendered euthyroid, the dose of ATD is tapered down gradually and continued for 12-18 months and discontinued if TSH is normal. This recommendation is based on a systematic review that looked at two studies which found that remission rates are not higher even if ATD are continued for longer than 18 months. However, it may be prudent to note that, by admission of the authors themselves, these studies had small number of subjects, had high drop out rates for follow up, and the confidence intervals were wide.[12] Patients with small goiters, mild disease, small maintenance dose of ATDs (5-10 mg of carbimazole/day), and negative TSHrAb are more likely to have remission. Males, smokers, patients with large goiters and persistently high TSHrAb have higher relapse rates. For patients with difficulty in access to radioablation, or patients who are poor candidates for surgery, long-term and low-dose continuous antithyroid use might be an option.[13]

Radioiodine Ablation

Radioiodine, when orally administered, is preferentially taken by the follicular cell under the influence of the stimulating TSH receptor antibody and stored in the colloid of the gland. The beta rays emitted by radioiodine decreases the function of the hyperfunctioning follicular cell and thus, induce remission.[14] Treatment with ^{131}I is an effective nonsurgical modality of treatment for patients with hyperthyroidism due to Graves' disease. This modality of treatment is ideal for patients who are poor candidates for surgery and those patients who are unable to tolerate ATD.

Possible side effects of ^{131}I therapy include mild anterior neck pain caused by radiation thyroiditis or worsening thyrotoxicosis for several days, owing to the release of preformed thyroid hormones from the damaged thyroid gland. The radiation thyroiditis was found to affect approximately 1% of patients.[15] Graves' ophthalmopathy may develop or worsen after treatment with ^{131}I, especially in smokers and in patients with active ophthalmopathy. Radioactive iodine is absolutely contraindicated during pregnancy and lactation and is avoided in children less than 5 years of age.[10]

There are various radioiodine treatment regimens in use, with the two most common being fixed dosing and calculated dosing. With fixed dosing, a fixed amount of ^{131}I is given as treatment (usually 10-15 mCi) to all patients, whereas calculated dosing is designed to deliver a fixed number of microcuries per gram of thyroid tissue, based on the measured volume of the thyroid gland and then adjusted for the radioiodine uptake.[14] There is little evidence to show that a calculated radioiodine dose is better than a fixed dose.[16,17] Hence, fixed dose of radioiodine administered to render patient hypothyroid is the goal of treatment.

Many studies from India have confirmed that fixed dose administered is a highly effective treatment option for Graves' disease, even in the long run.[18] A dose of 6 mCi was found to render 72% euthyroid and 25% hypothyroid with a mere 1.9% required a repeat dose of radioiodine.[19]

Most patients with Graves' disease receive ATDs first prior to radioablation. There is evidence to show that prior use of ATDs can decrease the efficacy of radioablation as reviewed here.

In a retrospective study that looked at men with Graves' disease, the success rate of a single dose of ^{131}I was significantly higher in patients without pretreatment than in patients who were pretreated with carbimazole (91.4% vs. 82.3%, P = 0.01).[20] In a more recent retrospective study involving 426 patients, prior use of ATD was found to be associated with a delay in remission (102 days vs. 253 days, p <0.001) post radioablation in patients with high uptake Graves'.[21] But a similar study with 5 mCi dose of radioablation found no difference in cure rates at the end of 6 months in patients who were drug naive (61.1% vs. 58.8%, p = 0.845). Higher baseline technetium (^{99m}Tc) uptake, male gender, body mass index (BMI), and higher baseline free thyroxine (fT4) level predicted treatment failure following radioiodine therapy.[22]

A study which looked at the acute changes in the thyroid post-radioablation in patients with pretreatment and those without concluded that pretreatment with antithyroid drugs does not protect against worsening thyrotoxicosis after radioiodine, but may allow such patients to start from a lower baseline level should an aggravation in thyrotoxicosis occur. The findings support the recommendation that most patients with Graves' disease do not require ATD pretreatment before receiving radioiodine.[23] It is pragmatic, that patients who are older, with cardiovascular comorbidities may be candidates who might warrant pretreatment with drugs to render them euthyroid prior to radioablation, to avoid thyroid storm after radioiodine ablation. If ATDs are used to pretreat patients before radioablation, they should be discontinued 4-5 days before treatment to avoid ATD-mediated interference of uptake.

Follow-up of Patients who Receive Radioiodine Ablation

If the patient who received radioiodine was on β-blockers prior to administration, he or she can continue to remain on the same. Most patients post ablation does not require

ATDs. Antithyroid drugs may be resumed 3 to 7 days after radioiodine administration in selected high-risk patients who would poorly tolerate a transient worsening of thyrotoxicosis after radioiodine treatment.[24] Patient is asked to follow up in 4–8 weeks with total T4 or free T4 and total T3 levels. The TSH levels can be suppressed for a few months even after the thyroid hormone levels normalize, hence TSH alone is not the best indicators of thyroid status immediately after radioablation. Once thyroid hormone levels are found to be low, thyroid hormone replacement can be initiated. Most patients respond by 2 months, although some patients may take up to 6 months after which a repeat dose of radioablation may be administered to patient who do not respond. Very rarely, transient hypothyroidism following radioablation which subsequent complete recovery or recurrent hyperthyroidism can occur.[25] Hence, the dose of T4 needs to be started carefully at a lesser than required dose and monitored.

Surgery—Thyroidectomy

A meta-analysis found that thyroidectomy cures hyperthyroidism in more than 90% of cases.[26] Near-total thyroidectomy is a preferred modality for patients who have compressive symptoms like dysphagia, difficulty breathing, or change in voice, or patients with large goiters, have a nodule suspicious of malignancy, patients who have moderate to severe active Graves' ophthalmopathy (where radioiodine can worsen condition), or patients planning pregnancy within 4–6 months are candidates ideal for surgery. All patients should ideally be rendered euthyroid by pretreatment with antithyroid drugs prior to surgery. Pretreatment with ATD for more than 12 months is associated with less thyroid vascularity on Doppler and with less intraoperative blood loss.[26] Preoperative potassium iodide is usually used to reduce vascularity of the thyroid gland and reduce intra-operative blood loss.[27] A study comparing surgical outcomes in 162 patients with Graves' disease with 102 patients with a toxic MNG in which neither group received potassium iodide (KI) solution showed similar intraoperative blood loss and rates of surgical complications.[28] Thus, there is debate over the routine use of preoperative KI in Graves' disease.[29] Patients with substantial coexisting comorbidities, previous history of neck surgery, or radiation make poor candidates for surgery.

The most common complications following near-total or total thyroidectomy are hypocalcemia (which can be transient or permanent), recurrent or superior laryngeal nerve injury (which can be temporary or permanent), postoperative bleeding, and complications related to general anesthesia. Most of these complications are low in the hands of an experienced surgeon.

PATIENTS' SELECTION FOR SURGERY, RADIOABLATION, AND MEDICAL TREATMENT

Patients who have compressive symptoms, like dysphagia, difficulty breathing, or change in voice, or patients with large goiters, have a nodule suspicious of malignancy, patients who have moderate to severe active Graves' ophthalmopathy, (where radioiodine can worsen condition) or patients planning pregnancy within 4–6 months are candidates ideal for surgery. Patients with substantial coexisting comorbidities make poor candidates for surgery.

Patients with substantial comorbidities making them poor candidates for surgery, patients with past history of neck surgery or irradiation (making surgery difficult), patients who develop adverse effects to ATD are suitable candidates for radioablation.

Pregnancy, breastfeeding, moderate-severe active Graves' ophthalmopathy, coexisting thyroid cancer or suspicion of the same, and patients who cannot comply with post-ablation safety regulations are contraindications for radioablation.

CHOICE OF THERAPY FOR GRAVES' THYROTOXICOSIS

The pragmatic approach for choice of therapy in Graves' disease is to discuss with the patient all the three choices of therapy and help making a decision regarding the choice. The patient should be informed about all three therapies, its advantages, disadvantages, consequences, and cost of therapy. It is advisable to record or document in the case file of the person that all three choices of therapy were discussed, relevant literature was provided to the patient, and after due consideration and discussion, the patient chose a particular therapy as the first choice.

RECENT ADVANCES

While we have discussed all three management options available, it is important to note that none of these methods are targeting the pathophysiology of Graves' disease revolving around the activating TSH-receptor antibody. Many advances in this avenue show promise.

In one such study, Rituximab, a monoclonal CD20 antibody, induced a sustained remission in patients with low TSH-receptor antibody levels as well as ameliorating the signs of thyroid eye disease.[30] Of course, the medication is expensive and has a serious adverse effect profile preventing it from routine use. Neumann et al. have described a family of novel small molecule ligands that bind to the transmembrane pocket of the TSH-receptor and inhibit the conformational change necessary for activation have been discovered.[31] While these ligands have emerged as promising targets, the studies are in the preclinical validation stages.

CONCLUSION

Thyrotoxicosis is a common clinical condition in India with Graves' thyrotoxicosis being the most common cause of hyperthyroidism. Radioiodine or Technetium[99] scans can aid diagnosis when a clinical diagnosis of Graves' is not straightforward. Antithyroid drugs are commonly used to treat Graves' disease, but fewer than 50% of patients treated with ATDs remain in long-term remission. Surgery is used in specific situations—patients who have a large goiter or active vision threatening ophthalmopathy. Radioactive iodine is the choice of therapy unless contraindicated. It is the most simple, economical, and safe therapy for Grave's thyrotoxicosis. Appropriate therapy is provided after factoring in patients' preferences and clinical scenario. Newer advances targeting TSH-receptor seem promising.

REFERENCES

1. Unnikrishnan AG, Menon UV. Thyroid disorders in India: an epidemiological perspective. Indian J Endocrinol Metab. 2011;15(6):78-81.
2. Abraham R, Srinivasa Murugan V, Pukazhvanthen P, Sen SK. Thyroid disorders in women of Puducherry. Indian J Clin Biochem. 2009;24(1):52-9.
3. Velayutham K, Selvan SSA, Unnikrishnan AG. Prevalence of thyroid dysfunction among young females in a South Indian population. Indian J Endocrinol Metab. 2015;19(6):781-4.
4. Canaris GJ, Manowitz NR, Mayor G, Ridgway EC. The Colorado thyroid disease prevalence study. Arch Intern Med. 2000;160(4):526-34.

5. Braverman EL, Cooper SD. Introduction to thyrotoxicosis. In: Braverman LE, Cooper D, editors. Werner & Ingbar's The Thyroid: A Fundamental and Clinical Text. 10th ed. Philadelphia: Lippincott Williams & Williams; 2012.
6. Jameson JL, Weetman AP. Disorders of thyroid gland. In: Fauci A, Braunwald E, Kasper D, editors. Harrison's Principles of Internal Medicine. 17th ed. New York: McGraw Hill Publications; 2008.
7. Summaria V, Salvatori M, Rufini V, Mirk P, Garganese MC, Romani M. Diagnostic imaging in thyrotoxicosis. Rays. 1999;24(2):273-300.
8. Bogazzi F, Vitti P. Could improved ultrasound and power Doppler replace thyroidal radioiodine uptake to assess thyroid disease? Nat Clin Pract Endocrinol Metab. 2008;4(2):70-1.
9. Costagliola S, Morgenthaler NG, Hoermann R, Badenhoop K, Struck J, Freitag D, et al. Second generation assay for thyrotropin receptor antibodies has superior diagnostic sensitivity for Graves' disease. J Clin Endocrinol Metab. 1999;84(1):90-7.
10. Bahn Chair RS, Burch HB, Cooper DS, Garber JR, Greenlee MC, Klein I. Hyperthyroidism and other causes of thyrotoxicosis: management guidelines of the American Thyroid Association and American Association of Clinical Endocrinologists. Thyroid. 2011;21(6):593-646.
11. Cooper DS. Antithyroid drugs. N Engl J Med. 2005;352(9):905-17.
12. Abraham P, Avenell A, Park CM, Watson WA, Bevan JS. A systematic review of drug therapy for Graves' hyperthyroidism. Eur J Endorinol. 2005;153(4):489-98.
13. Azizi F, Ataie L, Hedayati M, Mehrabi Y, Shiekholeslami F. Effect of long-term continuous methimazole treatment of hyperthyroidism: comparison with radioiodine. Eur J Endocrinol. 2005;152(5):695-701.
14. Muldoon BT, Mai VQ, Burch HB. Management of Graves' disease: an overview and comparison of clinical practice guidelines with actual practice trends. Endocrinol Metab Clin North Am. 2014;43(2):495-516.
15. Sundaresh V, Brito JP, Wang Z, Prokop LJ, Stan MN, Murad MH, et al. Comparative effectiveness of therapies for Graves' hyperthyroidism: a systematic review and network meta-analysis. J Clin Endocrinol Metab. 2013;98(9):3671-7.
16. De Rooij A, Vandenbroucke JP, Smit JW, Stokkel MP, Dekkers OM. Clinical outcomes after estimated versus calculated activity of radioiodine for the treatment of hyperthyroidism: systematic review and meta-analysis. Eur J Endocrinol. 2009;161(5):771-7.
17. Leslie WD, Ward L, Salamon EA, Ludwig S, Rowe RC, Cowden EA. A randomized comparison of radioiodine doses in Graves' hyperthyroidism. J Clin Endocrinol Metab. 2003;88(3):978-83.
18. Gopinath PG, Prassana KM, Padhy AK, Aggarwal SL. Thyroid status 10 years after I-131 therapy for toxic diffuse goitre. Indian J Nucl Med. 1989;4(1):8-10.
19. Prasanna Kumar KM, Dharmalingam M. Radioablation in Graves Thyrotoxicosis. Indian J Endocrinol Metab. 1997;1(1):1-2.
20. Shivaprasad C, Prasanna Kumar KM. Long-term carbimazole pretreatment reduces the efficacy of radioiodine therapy. Indian J Endocrinol Metab. 2015;19(1):84-8.
21. Subramanian M, Baby MK, Seshadri KG. The effect of prior antithyroid drug use on delaying remission in high uptake Graves' disease following radioiodine ablation. Endocr Connect. 2016;5(1):34-40.
22. Karyampudi A, Hamide A, Halanaik D, Sahoo JP, Kamalanathan S. Radioiodine therapy in patients with Graves' disease and the effects of prior carbimazole therapy. Indian J Endocrinol Metab. 2014;18(5):688-93.
23. Burch HB, Solomon BL, Cooper DS, Ferguson P, Walpert N, Howard R. The effect of antithyroid drug pretreatment on acute changes in thyroid hormone levels after (131)I ablation for Graves' disease. J Clin Endocrinol Metab. 2001;86(7):3016-21.
24. Lee SL. Radioactive iodine therapy. Curr Opin Endocrinol Diabetes Obes. 2012;19(5):420-8.
25. Uy HL, Reasner CA, Samuels MH. Pattern of recovery of the hypothalamic-pituitary-thyroid axis following radioactive iodine therapy in patients with Graves' disease. Am J Med. 1995;99(2):173-9.
26. Palit TK, Miller CC 3rd, Miltenburg DM. The efficacy of thyroidectomy for Graves' disease: A meta-analysis. J Surg Res. 2000;90(2):161-5.
27. Erbil Y, Giris M, Salmaslioglu A, Ozluk Y, Barbaros U, Yanik BT, et al. The effect of anti-thyroid drug treatment duration on thyroid gland microvessel density and intraoperative blood loss in patients with Graves' disease. Surgery. 2008;143(2):216-25.
28. Erbil Y, Ozluk Y, Giriş M, Salmaslioglu A, Issever H, Barbaros U, et al. Effect of lugol solution on thyroid gland blood flow and microvessel density in the patients with Graves' disease. J Clin Endocrinol Metab. 2007;92(6):2182-9.
29. Shinall MC, Broome JT, Baker A, Solorzano CC. Is potassium iodide solution necessary before total thyroidectomy for Graves disease? Ann Surg Oncol. 2013;20(9):2964-7.
30. El Fassi D, Nielsen CH, Bonnema SJ, Hasselbalch HC, Hegedüs L. B lymphocyte depletion with the monoclonal antibody rituximab in Graves' disease: a controlled pilot study. J Clin Endocrinol Metab. 2007;92(5):1769-72.
31. Neumann S, Eliseeva E, McCoy JG, Napolitano G, Giuliani C, Monaco F, et al. A new small-molecule antagonist inhibits Graves' disease antibody activation of the TSH receptor. J Clin Endocrinol Metab. 2011;96(2):548-54.

CHAPTER 3

Thyroid Disorders During Pregnancy

Vivek Mathew, Vageesh Ayyar S

INTRODUCTION

Women during their reproductive period do present with thyroid disorders. As pregnancy is also a hypermetabolic state, many a times, thyroid dysfunction is often overlooked because of its nonspecific manifestations. Physiological alterations in the thyroid functions during pregnancy further compounds the diagnosis of thyroid disorders during pregnancy. In fact, it becomes difficult for clinicians many a times to differentiate physiological alterations in the thyroid functions from the true thyroid disorder. Thyroid disorders in the mother can affect the growing fetus in the womb either directly by transplacental passage of maternal thyroid hormones or thyroid stimulating hormone (TSH)-receptor antibodies or indirectly, through the medications used to treat the maternal thyroid disorders (Table 1). It is also well-known that untreated thyroid disorders during pregnancy do result in increased adverse events. Therefore, appropriate knowledge is necessary for proper management of the thyroid disorders during pregnancy.

TABLE 1: Placental transfer

Complete transfer	Thyrotropin releasing hormone, thyroid antibodies, thionamides, and iodide
Some transfer	Thyroxine and triiodothyronine
No or negligible transfer	Thyroid stimulating hormone

EPIDEMIOLOGY

The prevalence of hypothyroidism in pregnancy is about 2–3% according to the Western literature. Among them, 0.3–0.5% are overt hypothyroid and 2–2.5% found to have subclinical hypothyroidism. The prevalence of hyperthyroidism is less common and it occurs in less than 0.4% of pregnant women.[1] The prevalence of hypothyroidism during pregnancy is between 4.8 and 13.3% and this is based on few reports and it is mainly from the secondary and tertiary hospitals.[2-4] Iodine deficiency continues to be major cause for thyroid disorders during pregnancy worldwide. The data regarding iodine sufficiency from India are scant. The prevalence is as high as 57% from older studies and from the rural areas whereas it is less than 2.5% from newer studies and from the tertiary centers. However, adequate supplementation with iodine is essential to prevent maternal hypothyroxinemia during pregnancy. Women of reproductive age need around 150 μg/day, and requirement increases to 250 μg/day during pregnancy and lactation.[5]

TABLE 2: Thyroid stimulating hormone reference ranges during pregnancy

Trimester	Thyroid stimulating hormone (mIU/L)
First	0.1–2.50
Second	0.2–3.00
Third	0.3–3.00

THYROID FUNCTION TEST IN PREGNANCY

Once women conceive, around 4–8 weeks, there is increase in the circulating thyroxine binding globulin (TBG) concentrations and total thyroxine (TT4) concentrations. Human chorionic gonadotropin (hCG) has thyrotropic activity and this results in decrease in serum TSH in the first trimester.[6,7] Hence, serum TSH concentrations are lower than nonpregnant women. Though theoretically free T4 (FT4) levels should be unaltered in gestation, there is substantial decrease in serum FT4 concentrations in gestation. It is further affected by the reliability of the immunoassay measurement of FT4 assays, which is affected by increased TBG and reduced albumin levels seen during gestation. Hence, trimester specific TSH levels (Table 2) should be applied during pregnancy, failure to understand these ranges certainly results in mismanagement of the thyroid disorders during pregnancy.[8,9]

CASE 1

A 27-year-old female, married for 3 years and being evaluated by obstetrician for primary infertility was presented with sensitive TSH (sTSH) value of 8 µIU/mL, the sole abnormality found while being evaluated for the infertility. She had regular cycles and workup for male factors and family history were not contributory. On examination, she had grade II diffuse firm goiter otherwise examination was normal. On evaluation, her TT4: 8 µg/mL was normal and thyroid peroxidase antibodies were positive. Based on above parameters, patient was started on 50 µg of levothyroxine (LT4) and came for follow-up after 3 months with sTSH of 1.4 µIU/mL. Patient was asked to continue work same dosage and was called after 3 months or on conception. Patient came after 2 months with missed period and on evaluation, her urinary pregnancy test was positive for pregnancy. She was asked to increase her dosage to 62.5 µg/day and was called after 4 weeks with TT4 and TSH. On follow-up, her TSH was 4.0 µIU/mL and TT4 was 12 µg/mL. Her dosage was further increased to 75 µg/day and was called after 4 weeks. On follow-up subsequently, her TSH remained less than 2.5 µIU/mL till delivery. Her delivery was uneventful and was discharged with 50 µg of LT4 with advice of regular follow-up.

OVERT HYPOTHYROIDISM

In overt primary hypothyroidism, one will find a low FT4 with high TSH levels. Iodine deficiency disorders continue to remain main reason across the globe. However, in countries where iodine intake is sufficient, the most frequent reason being autoimmune thyroiditis.[10,11]

If overt hypothyroidism (OH) is left untreated during pregnancy, it is associated with serious adverse outcomes. Reduced intelligence quotient (IQ) is one of the best known adverse outcomes. Children born to untreated hypothyroid mothers had 7 IQ scores less than the controls which was statistically significant. Even untreated mothers experience several obstetric complications. Important ones being spontaneous miscarriage, preterm

> **Box 1: Practical tips for the clinical management of hypothyroidism in pregnancy**
> - Serum TSH level should be checked as soon as pregnancy is diagnosed
> - Need to increase the dosage of LT4 by 25–40% based on the etiology
> - For overt hypothyroidism, administer 2 µg/kg/day of LT4
> - Need to monitor serum TSH every 4 weeks during first half of pregnancy and every 6 weeks thereafter
> - Maintain serum TSH less than 2.5 mU/L during first trimester and less than 3.0 mIU/L thereafter
> - Monitor serum TSH after 3–4 weeks of every dosage adjustment
> - LT4 ingestion should be at least 4 hours separated from calcium and iron supplements
> - Following delivery, reduce LT4 to prepregnancy dosage
>
> LT4, levothyroxine; TSH, thyroid stimulating hormone.

TABLE 3: Levothyroxine dosage based on thyroid stimulating hormone level

Thyroid stimulating hormone level (mIU/L)	Levothyroxine dosage (µg)
5–10	25–50
10–20	50–75
>20	75–100

delivery, stillbirth, fetal distress, and perinatal death. Many studies have also shown increased incidence of gestational hypertension, abruptio placentae, and postpartum hemorrhage. Adequate treatment ensures lesser complications than the untreated OH subjects.[11,12]

Diagnosis of OH during is very essential and it is also very crucial to restore euthyroidism as early as possible. Levothyroxine is the treatment of choice for the hypothyroidism. In women with preexisting hypothyroidism, one needs to increase the dosage of the LT4 by 25–40% depending on the etiology of the hypothyroidism (Box 1). In patients with Hashimoto's thyroiditis, the requirement is less than patient's having hypothyroidism following total thyroidectomy.[13,14] Dosages need to be adjusted to keep TSH less than 2.5 mIU/L before conception and during first trimester, and should not exceed 3.0 mIU/L during the second and third trimesters. Dose can be brought down to prepregnancy levels once patient delivers (Table 3).[15-17]

SUBCLINICAL HYPOTHYROIDISM

Subclinical hypothyroidism (SH) is the common thyroid dysfunction encountered during pregnancy. It is defined when TSH is slightly elevated and FT4 within normal limits. It has variable prevalence from one study to another, based on the definition, iodine sufficiency and ethnicity. Overall prevalence is between 1.5 and 4.0%. Similar to OH, SH also has several obstetrical and perinatal outcomes associated with the condition. However, results from various studies are perplexing, perhaps due to differences in study design, power of the study, and the population studied. One of the most frequent outcomes noticed in many studies is pregnancy loss.[18,19]

Several retrospective studies have shown that SH is linked with heightened risk of adverse obstetrical and perinatal outcomes. Two prospective studies have shown benefit of treating SH during pregnancy. Hence, it is better to intervene and treat SH during pregnancy as there are no documented adverse effects of LT4 therapy either to mother or fetus as long as pregnancy specific TSH ranges are followed.[13,14,20,21]

Disorders of Thyroid

> **CASE 2**
>
> A 28-year-old female was referred with 6 weeks gestation in view of her sTSH: 0.1 µIU/mL (0.34–4.1) and TT4:16 µg/mL (6.09–12.23). Patient had mild morning sickness symptoms otherwise asymptomatic. She gave a history of being treated for Graves' disease 3 years ago and in remission since then with regular follow-up with her physician and TSH done 6 months ago was 1.5 µIU/mL. Her sister 5 years elder to her was also suffering from hypothyroidism. On clinical examination, she had a grade II goitre—soft in consistency with no bruit, no eye signs or dermopathy. She was counseled and was asked to come back after 4 weeks with thyroid function tests. Patient came after 2 weeks with worsening of her morning sickness symptoms with increasing tiredness with weight loss of 1 kg in 2 weeks. Her evaluation this time revealed heart rate of 96 beats/min, tachycardia, and tremulousness of extended hands. Laboratory tests showed sTSH: 0.03 uIU/mL and TT4: 20 µg/mL, and ultrasound of the thyroid with Doppler showing increased blood flow. With the above reports, patient was diagnosed to have relapsed Graves' disease and started on propylthiouracil (PTU) 25 mg thrice daily and was asked to follow-up after 4 weeks. After follow-up, patient was symptomatically better and no further weight loss was observed, and her TSH was 0.4 µIU/mL and TT4 was 16 µg/mL. As patient had completed her first trimester, her antithyroid medication was changed to methimazole (MMI) 5 mg once daily as it is safe to change over to MMI after first trimester. Patient was followed up every 4 weeks and anomaly scan was carried out around 22nd week and it revealed no fetal goiter and no signs of fetal toxicosis. She remained euthyroid on regular 4 weekly follow-up and her MMI was tapered and stopped by 30th week of gestation and patient remained euthyroid clinically and also on laboratory evaluation till her delivery. She was sent home with the advice of possible recurrence of her Graves' disease in puerperium and was asked to come with TSH after 12 weeks.

HYPERTHYROIDISM IN PREGNANCY

Excessive production of thyroid hormones by the thyroid gland results in the hyperthyroidism. The prevalence of hyperthyroidism during pregnancy ranges from 0.1 to 0.4%. In pregnancy, the causes of hyperthyroidism may be immune and/or nonimmune mediated. Graves' disease accounts for 85% of cases of hyperthyroidism during pregnancy and it is an autoimmune disease. The most common cause of nonimmune hyperthyroidism is transient hyperthyroidism of hyperemesis gravidarum (THHG), which is typically seen in the first trimester of the pregnancy and characterized by elevated serum FT4 and suppressed or undetectable TSH, in the absence of thyroid autoimmunity. Toxic adenoma, toxic multinodular goiter, and subacute thyroiditis occur with lesser frequency during pregnancy, whereas hydatidiform molar disease are extremely rare.

Transient Hyperthyroidism of Hyperemesis Gravidarum

Transient hyperthyroidism of hyperemesis gravidarum diagnosed by suppressed or undetectable serum TSH levels in the presence of elevated FT4. Elevated FT4 levels are essential for the diagnosis as TSH can be as low as 0.03 mIU/L during first trimester of the pregnancy. Research strongly points to that the high serum concentrations of hCG during early pregnancy have the ability to stimulate or activate the TSH receptor. Usually, THHG is not severe but rarely it may require hospitalization. Whether symptomatic or not, THHG usually resolves spontaneously by 20 weeks gestation when hCG declines. Neonatal and obstetrical consequences are almost nil. Differentiating THHG from Graves' disease may be difficult or challenging if goiter and ophthalmopathy are absent, and if markers of autoimmunity like thyroid peroxidase (TPO) antibodies and thyroid receptor antibodies (TRAb) are negative. Treatment with antithyroid agents (ATA) is generally not needed. If THHG continues even after 20 weeks, one needs to reevaluate for other causes of hyperthyroidism.[10,22]

Graves' Disease

The most common cause of hyperthyroidism during pregnancy is Graves' disease. There are many ways it can present during pregnancy. There can be exacerbation of the Graves' disease in someone who is stable on antithyroid medication during beginning of the pregnancy, or it may present *de novo* first time during pregnancy or there can be relapse of the Graves' disease who is in remission. Even the cause of the disease is quite variable like other autoimmune diseases with exacerbations during first trimester with gradual betterment during later part of the pregnancy, with even possibility of exacerbation during postpartum.[23]

Diagnosis of the Graves' disease often poses challenge during pregnancy as symptoms and some signs do overlap with hypermetabolic features of pregnancy. Graves' disease often presents with goiter with or without bruit which makes the diagnosis of Graves' more likely. However, other signs of autoimmunity like ophthalmopathy or dermopathy are quite rare.[23,24]

Laboratory investigations are helpful in diagnosis which reveal suppressed TSH levels with elevated total and free thyroid hormones. One needs to be careful in interpreting laboratory values as it overlaps with THHG. Finally, measurement of TSH receptor antibody (TRAb) may help in confirming the diagnosis as it is usually elevated in patients with Graves' disease.[9,23]

Pregnancy outcomes are related to the duration and degree of the maternal hyperthyroidism. Both mother and fetus are at risk of complications. Preterm labor, stillbirth, and preeclampsia are seen with increasing frequency in women with untreated or uncontrolled hyperthyroidism. It has been shown that children born to women with uncontrolled Graves' disease during pregnancy more frequently have small for gestational age and congenital malformations which are unrelated to thionamide therapy.[10,24]

Efficient and appropriate treatment of the hyperthyroid state is of utmost importance to not only prevent maternal and fetal complication but also have good neonatal outcome. Antithyroid agents remains the mainstay of the treatment. The aim is to use the smallest possible dose of the ATAs with frequent monitoring. Excessive dosage need to be avoided as it results in fetal goiter or fetal hypothyroidism.[13,25]

Thionamides, PTU, and MMI are the drugs used to treat Graves' disease during pregnancy. These drugs reduce thyroid hormone production by inhibiting the organification of the iodine and coupling of the iodotyrosine by TPO. Median time to achieve normalization of the maternal thyroid function is around 7 weeks by PTU and 8 weeks by MMI. Propylthiouracil and MMI are equally efficacious in achieving euthyroidism. Propylthiouracil has a higher incidence of hepatotoxicity, whereas MMI has been associated with "MMI embryopathy" which has several congenital defects including aplasia cutis. The current recommendation by the American Thyroid Association is restrict use of PTU to first trimester, then switch to MMI during second and third trimester. Maternal side effects from ATAs are seen in less than 5% of the patients and it is mainly pruritus and skin rashes, and rarely leads to discontinuation of the medication (Box 2).[25,26]

Fetal and neonatal outcomes are dependent on the degree of hyperthyroidism, overtreatment with antithyroid drugs (ATDs), and maternal TRAb levels. To achieve best

> **Box 2: Practice points about hyperthyroidism in pregnancy**
> - "Euthyroid" hyperthyroidism seen in pregnancy by itself is not an indication for treatment
> - Gestational hyperthyroidism should be differentiated from Graves' disease
> - Monitoring of maternal status with thyroid-stimulating hormone and free thyroxine for initiation and adjustment of antithyroid drugs
> - Fetal thyroid status should be screened by ultrasonography and thyroid-stimulating hormone-receptor antibody at 24 to 28 weeks
> - Propylthiouracil should be used in first trimester and the methimazole subsequently.

outcomes, one needs to monitor maternal T4 once in 2–4 weeks based on severity of the hyperthyroid state and maintain the T4 levels in the upper tertile or above the upper limit of the normal range suggested for the pregnancy. Thyroid stimulating hormone receptor antibody crosses placental barrier and stimulates fetal thyroid gland. Maternal TRAb 3–5 times above the normal range in the second half of the pregnancy is a risk factor for the fetal hyperthyroidism. Hence, measurement between 26 and 28 weeks has been recommended by ATA. Signs of fetal hyperthyroidism are fetal goiter, fetal tachycardia, fetal growth retardation, hydrops fetalis, and advanced bone maturation. Serial fetal ultrasound along with fetal nonstress test to assess fetal well-being is been recommended in affected pregnancies.[25,26]

Beta-blocking agents like, propranolol or atenolol, to control hyperadrenergic symptoms are recommended, however, it carries a small risk of increased first trimester miscarriage.[27]

Use of iodide alongside of thionamides has fallen out of favor in view of fetal goiter and fetal hypothyroidism.[26,27]

Subtotal thyroidectomy for Graves' disease during pregnancy is reserved only for specific situations, when high doses of thionamides (PTU >600 mg and MMI >40 mg/day) are required to control maternal state, or patient is allergic to both PTU and MMI, or if compressive symptoms appear in the mother due to goiter size. Second trimester before 24 weeks is ideal time to subject to the surgery.[28,29]

Radioactive iodine therapy is contraindicated for the treatment of hyperthyroid state during pregnancy and lactation.[14,24]

POSTPARTUM CARE

Recurrence of hyperthyroidism may happen to many patients within 1 year after delivery. Hence, thyroid functions should be monitored starting from 6 weeks postpartum regularly till the end of 1 year. It is essential to distinguish between hyperthyroid state of postpartum thyroiditis and relapsed Graves' hyperthyroidism, as one can avoid using ATDs in postpartum thyroiditis. Use of nuclear uptake scan is dependent on the breastfeeding status of the mother.[30,31]

EUTHYROIDISM WITH AUTOIMMUNE THYROID DISEASE

Positivity of thyroid auto antibodies are quite common in otherwise normal euthyroid women of reproductive age group. These women may be at an increased risk for poor pregnancy outcomes including spontaneous miscarriage and postpartum thyroiditis. Possible explanation for the spontaneous miscarriage may be an unfavorable auto-immune environment or reduced functional thyroid reserve. This observation is not uniform and consistent with the other studies.[32,33]

Given conflicting data across the studies regarding euthyroid autoimmunity and poor pregnancy outcomes, two treatment lines have been suggested. These include intravenous immunoglobulin (IVIg) and LT4 administration. Data from these studies are considered preliminary and cannot be recommended to all.[34]

PREGNANCY AND THYROID NODULES

Incidence and prevalence of nodular thyroid disease is higher in women compared to men and it increases with age, pregnancy and with the use of ultrasonography as investigational tool. There is significant increase in new nodule and increase in size of existing nodules during pregnancy. However, this increase in size and number does not translate into *de novo* increase in thyroid malignancy during pregnancy. Thyroid nodule detected during pregnancy should be evaluated on similar lines of nonpregnant state.[13,35] Laboratory tests of the thyroid should be interpreted keeping in view of altered normal physiology of thyroid functions during pregnancy. Nodule should be characterized sonologically and fine needle aspiration should be obtained if required with or without sonological guidance. Cytological interpretation is similar to nonpregnant state. Evidence and approach is divided regarding the approach to the management of thyroid cancer discovered during pregnancy as they are not more aggressive compared to nonpregnant state of similar age. Hence, surgery may be postponed to after delivery. If surgical intervention decided, it is suggested to carry out before 24 weeks during second trimester to minimize risk of miscarriage and radionuclear studies should be postponed till after delivery as it is contraindicated during pregnancy.[14,36]

CONCLUSION

Thyroid disorders are quite frequent in women during childbearing age. Thyroid functions do get altered physiologically during normal pregnancy. Interpretation of thyroid functions during pregnancy requires specific pregnancy ranges otherwise leads to misdiagnosis and improper institution of therapy. Adequate screening programs need to be instituted for early detection of the thyroid dysfunction in predisposed individuals so that proper therapy can be initiated and adverse outcomes associated with thyroid dysfunction can be prevented.

REFERENCES

1. Negro R, Mestman JH. Thyroid disease in pregnancy. Best Pract Res Clin Endocrinol Metab. 2011;25(6):927-43.
2. Dhanwal DK, Bajaj S, Rajput R, Subramaniam KA, Chowdhury S, Bhandari R, et al. Prevalence of hypothyroidism in pregnancy: an epidemiological study from 11 cities in 9 states of India. Indian J Endocrinol Metab. 2016;20(3):387-90.
3. Menon VU, Chellan G, Sundaram KR, Murthy S, Kumar H, Unnikrishnan AG, et al. Iodine status and its correlations with age, blood pressure, and thyroid volume in South Indian women above 35 years of age (Amrita Thyroid Survey). Indian J Endocrinol Metab. 2011;15(4):309-15.
4. Rajput R, Goel V, Nanda S, Rajput M, Seth S. Prevalence of thyroid dysfunction among women during the first trimester of pregnancy at a tertiary care hospital in Haryana. Indian J Endocrinol Metab. 2015;19(3):416-9.
5. Grewal E, Khadgawat R, Gupta N, Desai A, Tandon N. Assessment of iodine nutrition in pregnant north Indian subjects in three trimesters. Indian J Endocrinol Metab. 2013;17(2):289-93.
6. Glinoer D. The regulation of thyroid function in pregnancy: pathways of endocrine adaptation from physiology to pathology. Endocr Rev. 1997;18(3):404-33.
7. Glinoer D Spencer CA. Serum TSH determinations in pregnancy: how, when and why? Nat Rev Endocrinol. 2010;6(9):526-9.

8. LeBeau SO, Mandel SJ. Thyroid disorders during pregnancy. Endocrinol Metab Clin North Am. 2006;35(1):117-36.
9. Krassas G, Karras SN, Pontikides N. Thyroid diseases during pregnancy: a number of important issues. Hormones (Athens). 2015;14(1):59-69.
10. Galofre JC, Davies TF. Autoimmune thyroid disease in pregnancy: a review. J Womens Health (Larchmt). 2009;18(11):1847-56.
11. Vissenberg R, van den Boogaard E, van Wely M, van der Post JA, Fliers E, Bisschop PH, et al. Treatment of thyroid disorders before conception and in early pregnancy: a systematic review. Human Reprod Update. 2012;18(4):360-73.
12. Haddow JE, Palomaki GE, Allan WC, Williams JR, Knight GJ, Gagnon J, et al. Maternal thyroid deficiency during pregnancy and subsequent neuropsychological development of the child. N Engl J Med. 1999;341(8):549-55.
13. Stagnaro-Green A, Abalovich M, Alexander E, Azizi F, Mestman J, Negro R, et al. Guidelines of the American Thyroid Association for the diagnosis and management of thyroid disease during pregnancy and postpartum. Thyroid. 2011;21(10):1081-125.
14. De Groot L, Abalovich M, Alexander EK, Amino N, Barbour L, Cobin RH, et al. Management of thyroid dysfunction during pregnancy and postpartum: an Endocrine Society clinical practice guideline. J Clin Endocrinol Metab. 2012;97(8):2543-65.
15. Alexander EK, Marqusee E, Lawrence J, Jarolim P, Fischer GA, Larsen PR. Timing and magnitude of increases in levothyroxine requirements during pregnancy in women with hypothyroidism. N Engl J Med. 2004;351(3):241-9.
16. Yassa L, Marqusee E, Fawcett R, Alexander EK. Thyroid hormone early adjustment in pregnancy (the THERAPY) trial. J Clin Endocrinol Metab. 2010;95(7):3234-41.
17. Poppe K, Glinoer D. Thyroid autoimmunity and hypothyroidism before and during pregnancy. Hum Reprod Update. 2003;9(2):149-61.
18. Mascarenhas JV, Ayyar SV, Bantwal G. Subclinical hypothyroidism and conception in a woman with primary infertility. J Clin Sci Res. 2012;1:94-6.
19. Mascarenhas JV, Anoop HS, Patil M, Kulkarni S, George B, Ananthraman, et al. Improvement in fertility outcome follows initiation of thyroxine for women with subclinical hypothyroidism. Thyroid Res Pract. 2011;8(3):3-6.
20. Negro R, Stagnaro-Green A. Diagnosis and management of subclinical hypothyroidism in pregnancy. BMJ. 2014;349:4929.
21. Vaquero E, Lazzarin N, De Carolis C, Valensise H, Moretti C, Ramanini C. Mild thyroid abnormalities and recurrent spontaneous abortion: diagnostic and therapeutic approach. Am J Reprod Immunol. 2000;43(4):204-8.
22. Mestman JH. Hyperthyroidism in pregnancy. Best Pract Res Clin Endocrinol Metab. 2004;18(2):267-88.
23. Patil-Sisodia K, Mestman JH. Graves hyperthyroidism and pregnancy: a clinical update. Endocr Pract. 2010;16(1):118-29.
24. Marx H, Amin P, Lazarus JH. Hyperthyroidism and pregnancy. BMJ. 2008;336(7645):663-7.
25. Luton D, Le Gac I, Vuillard E, Castanet M, Guibourdenche J, Noel M, et al. Management of Graves' disease during pregnancy: the key role of fetal thyroid gland monitoring. J Clin Endocrinol Metab. 2005;90(11):6093-8.
26. Zimmerman D. Fetal and neonatal hyperthyroidism. Thyroid. 1999;9(7):727-33.
27. Mandel SJ, Cooper DS. The use of antithyroid drugs in pregnancy and lactation. J Clin Endocrinol Metab. 2001;86(6):2354-9.
28. Mandel SJ, Brent GA, Larsen PR. Review of antithyroid drug use during pregnancy and report of a case of aplasia cutis. Thyroid. 1994;4(1):129-33.
29. Laurberg P, Bournaud C, Karmisholt J, Orgiazzi J. Management of Graves' hyperthyroidism in pregnancy: focus on both maternal and fetal thyroid function, and caution against surgical thyroidectomy in pregnancy. Eur J Endocrinol. 2009;160(1):1-8.
30. Benhaim RD, Davies TF. Increased risk of Graves' disease after pregnancy. Thyroid. 2005;15(11):1287-90.
31. Rotondi M, Pirali B, Lodigiani S, Bray S, Leporati P, Chytiris S, et al. The post partum period and the onset of Graves' disease: an overestimated risk factor. Eur J Endocrinol. 2008;159(2):161-5.
32. Abramson J, Stagnaro-Green A. Thyroid antibodies and fetal loss: an evolving story. Thyroid. 2001;11(1):57-63.
33. Stagnaro-Green A, Glinoer D. Thyroid autoimmunity and the risk of miscarriage. Best Pract Res Clin Endocrinol Metab. 2004;18(2):167-81.
34. Toulis KA, Goulis DG, Venetis CA, Kolibianakis EM, Negro R, Tarlatzis BC, et al. Risk of spontaneous miscarriage in euthyroid women with thyroid autoimmunity undergoing IVF: a meta-analysis. Eur J Endocrinol. 2010;162(4):643-52.
35. Tan GH, Gharib H, Goellner JR, van Heerden JA, Bahn RS. Management of thyroid nodules in pregnancy. Arch Intern Med. 1996;156(20):2317-20.
36. Kung AW, Chau MT, Lao TT, Tam SC, Low LC. The effect of pregnancy on thyroid nodule formation. J Clin Endocrinol Metab. 2002;87(3):1010-4.

CHAPTER 4

Approach to the Solitary Thyroid Nodule and Cancer

Krishna G Seshadri

INTRODUCTION

A thyroid nodule may be defined as a discrete lesion within the thyroid gland that is radiologically distinct from the surrounding gland.[1] Palpable thyroid nodules are present in approximately 5% of women and 1% of men in iodine sufficient areas. If high resolution ultrasound (USG) was used, up to 68% of randomly selected individuals may have nodules—more in women and increasing with age in both sexes.[2] There is a linear increase in prevalence from almost none at age 15 to 50% by age 65.[3]

> **CASE STUDY**
>
> A 32-year-old woman was evaluated for a solitary nodule of the thyroid. She had noticed this swelling 6 months ago while examining a necklace with a mirror. She had no other complaints. There was no family history of thyroid cancer. There was no history of childhood irradiation. The swelling was approximately 2.0 cm in the transverse direction and moves with deglutition. There was no fixity to the surrounding tissue. There was no lymphadenopathy.
>
> A USG done elsewhere revealed a 2.0 cm × 2.0 cm × 2.5 cm nodule isoechoic nodule with normal contour and border with normal vascularity. Serum thyroid stimulating hormone (TSH) was 2.0. A fine needle aspiration cytology (FNAC) done outside stated that the slide had increased atypia of unknown significance. The patient had a previous opinion with a recommendation for surgery. A second opinion had been sought.

PATHOPHYSIOLOGY

Thyroid Nodules

The principal causes of thyroid nodules are summarized in table 1. Thyroid nodules are the clinical manifestation of a myriad of pathologic processes. Non-neoplastic nodules are the result of glandular hyperplasia arising spontaneously or following partial thyroidectomy.[5] Hashimoto's thyroiditis (HT) may present with a nodular feel but do not represent an example of true nodule formation. Adenomas are characterized by orderly architecture and few mitosis with no lymphatic or vascular invasion. Necrosis is common in nodules resulting in cyst formation. Nodules are monoclonal and grow slowly reflecting the long time taken by thyroid cells to divide. They may increase in pregnancy; new nodules may also develop in pregnancy. Most nodules are detected

TABLE 1: Classification of thyroid nodules[4]

Adenomas	Malignant tumors	Others

• Follicular
  ○ Colloid variant
  ○ Embryonal
  ○ Fetal
  ○ Hurthle cell variant
• Teratoma
	• Differentiated adenocarcinoma
	  ○ Papillary
	  ○ Follicular
	• Medullary carcinoma
	• Undifferentiated
		• Lymphoma
		• Squamous cell epidermoid carcinoma
		• Fibrosarcoma
		• Mucoepithelial carcinoma
		• Metastatic tumor

incidentally. Symptoms of growth and invasion, such as dysphagia, dystonia, and stridor, are rare. Bleeding into the nodule occurs rarely and presents with increase in size, pain, and tenderness, or even transient thyrotoxicosis.

Most nodules are functionally inactive leading to the classic "cold" appearance on functional imaging. This may be due to a specific defect in iodide transport. The sodium iodide symporter (NIS) appears to be underexpressed in both benign and malignant cold nodules.[6] Some nodules appear to have intact iodide transport but lack peroxidase. These nodules appear hot on technetium-99m (Tc-99m) but cold on iodine (see later).[7] About 10% of follicular adenomas are "hot" and produce sufficient thyroxine to cause subclinical or overt thyrotoxicosis. Autonomously functioning thyroid nodules (AFTNs) are more common in areas with a high prevalence of endemic goiters. Activating thyroid stimulating hormone receptor (TSHR) mutations appear too common in AFTN; some patients have mutations in the stimulatory guanosine triphosphate-binding protein subunit.

Thyroid Cancer

Thyroid cancers are uncommon and account for less than 0.5% of cancer deaths.[8] However, the incidence of thyroid cancer is increasing rapidly and currently appears to be the most rapidly increasing malignancy among men and women in the general population.[9] This appears to be a worldwide phenomenon.[10] The mortality rates appear to be unchanged largely reflecting the fact that the increase is primarily in early stage papillary carcinoma. In part, this increase may be attributed to greater use of imaging since the early 1990s. Thyroid carcinoma (TC) is more common in women than men; the ratio being highest after puberty and declining thereafter. The median age of occurrence is 49 years. There are significant ethnic variations. The most common histologic type is papillary thyroid cancer (PTC).[11]

Radiation

Radiation exposure during childhood is the clearest pathogenetic factor. A consistent and strong relationship between doses as low as 0.05 Gy and TC can be demonstrated. The risk above an age of 15 years is not consistent. In atomic bomb survivors, the risk of malignancy is reduced after an age of 10 years but is clearly present. Women appear to be more vulnerable; the risk is constant for up to 30 years after exposure. Thyroid carcinoma in patients with radiation exposure increases the risk that a nodule in a gland is malignant. Most are PTC or its follicular variant. There is a greater risk of multifocal carcinoma and more frequent local residual carcinoma. Recurrence and mortality rates are not different.

Exposure to radioactive iodine (RAI) in childhood, particularly ^{131}I, after nuclear fallout (for instance, after the Chernobyl incident) confers an increased risk for TC. Particularly in childhood, the latency is shorter than due to external radiation; the majority of patients present with a rapidly growing aggressive solid variant of PTC with infiltration beyond the capsule and lymph node involvement. These are associated with distinct rearrangements of the *RET* oncogene. A small increase in the risk of TC but no increase in mortality has been reported in patients who have ^{131}I for toxic multinodular goiters but not Graves' disease. Diagnostic ^{131}I use for thyrotoxicosis, similarly, is not associated with increased risk of thyroid carcinoma.

Genetic and Familial Syndromes

Thyroid carcinoma may be a part of genetic syndromes. It may develop in as many as 12% of patients with familial adenomatous polyposis (FAP) with a risk of TC being 100-fold over the general population. Papillary thyroid cancer occurs early and a cribriform pattern with spindle cells is a characteristic. Germline mutations with TC tend to cluster in a region of the *APC* gene associated with congenital hypertrophy of retinal pigment epithelium. The *RET/PTC1* activation but not *BRAF* is common. Screening may be useful in families with FAP from 15 years of age.

The *PTEN* hamartoma tumor syndromes (Cowden's and other related syndromes) are rare autosomal recessive conditions resulting from inactivating mutations of the tumor suppressor gene. Thyroid abnormalities are found in approximately two-thirds of patients with Cowden's syndrome. Multiple adenomatous nodules in a background of lymphocytic thyroiditis are characteristic. Papillary carcinomas and follicular thyroid carcinomas/cancer (FTC) are found in approximately half of the abnormal thyroid. Screening is warranted. Other familial syndromes with specific gene mutations and TC include Carney complex, Pendred's syndrome, and Werner syndrome.

The prevalence of familial nonmedullary TC based on retrospective studies is approximately 2.6%. The literature is inconsistent with regards to differences in presentation, metastasis, aggressiveness, and recurrence when compared with sporadic TC.

Others

A previous history of goiter or thyroid nodules may confer an increased risk of TC. It is unclear if either Graves' disease or HT confers increased risk; it is clear, however, that they often occur together. Increase in body mass index (and consequently increase in insulin resistance) seems to confer increased risk of TC. In women, increased parity, greater age at first pregnancy and increased age of menopause seem to increase the risk of TC. Similarly, current oral contraceptive use seems to confer increased risk as are drugs used to suppress lactation. The incidence of FTC is higher in iodine deficiency whereas PTC is higher in areas of iodine excess. Fish consumption in iodine-sufficient areas appears to increase the risk of TC.

Molecular Genetics

Thyroid neoplasms are clonal cell populations. Tumor development begins with a somatic mutation that confers a growth advantage. Gain of function of genes involved in growth stimulation and loss of function mutations of genes involved in growth inhibition, cell cycle check points, or cell survival are the principal changes involved. In thyroid cancer, this includes the activation of the MAPK and PI3K signaling pathways which appear to be crucial for tumor initiation and progression. Specific etiologic factors are involved and cause point mutations and chromosomal rearrangements. Other changes include alteration in gene expression patterns, dysregulation of microRNAs, and aberrant gene methylation.

Thyroid stimulating hormone is an important facilitator of tumor growth and mitosis. There appears to be an association with higher levels of TSH and the risk of thyroid cancer in thyroid nodules. BRAF (see later) requires TSH simulation to transform thyroid cells and initiate tumor development. Somatic mutations of the TSHRs are observed in AFTN but are generally not associated with malignant transformation. Downstream to the TSHR, mutations in the components of the cyclic adenosine monophosphate signal cascade can function as oncogenes. Activating point mutations of *Gsα* are associated with AFTN. Growth factors and eicosanoids are also involved in tumor formation and progression.

Peroxisome proliferator-activated receptors (PPARs) are nuclear receptors that bind to deoxyribonucleic acid (DNA) as heterodimers with retinoid X receptors. Mutations of *PPAR-γ* are seen in approximately 35% of patients with FTC, a small proportion of follicular variants of PTC and follicular adenomas.[12] These mutations result in the fusion of the DNA-binding domain of the thyroid transcription factor PAX8 to domains A to F of *PPAR-γ*. *PAX8/PPAR-γ* positive tumors are present in younger patients, appear to be smaller, show solid growth pattern, and greater vascular invasion.

Mutations in *RAS* are found in thyroid follicular cell-derived tumors including FTC, follicular adenomas, and follicular variant of PTC (FVPTC). Mutations in *RAS* are associated with tumor dedifferentiation and less favorable prognosis, metastasis (particularly bone) on the one hand and encapsulated FVPTC (an indolent tumor) on the other hand. *RAS* mutations and *PAX8/PPAR-γ* are never found together indicating two distinct pathways of tumorigenesis.[12]

Mutations of receptors of extracellular ligands most significantly of the tyrosine kinase receptors RET and NTRK1, TET/PTC and TRK oncogenes are involved.

Rearrangements of *RET* resulting in its constitutional activation are implicated in a significant proportions of TCs.[14] Several types of *RET/PTC* have been identified depending on the 5′ partner gene involved in the rearrangement of the most common of these being the *RET/PTC1* and *RET/PTC3*. *RET/PTC* appears to be involved in the earliest steps of carcinogenesis since they are seen in microcarcinomas.[15] *RET/PTC1* is particularly found in PTC with classic papillary architecture; *RET/PTC3* is seen with solid variants. The *RET/PTC1* rearrangement is associated with favorable outcomes when compared to other mutations such as RAS and BRAF. Radiation exposure (such as the one that occurred in Chernobyl) is associated with increased frequency of *RET/PTC3*. This is associated with aggressive behavior and progression to dedifferentiation.

Mutations in the B isoform of the serine-threonine kinase RAF (*BRAF*) are found in up to 45% of PTC and represent the most common genetic alterations seen in thyroid tumors. A transversion of thymine to adenine at nucleotide position 1799 leading to a valine to glutamate substitution at residue 600 (V600E) accounts for up to 99% of all *BRAF* mutations in thyroid cancer. The mutation leads to aberrant expression of the sodium iodide symporter (NIS) and other genes involved in iodine metabolism. *BRAF* V600E and other mutations of the *BRAF* lead to the activation of BRAF kinase, increase MEK phosphorylation and stimulate the MAPK pathway. *BRAF* requires TSH stimulation to initiate PTC development.[16] *BRAF* V600E mutation is found in all important variants of PTC. They are also seen in tumors that dedifferentiate and those PTCs that have apparently undergone anaplastic transformation. These mutations are not found in benign thyroid tumors or FTC and are thus a specific marker of PTC. It is associated with extrathyroidal extension, advanced stage at presentation, lymph node, and distant metastases.[17] *BRAF* is an independent predictor of treatment failure, recurrence, and death.[18] There is no overlap between *PTC* with *RET/PTC*, *RAS*, or *BRAF* indicating involvement of a single pathway of tumorigenesis in PTC. There is some suggestion of a relationship with high iodine content in drinking water[19] but also of metals and chemicals such as boron, iron, vanadium, and manganese.[20]

The PI3K protein kinase B (AKT) pathway, which plays a role in cell survival, proliferation, and migration, can be stimulated by activating mutations including *RAS*, *PIK3CA,* and *AKT* genes or inactivating mutations including the *PTEN* tumor suppressor gene. Mutations affecting this pathway are found in 5–10% of FTC and are rarely found in PTC. They are frequently found together with *BRAF* or *RAS* mutations. They are more common in anaplastic and poorly differentiated carcinomas and appear to represent a late event in cancer transformation. In addition, these mutations may be present in metastatic lesions while being absent in primary tumors. There is data to support the role of *AKT* activation in the development of metastases.

Other oncogenes which may be involved in TC include *β catenin ALK tyrosine kinase receptor* gene and *isocitrate dehydrogenase (IDH1)* gene. Tumor suppressor (Ts*)* genes may also be involved. The most well-studied Ts gene, the *TP53* gene is commonly seen in anaplastic and poorly differentiated TC but not in well-differentiated TC.[21]

Epigenetic changes may be important contributors. Hypermethylation of metalloproteinase inhibitor TIMP3 is frequently observed in *BRAF* V600E positive TC. Microsatellite instability, loss of heterozygosity of chromosomes, and chromosomal instability are other factors that may be involved.

CLINICAL APPROACH TO THYROID NODULES

The clinician's approach to the thyroid nodule over the years is to primarily distinguish the small number of nodules that harbor a malignancy from the majority that do not. At autopsy up to 30% of thyroid glands will harbor malignant nodules which are under 1 cm (microcarcinomas); many but not all of them will have an indolent course.

A detailed history and physical examination is invaluable in the clinical approach to a thyroid nodule and is focused upon stratifying the risk for malignancies. Nodules in the young (<20 years), elderly (>65 years), or in men are more likely to be malignant. Between 4 and 8% of patients with PTC will have a family history of the same tumor. Papillary thyroid cancer is also increased in patients with familial tumor syndromes. Medullary cancer of the thyroid (MTC) can be familial especially as part of the multiple endocrine neoplasia 2 (MEN2) syndrome. Exposure to head and neck radiation, total body irradiation for bone marrow transplant (especially in childhood) or nuclear fallout, are other risk factors.

It is unclear if the size of the nodule confers an increased risk of malignancy. The risk of malignancy also appears to be independent of the number of nodules. Rapid growth of the nodule and signs of fixity to the surrounding structures are suggestive of higher risk. Change in voice due to compression or infiltration of the recurrent laryngeal nerve and presence of nontender cervical lymphadenopathy confer a higher risk. Nodules that are incidentally discovered on 18-fluorodeoxyglucose positron emission tomography (18 FDG-PET) have up to 30% risk of malignancy;[22] some studies suggest a higher risk of malignancy in nodules identified on Tc99m sestamibi scans used in cardiac and parathyroid imaging. These are summarized in table 2.

TABLE 2: Clinical risk stratification of thyroid nodules

Risk for cancer	Clinical features
Low	• No suspicious symptoms or signs
Moderate	• Age <20 or >60 years • History of head or neck irradiation in childhood • Family history of thyroid cancer or familial syndromes with thyroid cancer • Exposure to nuclear fallout • Male sex • Nodule detected on 18 FDG-PET or sestamibi
High	• Rapid tumor growth • Very firm nodule • Fixation to adjacent structures • Vocal cord paralysis • Nontender lateral lymphadenopathy

18 F DG-PET, fluorodeoxyglucose positron emission tomography.

Thyroid Stimulating Hormone

A serum TSH is essential in all patients with thyroid nodules. A suppressed TSH (with elevated free thyroxine and free triiodothyronine) is indicative of thyrotoxicosis. A radionuclide scan is recommended in this instance and will help determine if the nodule is:
- Autonomously functioning with suppression of the surrounding gland (hot)
- A nonfunctioning area in a gland with Graves' disease (cold), or
- Having the same function of the surrounding gland (warm).

When available, a radioiodine scan is preferred. While both Tc99m and ^{131}I or ^{123}I are taken up by the thyroid, only radioiodine is organified and stored in the thyroid follicles. While most benign and almost all malignancies appear "cold" on radioisotope scans, up to 5% of thyroid cancers are discordant, viz., they take up pertechnetate but not radioiodine. Patients with nodules that are functioning on Tc99m should undergo radioiodine imaging to confirm if they are concordant.

Higher TSH values appear to confer a greater risk of malignancy. When the TSH is higher than 5.5 mU/L, for instance, the prevalence of malignancy was 29.7% versus a prevalence of 2.8% with TSH concentration of less than 0.4 mU/L. A higher TSH was also associated with a more advanced stage of cancer when diagnosed.

Serum thyroglobulin can be elevated in many thyroid diseases and does not help differentiate benign from malignant disease. Its use is not recommended.

Some studies have suggested the routine use of calcitonin in patients with nodules as a screen for MTC. Calcitonin is superior to FNAC in detecting MTCs. Calcitonin levels above 60 are typically indicative of MTC; levels between 10 and 60 are inconclusive. Basal calcitonin is plagued by confounders including drug interference (chronic proton pump inhibitor, β-blocker, and glucocorticoid use) and other conditions including hypergastrinemia, neuroendocrine tumors, real insufficiency, differentiated thyroid cancer (DTC), thyromegaly, and autoimmune thyroiditis. Pentagastrin stimulation when available appears to improve the reliability of calcitonin measurements. There is no high level evidence or consensus that recommends the routine use of calcitonin at this time.

Imaging

Ultrasound

A diagnostic ultrasound should be performed in all patients with a suspected thyroid nodule. This includes patients who have a nodule detected by another imaging procedure [computed tomography (CT), magnetic resonance imaging (MRI), or 18 FDG-PET scan]. An ultrasound should evaluate the homogeneity of the thyroid parenchyma, gland size, location, size (in three dimensions), composition (solid, cystic, or mixed), echogenicity, margins, presence and size of calcifications, shape (if taller is more than wider), and vascularity. The USG should also evaluate the presence of lymph nodes. High risk features for malignancy in nodules have been identified.

Several USG features have been identified in multivariate analysis as associated with malignancy, specifically PTC. These include the presence of microcalcifications, nodule hypoechogenicity when compared with strap muscles, irregular margins (infiltrative microlobulated and spiculated), shape taller than white on transverse view, central vascularity and twinkling on B-flow imaging.[23] Follicular thyroid carcinomas has somewhat different features. They are more often iso- or hyperechoic, noncalcified, round with greater anteroposterior dimensions and regular smooth margins. Follicular variant of PTC has similar dimensions.[24]

Similarly, there are features on USG that are associated with a low risk of DTC. A spongiform appearance defined as the aggregation of multiple microcystic components in more than 50% of the volume of nodule is strongly suggestive of a benign nodule. Other USG features include hyperechogenicity, large coarse calcifications or peripheral calcifications, puff pastry appearance, and Comet-tail shadowing.

Several risk scoring systems have been developed which aim to reduce interobserver variability and allow clinicians to make decisions regarding further workup and follow-up. The most useful of these is the Thyroid Image Reporting and Data System (TIRADS) classification (Table 3). Similar to the Breast Imaging, Reporting and Data System (BIRADS) for breast lesion, the TIRADS system allows the user understand and explain to the patient the risk of malignancy in a nodule and the need for further workup including aspiration.[25] In the author's experience, the TIRADS system correlates exceptionally well with the Bethesda system for cytology. The American Thyroid Association (ATA) uses a

TABLE 3: Thyroid Image Reporting and Data System scoring system[24,25]

TIRADS	Feature	Description	Risk of malignancy
TIRADS 1	Normal thyroid gland	–	–
TIRADS 2	Benign lesion	–	0
TIRADS 3	Probably benign lesions	No suspicious features of malignancy	<5%
TIRADS 4 4a 4b 4c	Suspicious lesions	 One suspicious feature Two suspicious features Three to four suspicious features	 5–10% 10–80%
TIRADS 5	Probably malignant	All five suspicious features	–
TIRADS 6	Proven malignancy	–	–

TIRADS, Thyroid Image Reporting and Data System.

TABLE 4: The American Thyroid Association's risk scoring system[1]

Category	Description	Risk of malignancy
Benign	Purely cystic nodules with no solid component	<1%
Very low suspicion	Spongiform or partially cystic lesions with no other features described in rows below	<3%
Low suspicion	Isoechoic or hyperechoic lesions with no suspicious features	5–10%
Intermediate suspicion	Hypoechoic lesion with no other suspicious findings	10–20%
High suspicion	Hypoechoic lesion with one or more suspicious findings	>70–90%

different system based on an estimated risk of malignancy from centers that deal with a high volume of patients with thyroid nodules and malignancy (Table 4). There is significant correlation between both systems. However, nodules that do not meet the criteria for malignancy in the ATA guidelines appeared to have increased risk of malignancy (18.2%).[26]

Ultrasound elastography (USE) has emerged as a useful adjunct to ultrasound. Despite initial promise, its performance appears too variable and is affected by multiple factors. In the author's opinion, a high risk USE adds a cautionary note for increased malignancy in otherwise benign-appearing nodules.

Radionuclide Imaging

Radionuclide imaging is seldom used today in the evaluation of thyroid nodules. It is used predominantly in AFTN which must be suspected when the TSH is suppressed (see earlier). Some authorities recommend ^{123}I scintigraphy in a subset of nodules with follicular neoplasm cytology if the TSH is in the low normal range. Some AFTNs, especially those with diameter less than 2.5 cm, may have this cytology but do not produce sufficient thyroxine to suppress TSH. These appear "hot" on scintigraphy. The risk of carcinoma is low in this subset of patients.

Fine Needle Aspiration Cytology

Fine needle aspiration cytology of the thyroid is the confirmatory procedure of choice in thyroid nodules. It reduces the number of unnecessary surgeries and, at this time, is most accurate among tests or combination of tests to determine if a nodule requires surgery or not. Ultrasound-guided FNAC with real-time visualization of needle placement decreases false negative rates.[27] A 23-27 G needle is used with or without local anesthesia. In experienced hands, adequacy of sample is seen in up to 97% of aspirates (see later). The capillary action technique in which no suction is applied appears to have lower nondiagnostic rates.[28] Complications are rare. The occasional patient may have mild pain radiating to the jaw or ear for a day or two. Infection is uncommon. Seeding of carcinoma cells in the needle track has been reported in two patients who have had large needle biopsies and one who had a fine needle biopsy. Thyroglobulin levels may be elevated for a few days after FNAC.[29]

Both clinical and sonographic features are used to determine if FNAC is required. Fine needle aspiration cytology is recommended for nodules with high and intermediate risk for malignancy whose greatest diameter is larger than 1 cm and in nodules with low risk of malignancy whose greatest diameter is larger than 1.5 cm. In the presence of suspicious lymph nodes, nodules of any size must be aspirated. The lymph node itself may be aspirated first and the nodule subsequently. Spongiform nodules on USG have a very low risk for malignancy and may be followed without an FNAC. Patients with multiple nodules greater than 1 cm should be evaluated in the same fashion as those with solitary nodules. Sonographic features suggestive of malignancy must be the determining factor for which nodule requires FNAC since the malignancy may not be in the dominant nodule in over a third of patients.[30] If the TSH is low in a patient with multinodular goiter, then a radionuclide scan (iodine is preferred) may be obtained and compared with the USG. Nodules that are greater than 1 cm and isofunctioning or nonfunctioning may be aspirated. Spongiform-appearing nodules have very low malignant potential and may be carefully followed without FNAC. Fine needle aspiration cytology is also not recommended for purely cystic lesions.

Cytology

The diagnostic groups reported under the six-tiered Bethesda system for reporting thyroid cytopathology has gained widespread acceptance[31] (Table 5). An adequate specimen is defined as composing of at least six groups of cells each having 10–15 cells. When this is not present, the FNAC is deemed inadequate or nondiagnostic. Approximately 5% of all aspirations in experienced hands will fall into this category. Several factors contribute to nondiagnostic specimens including nodule component and FNAC technique.

Adequate specimens are categorized as benign, malignant, or indeterminate with the latter being divided into three specific categories each correlating with a different malignancy risk. These include atypia of undetermined significance, follicular or Hurthle cell neoplasms and suspicious for malignancy (Table 5). About 2–3% of benign nodules as determined by FNAC will subsequently prove to be malignant. Conversely, the same amount of malignant nodules on FNAC will prove to be benign.[32] Large studies show a high degree of concordance between the system and pathology, especially in the definitively benign and the definitively malignant categories with variability in the intermediate categories. Despite limitations, the adaptation of the system allows clinicians to explain malignancy risk better to patients.

TABLE 5: The Bethesda scoring system[31]

Bethesda class	Diagnostic category	Cancer risk
I	Nondiagnostic	1–4%
II	Benign	0–3%
III	Atypia of undetermined significance or follicular lesion of undetermined significance	5–15%
IV	Follicular neoplasm	15–30%
V	Suspicious for malignancy	60–75%
VI	Malignant	97–99%

MANAGEMENT

Nondiagnostic Cytology

Nondiagnostic FNAC (Bethesda I) warrants repetition especially with USG guidance and if available on-site cytology can be examined. In patients with repeated nondiagnostic results, surgery may be offered if the USG is suspicious or if growth (>20% in two dimensions) is demonstrated on follow-up.

Benign Cytology

When a combination of USG and FNAC are used to guide the diagnosis, a low suspicion on USG and benign cytology (Bethesda II) warrants a strategy of clinical observation. This may be true even of lesions greater than 4 cm where low risk USG and benign cytology appear to confer negligible mortality despite a risk of false negatives (approximately 1.1%). In cytologically benign nodules with high suspicion USG pattern, a repeat FNAC within 12 months is warranted. In nodules with low or intermediate suspicion pattern, relate USG is warranted at 12-24 months. An increase in size of more than 2 mm in more than two dimensions or a more than 50% change in volume (measured by the formula 0.52 times the three nodule dimensions) or the development of new suspicious sonographic features warrants repeat aspiration.[33] Based on these criteria, only 4-10% of nodules will increase in size over a 18-month period. Suspicious sonographic features rather than size per se appear to predict a malignant cytology in a subsequent aspiration. Nodule growth does not necessarily indicate malignancy. In nodules that appear benign on USG, subsequent growth does not appear to influence the low risk of malignancy.[34] Some authorities advocate a selective sampling approach in this setting.

Thyroid suppression is not warranted in benign nodules. Modest reduction is size with TSH suppression has been documented in areas with borderline iodine deficiency but the trade-off has been an increased risk of cardiac arrhythmias and osteoporosis. Surgery may be considered in benign nodules if they are large or cause compression. Laser thermal ablation has been applied to benign nodules. The procedure is cumbersome but offers a nonsurgical option in some patients who require or desire reduction in nodule size.

Cystic nodules that are cytologically benign can also be monitored. Fluid reaccumulation after aspiration occurs in 60-90% of these patients. If symptomatic, these patients may be offered hemithyroidectomy or percutaneous ethanol instillation. This may be an option in predominantly cystic nodules that are benign on cytology.

Nodules that do not meet the criteria for aspiration which are classified as low or intermediate risk for malignancy may be followed by USG at 12 months. Longer times may be warranted for spongiform or pure cystic nodules.

Indeterminate Cytology

Atypia of Undetermined Significance or Follicular Lesion of Undetermined Significance

Nodules that are reported as Bethesda III–atypia or follicular lesion of unknown significance (AUS/FLUS)–constitutes up to 27% of all reported FNACs and has a mean malignancy risk of 16%. The diagnostic category includes specimens that cannot be classified as benign or as follicular neoplasm because of increased cellularity, atypia, or fixation artefacts. A second opinion with an experienced thyroid cytopathologist is recommended. A repeat aspiration may yield a more definitive diagnosis with up to 60% being reported as benign, 10-15% reported as follicular neoplasm and 5-10% reported as suspicious for PTC.[35] Molecular testing has been attempted to improve certainty but is fraught with inconsistencies and hence is not routinely recommended. Correlation of the cytology with ultrasound findings (with the additional use of USE) is useful. The presence of one suspicious feature of malignancy in USG increases the risk of malignancy in Bethesda III nodule significantly (proportional to the pretest probability).

Follicular Neoplasm

Nodules that are Bethesda IV (follicular neoplasm, suspicious for follicular neoplasm or Hurthle cell neoplasm) describes a cellular aspirate characterized by follicular cells arranged in an altered architectural pattern with cell crowding and/or microfollicle formation and lacking clear features of PTC or composed exclusively of Hurthle cells. This category is associated with a 15-30% estimated risk of malignancy and constitutes 6-12% of the specimens. Nodules larger than 4 cm with this cytologic diagnosis appear to have a higher risk of malignancy.[36] Ultrasound elastography has been suggested as a tool in discriminating malignancy in this setting but the initial promise of high negative predictive value of 99%[37] has not been reproduced in subsequent studies.[38] Imaging with ^{123}I may be used in follicular but not Hurthle cell neoplasm if the TSH is low normal. If the nodule is hyperfunctioning and suppresses the extranodular tissue, the risk of malignancy is low and surgery is not required. Other imaging including the use of molecular markers in this setting has been recommended. Testing for a seven panel of genes has a negative predictive value of 79-86% and a positive predictive value of 87-100%. Molecular testing with the gene expression classifier (GEC) has a 94% negative predictive value. If molecular testing is unavailable or inconclusive, surgery is recommended.

Suspicious for Malignancy

Nodules that are Bethesda V [suspicious for papillary carcinoma (SUSP)] demonstrate cytologic features that are suspicious for malignancy but not conclusive for malignancy. Up to 6% of nodules are in this category with a mean risk of malignancy of 75%. A USG assessment of the neck to discover metastatic nodes and confirmation of malignancy upon aspiration reduces uncertainty in this setting. Molecular testing for *BRAF* confers a high predictive value when positive and can guide surgery. Total thyroidectomy is recommended in the following situations: Bethesda V, positive molecular testing, suspicious USG findings, tumor larger than 4 cm, family history of thyroid cancer, and may be considered in the presence of contralateral nodules and coexistent thyrotoxicosis. Lobectomy or hemithyroidectomy may be considered in other indeterminate nodule with intraoperative frozen section and/or cytologic assessment which identifies between 50 and 80% of thyroid cancers and leads to definitive surgery.[39]

Malignant Cytology

Surgery is recommended in patients with a diagnosis of malignancy on cytology (Bethesda VI) and is discussed in detail in the section on management of DTC. Surveillance as opposed to surgery may be an option in patients with papillary microcarcinomas (tumors less than 1 cm) with no evidence of local, regional, or distant metastasis since there appears to be a low rate of clinical progression. However, this option is seldom offered to patients outside of Japan.

INITIAL MANAGEMENT OF DIFFERENTIATED THYROID CANCER

Surgery

Differentiated thyroid cancers are malignancies arising from follicular epithelial cells and constitute the vast majority of thyroid cancers. The PTCs makeup up to 85% with rest being follicular (12%) and poorly differentiated cancers (<3%). Preoperative USG of the neck with a special emphasis on the central and lateral compartments is imperative since cervical lymph node metastasis is seen in 20–50% of most series; metastasis may be seen irrespective of tumor size and location. Sonographic features that are highly suggestive of metastasis include the absence of a hilum and the presence of microcalcifications. A USG-guided aspiration is recommended. Measurement of thyroglobulin in the FNAC needle washout may be helpful but is limited by availability and standardization issues. Symptoms or USG features suggestive of extrathyroidal invasion warrants additional imaging (CT with contrast). Positron emission tomography scanning has no role.

Similarly, routine preoperative thyroglobulin or antithyroglobulin antibodies are not recommended. Preoperative assessment of voice is recommended in all patients.

The purpose of surgery is to remove the primary tumor and disease that has extended beyond the thyroid capsule and significant lymph node metastasis. In patients with unifocal tumors less than 4 cm and no evidence of extrathyroidal extension or lymph node metastasis, the extent of initial surgery appears to have little impact on disease-specific survival. Total thyroidectomy, however, is preferred by most. Lesions larger than 4 cm, extrathyroidal extension, and regional and distant metastasis warrant total or near total thyroidectomy. Lesions 1–4 cm in older patients (>45 years), contralateral nodules, history of radiation to head and neck, or familial DTC also require total or near total thyroidectomy. Lesions 1–4 cm in others may be offered either total/near total thyroidectomy or lobectomy. Adequate surgery is the most important treatment variable that determines the outcome. Visual identification of the right laryngeal nerve and preservation of the external branch of the superior laryngeal nerve is important during surgery. Similarly, every attempt must be made to preserve the parathyroid glands and their blood supply.

Completion thyroidectomy may be necessary when the diagnosis of malignancy is made after lobectomy. Ablation of the remnant lobe with radioiodine is not recommended.

The most common site of nodal involvement in DTC is the central compartment (level VI); in many patients, this area appears normal on preoperative imaging. Dissection of the central compartment is recommended for patients with involved level VI nodes and prophylactically in patients with large primary tumors (triiodothyronine and thyroxine), with lateral neck node involvement or when prognostic features associated with increased metastasis and recurrence including *BRAF* V600E positivity.

Histology

The histopathologic classification of TC is summarized. Up to 10 microscopic variants of PTC have been described that differ in outcomes. The tall-cell variant, in particular, is found in older patients, tends to be more advanced and is associated with higher recurrence greater lymph node metastasis and decreased disease-free survival.[40] The *BRAF* V600E mutation is found in up to 80% of these tumors.[41] Other variants include the columnar and the hobnail variants both linked to increased risk of metastatic disease and *BRAF* V600E mutations.[42,43] The solid variant of DTC was seen particularly in the post Chernobyl fallout.[44] It must be distinguished from poorly differentiated PTC which has a worse prognosis. The diffuse sclerosing variant of PTC is seen in younger patients with higher rate of local and distant metastases particularly the lung but with lower overall mortality.[45] The encapsulated FVPTC is characterized by follicular growth pattern with no papillae formation but with characteristic nuclear features of PTC. These tumors frequently have *RAS* mutations[46] and appear to constitute two-thirds of all FVPTCs.[47] The risk of lymph node and distant metastases is extremely low.[48] The cribriform-morular variant of PTC is associated with FAP and is seen in patients with a germline mutation in the adenomatous polyposis coli gene.[49]

Follicular carcinomas are subdivided into the minimally invasive (encapsulated) and widely invasive. Angioinvasive tumors have been recently placed in a separate category since the mortality from these may be up to 30%.[50] Clinical outcomes are excellent when there is capsular invasion without vascular invasion.[51] Follicular thyroid carcinomas may develop as a part of the PTEN hamartoma tumor syndrome.[52]

Staging

Postoperative staging is recommended for all patients with DTC. Postoperative staging allows for risk stratification for surveillance and prognostic information. Many staging systems are available, the American Joint Committee on Cancer/Union for International Cancer Control TNM staging system is the most commonly used. None of the staging systems used adequately predicts risk of recurrence in DTC (Tables 6 and 7). The modified ATA risk stratification system may therefore be used after thyroidectomy to predict disease recurrence/persistence. This system classifies patients into low, intermediate, and high risk of recurrence (Table 8). A global composite scoring based on four response to initial therapy has been proposed to reflect the clinical status of the patient (Table 9).[53] These include:

1. Excellent response with no clinical biochemical or structural evidence of disease. This is usually defined as a TSH stimulated thyroglobulin of less than 1 ng/mL. An equivalent nonstimulated TSH of less than 0.2 ng/mL. In this scenario, the risk of recurrence over 5-10 years is 1-4%
2. Biochemical incomplete response with abnormal thyroglobulin or rising antithyroglobulin antibodies in the absence of localizable disease. Nonstimulated thyroglobulin values of more than 1 ng/mL or TSH stimulated values of more than 10 ng/mL define this category and is seen in up to 20% of patients based on their risk. Up to 68% of patients will be reclassified as no evidence of disease upon follow up; up to 27% will have persistent abnormal thyroglobulin values with no structural correlate and up to 17% develop structurally identifiable disease over 5-10 years follow-up. No deaths have been reported in patients with biochemical incomplete response to therapy in 10 years of follow-up
3. Structural incomplete response with persistent or newly identified locoregional or distant metastasis
4. Indeterminate response with nonspecific structural or biochemical findings that cannot be confidently classified as benign or malignant. This category includes patients with subcentimetric atypical non-biopsies nodules, faint uptake in the thyroid bed with undetectable stimulated thyroglobulin on follow-up imaging or nonspecific abnormalities on functional or cross sectional imaging, or patients with nonstimulated thyroglobulin detectable but less than 1 ng/mL or stimulated thyroglobulin values between 1 and 10 ng/mL or stable/declining thyroglobulin antibodies in the same

Disorders of Thyroid

TABLE 6: TNM classification for differentiated thyroid carcinoma[78]

Class	Definition
T0	No evidence of primary tumor
T1a	Tumor <1 cm; no extrathyroidal extension
T1b	Tumor >1 cm but <2 cm no extrathyroidal extension
T2	>2 cm but <4 cm no extrathyroidal extension
T3	Tumor >4 cm no extrathyroidal extension or any size with minimal extrathyroidal extension
T4a	Tumor of any size extending beyond the thyroid capsule including subcutaneous soft tissue and aerodigestive structures
T4b	Tumor of any size invading prevertebral fascia, or encasing carotid or mediastinal vessels
N0	No metastatic nodes
N1a	Metastases to level VI
N1b	Metastases to level I, II, III, IV, V, or VII
M0	No distant metastases
M1	Metastases

Stage	T	N	M
Age <45			
I	Any	Any	M0
II	Any	Any	M1
Age >45			
I	T1a/b	N0	M0
II	T2	N0	M0
III	T1-3	N0/1a	M0
IVa	T1a-3	N1b	M0
	T4a	N0-N1b	M0
IVb	T4b	Any N	M0
IVc	Any T	Any N	M1

TABLE 7: Risk of structural disease recurrence[1]

Risk	Dominant features	Others
High risk	Gross extrathyroidal extension, incomplete tumor resection, distant metastasis, lymph node >3 cm	FTC, extensive vascular extension, PTC >1 cm with *BRAF/TERT* mutation
Intermediate risk	Aggressive histology, minor thyroid all extension, vascular invasion, >5 involved lymph nodes	PTC with vascular invasion, clinical N1, intrathyroidal PTC <4 cm + *BRAF* mutation
Low risk	Intrathyroidal DTC, <5 lymph nodes (<0.2 cm)	Minimally invasive FTC, intrathyroidal <4 cm not *BRAF* mutated, intrathyroidal unifocal *PTMC BRAF* mutated, intrathyroidal encapsulated follicular variants of PTC, unifocal PTMC

DTC, differentiated thyroid cancer; FTC, follicular thyroid cancer; PTC, papillary thyroid cancer; PTMC, papillary thyroid microcarcinoma.

assay over time in the absence of structural disease. This category of response in up to 29% of low risk patients with lower numbers in intermediate and high risk patients with up to 20% of patients being reclassified as having persistent or recurrent disease in 10 years of follow-up. The majority remain disease free.

TABLE 8: Modified American Thyroid Association 2009 risk stratification[1]

Risk category	Features
Low risk	- PTC with no local or distant metastasis, complete macroscopic tumor resection, no locoregional extension, absence of histologically aggressive features, no post ablative RAI foci outside the thyroid bed, no vascular invasion, N0 or <5 lymph nodes <0.2 cm (N1) - Intrathyroidal encapsulated follicular variant of PTC - Intrathyroidal well-differentiated FTC with capsular invasion and <4 foci of vascular invasion - Intrathyroidal PTMC irrespective of *BRAF* status
Intermediate risk	- Microscopic perithyroidal invasion - RAI avid neck foci post ablation - Aggressive histology (see text) - N1 with >5 pathological nodes <3 cm - Multifocal PMTC with extrathyroidal invasion and *BRAF* positive
High risk	- Macroscopic perithyroidal invasion - Incomplete tumor resection - Distant metastases or postoperative thyroglobulin suggestive - N1 with lymph node >3 cm - FTC with >4 foci of vascular invasion

FTC, follicular thyroid cancer; PTC, papillary thyroid cancer; PTMC, papillary thyroid microcarcinoma; RAI, radioactive iodine

TABLE 9: Clinical implications of initial response to therapy[1]

Category	Definition	Implications
Excellent	Negative imaging and suppressed Tg <0.2 ng/mL or stimulated Tg <1 ng/mL	- <4% recurrence with <1% disease specific death leading to decrease in TSH suppression and intensity of follow-up
Incomplete biochemical response	Negative imaging with suppressed Tg >1 ng/mL or stimulated Tg >10 ng/mL or rising anti-Tg level	- No evidence of disease state may be seen spontaneously in 30% and with additional therapy in 20%. About 20% will progress to structural disease - Stable values may warrant follow-up. Progression or increase in titers may require further investigations and therapy
Structural incomplete response	Structural or functional evidence of disease with any level of Tg or anti-Tg antibodies	- Disease specific death rates increase with locoregional (11%) and distant metastasis (50%). Requires additional investigations and treatment
Indeterminate response	Nonspecific finding on imaging, faint uptake in thyroid bed, detect all but <1 ng/mL nonstimulated or <10 ng/mL stimulated Tg	- Structural disease seen in up to 20% on follow-up with resolution or stability seen in the rest - Warrants continued observation

Postoperative thyroglobulin levels and USG are invaluable in planning additional therapy. The postoperative thyroglobulin reaches its nadir by 3–4 weeks postoperatively. A thyroglobulin value of less than 1 ng/mL confers low risk of recurrence while a value greater than 10 ng/mL warrants additional evaluation since it increases the likelihood of persistent disease, failing RAI ablation, having distant metastases and death from thyroid cancer. Low post operative non stimulated (<0.4 ng/mL) or post thyroid hormone withdrawal (<1 ng/mL) negated the chance of finding RAI avid foci outside the thyroid bed in low risk patients.[54] This did not hold true for intermediate or high risk patients. Postoperative thyroglobulin levels may help identify patients who require additional therapy. A patient who is otherwise classified as low risk may require RAI ablation if the thyroglobulin value is more than 5 ng/mL. A TSH-stimulated Tg more than 6 ng/mL was also associated with a five-fold increase in the risk of failing ablation with 30 mCi of radioiodine.[55]

Radioactive Iodine Therapy

Treatment with ^{131}I has been used for more than 50 years to deliver therapeutic radioactivity to the thyroid bed, nodal and distant metastases in DTC. It depends on the presence of Na-I symporter and other mechanisms of iodine transport.[56] When tumors dedifferentiate some or when much of this mechanism is lost, their ability to respond to radioiodine ablation decreases. Radioiodine may be given (Table 10):
- To ablate residual normal thyroid tissue
- As an adjuvant to destroy residual microscopic cells
- To treat locoregional disease
- To treat distant metastatic disease.

Radioactive iodine ablation of the remnant (RA) is recommended after thyroidectomy to facilitate detection of recurrent disease by thyroglobulin measurements and to improve disease-free survival by destroying residual malignant cells. Since Tg is only produced by thyroid follicular cells, in the absence of normal thyroid tissue detectable thyroglobulin levels are highly specific for residual or recurrent disease. Since there are no reliable cutoffs for distinguishing thyroglobulin originating from residual or recurrent cancer from persistent normal tissue, elimination of persistent thyroid tissue, is critical to use of thyroglobulin in the follow-up patients. Similarly, whole-body RAI scans may not detect distant metastases when appreciable normal thyroid tissue remains after

TABLE 10: Postoperative radioactive iodine[1]

American Thyroid Association class	Modifier	Consideration for radioactive iodine
Low	Tumor <1 cm no nodes or metastasis	No
	Tumor <1–4 cm no nodes or metastases	Consider for aggressive histology or vascular invasion
Low to intermediate	Tumor >4 cm with no nodes or metastasis	Preferred
	Microscopic extrathyroidal extension, no nodes, or metastasis	Preferred
	Above with central compartment lymph nodes	Preferred
	Above with lateral or mediastinal lymph nodes	Preferred
High risk	–	Yes

surgery. The increasing use of USG in this situation has challenged the traditional paradigm presented here. A USG (in a trained hand) appears to have greater sensitivity, specificity, and negative predictive value in detecting residual or recurrent neck disease, and in combination with serial thyroglobulin measurements,[57] it is displacing whole-body scanning (WBS) as a primary follow-up modality.

Traditionally, thyroid hormone treatment is withheld or withdrawn for at least 3 weeks prior to RA to permit elevation of TSH to more than 30 mU/L. This permits maximum uptake and organification of ^{131}I by the thyroid. There appears to be no added benefit in adding liothyronine for the first 2 weeks.[58] An alternative to the unpleasant symptoms associated with thyroxine withdrawal is to use recombinant TSH (rTSH) prior to ablation. Though expensive, this provides comparative results to RA after thyroxine withdrawal.[59] At the present time, there is sufficient evidence to support the use of rTSH in lieu of thyroxine withdrawal in both low risk and intermediate risk patients.[60] Further evidence is required to recommend this approach in high risk patients.

Diagnostic whole body ^{131}I was done in the past prior to RA to verify the complete of surgical excision, detect any focus of uptake outside the thyroid bed and determine ^{131}I dosing.[61] Its utility has been questioned, as it appears to have a low impact on decision making. In addition, pre-ablation scanning appears to reduce the iodine trapping effect of the thyroid cancer cells (stunning) reducing the effectiveness of RA.[62] The current recommendation is to perform ^{131}I WBS post-treatment.

With accumulating evidence that high doses of ^{131}I are not necessary, for low risk patients doses between 30 and 100 mCi (1100–3700 MBq) appear to be sufficient. Large doses are recommended for documented or suspected residual disease.

There is no doubt that RAI is associated with significant improvement in disease-free and overall survival. However, there is a trend toward more selective use of RAI in clinical practice. Similarly, the role of RA in reducing the risk of cancer recurrence has been challenged. In a prospective large multicentric study, clear benefit with significant improvements in overall survival were seen in advanced (stage III and IV) disease but less so in stage II and none whatsoever in stage I disease.[63] RAI is unlikely to improve disease-free survival in tumors less than 1 cm in the absence of other high risk features. At this time, the available data seems to suggest against routine RA in low risk patients.[64] Radioactive iodine appears to be beneficial for aggressive variants of PTC.[65] In patients with intermediate risk, the greatest potential benefit may be observed with adverse thyroid cancer histologies, increasing volume of nodal disease, lymph node disease outside the central neck, and advancing patient age with questionable benefit in others. In high risk patients, the data is clearly in favor of RAI.[66] The role of molecular testing in guiding RAI is unclear.

Sufficient evidence supports the use of lower than conventional doses for RA.[67] At this time, low dose ablation with 30 mCi is recommended for low risk thyroid cancer or intermediate disease with low risk features. Higher doses are reserved for larger remnants or as adjuvant therapy. As adjuvant therapy, doses greater than 150 mCi are seldom recommended. A low-iodine diet for 1–2 weeks may be considered for patient undergoing RAI.

A post therapy scan whole body scan with or without single photon emission computed tomography (SPECT/CT) is recommended after RAI ablation. There is no role for routine adjuvant external beam radiation therapy (EBRT). There is no role for routine systemic adjuvant therapy in patients with DTC beyond RAI ablation and TSH suppression.

Thyroxine Therapy following Differentiated Thyroid Cancer

Differentiated thyroid cancer responds to TSH stimulation by increasing expression of several thyroid specific proteins and with increased rates of growth.[68] Thyroxine is therefore used to suppress TSH in an effort to decrease the risk of recurrence. Thyroid suppression is recommended in all patients. Thyroid stimulating hormone suppression below 0.1 mU/L may improve outcomes in high risk DTC but this evidence is lacking in low risk patients.[69] Further suppression to undetectable levels does not confer additional benefit[70] and may instead increase the risk of osteoporosis, angina, and atrial fibrillation. In high risk patients, initial TSH suppression to below 0.1 mU/mL is recommended, for intermediate risk patients, suppression to 0.1–0.5 mU/mL, and for low risk patients, suppression to 0.5–2 mU/mL (with an aim to keep it at the lower end of the reference level) is recommended (with and without ablation). It is unclear if patients who have only had lobectomies performed require TSH suppression.

During follow-up, a constantly suppressed TSH is associated with better outcomes with overall survival improving significantly if the TSH is less than 0.1 mU/L in state III /IV disease and between 0.1 and 0.5 mU/L in stage II disease. Cardiovascular mortality in DTC appears to be increased in patients with DTC and is associated with TSH less than 0.02. Therefore, an approach that balances the risk of tumor recurrence and adverse effects of TSH suppression is appropriate.

Surveillance

When disease free after thyroidectomy and/or RAI, lifespan is not reduced; in contrast, persistent disease reduces lifespan up to 60% of the population.[71] Measurement of serum thyroglobulin levels is an important modality to monitor patients for residual or recurrent disease. thyroglobulin is measured by immunometric assays and must be calibrated against the Certified Reference Material 457 (CRM-457) international standard. Given interassay variations, it is recommended that measurements in individual patients be performed with the same assay over time. Immunometric assays are prone to interference from anti-thyroglobulin autoantibodies which cause falsely low serum thyroglobulin levels. This must be particularly suspected when the surgical pathology indicates the presence of background HT. Anti-thyroglobulin antibodies may transiently rise postoperatively and after RAI.[72] Rising thyroglobulin antibodies after an initial fall may indicate recurrence. In the absence of interfering antibodies, thyroglobulin is highly sensitive and specific for recurrent cancer.

Follow-up for low risk patients who have undergone thyroidectomy and RA may be based on TSH suppressed thyroglobulin and USG. If the thyroglobulin is undetectable and the thyroglobulin assay does not have a functional sensitivity of 0.1–0.2 ng/mL, a TSH-stimulated assay (conventional or rTSH) may be warranted. A thyroglobulin of less than 0.15 ng/mL had 95.6% negative predictive value for residual or recurrent disease.[73] About 1 g of neoplastic thyroid tissue will increase the serum thyroglobulin by approximately 1 ng/mL during levothyroxine treatment and by approximately 2–10 ng/mL following TSH stimulation.[74] If a sensitive assay is used, in a low risk patient with a TSH suppressed thyroglobulin of less than 0.2–0.3 ng/mL may be followed with annual thyroglobulin and USG.

Cervical USG is recommended at 6 and 12 months and then periodically, depending on the risk and thyroglobulin status. Cervical USG with a high frequency probe is very sensitive in determining metastasis. Lymph nodes which are larger than 7 mm in the smaller dimension, cystic and with hyperechoic punctuation and peripheral vascularity are suggestive of thyroid cancer. The risk of lymph nodes recurrence is low in patient with low- and intermediate-risk patients and is usually higher in patient with elevated thyroglobulin. Recurrence is closely related to the initial lymph node status and commonly occurs in previously involved compartments.[75] Fine needle aspiration cytology is recommended for suspicious lymph nodes greater than 8 mm. Smaller lymph nodes may be followed up serially with biopsy reserved for increasing size. Measurement of thyroglobulin in the aspirate is useful. Levels higher than 10 ng/mL are highly suspicious for malignancy while levels between 1 and 10 ng/mL are moderately so.[76]

Low- and intermediate-risk patients with undetectable thyroglobulin on thyroxine, negative anti-thyroglobulin and normal USG do not require follow-up WBS. Diagnostic WBS may be required 6–12 months after adjuvant RAI in patients with higher risk or with thyroglobulin antibodies where risk of false negative thyroglobulin is high. A SPECT/CT RAI imaging is preferred over planar imaging.

An 18 FDG-PET is recommended in patients with elevated thyroglobulin (>10 ng/mL) and negative RAI imaging, and has a sensitivity and specificity of 83 and 84%, respectively. Positron emission tomography scanning may also be considered as part of initial staging in poorly differentiated cancers. In this setting, it predicts poor response to RAI and also poor prognosis. The sensitivity of this modality is low in patients with thyroglobulin less than 10 ng/mL. Computed tomography or MRI may be considered in patients with recurrent nodal disease and when invasive disease, especially aerodigestive invasion is suspected.

Management of Metastatic Disease

When metastasis is detected, surgery is most appropriate in locoregional disease in potentially curable patients. Compartmental neck dissection is recommended in patients with persistent neck nodes (central nodes >8 mm or lateral >10 mm). Basal thyroglobulin levels decrease by up to 90% but become undetectable only in 30–50% after dissection. A combination of surgery and RAI may be used depending on the extent and location of the disease. Percutaneous ethanol ablation may be considered in patients who are poor surgical candidates. Radiofrequency or laser ablation is another option in this setting. Multiple sittings are required in both these modalities. Other options include EBRT or stereotactic body radiotherapy (SBRT). These are reserved for surgically inappropriate patients with logoregional disease.

The prognosis of patients with DTC is usually favorable, even when metastatic RAI-avid disease is present. For this reason, ^{131}I is considered the gold standard in the treatment of metastatic disease. Radioactive iodine is preferred for metastatic disease that is iodine avid. Predictive factors to tumor response include presence of RAI uptake; among these younger age, lower 18-FDG uptake, well-differentiated histology and small metastasis predict better response. There is no evidence to support superiority of empiric or dosimetric approaches to therapy. Many centers prefer an empiric approach with dosimeter being reserved for renal insufficiency, distant metastasis, the elderly, and those with extensive pulmonary metastasis. Recombinant TSH stimulated RAI is not recommended for metastatic disease at this time as is lithium. It must be remembered that doses exceeding 150 mCi exceed the maximum tolerable tissue dose and must be avoided especially in patients over 70 years of age. A baseline complete blood count, renal function, and a pregnancy test (in premenopausal women) must be performed. Pregnant and nursing women must not be administered RAI. Pregnancy must be avoided for 6–12 months after therapy.

Pulmonary micrometastases are lesions that are less than 2 mm and not seen on anatomic imaging but are RAI avid. They have high rates of complete remission and are treated with repeated doses of RAI until the disease remits. Doses vary between 100 and 200 mCi. Macro-ocular metastasis are less responsive but may be treated with RAI, if found to be iodine avid.

Bone metastasis that is radioiodine avid must be treated with RAI. This is rarely curative but associated with improved survival. Other local modalities including surgery, EBRT, etc., may be used as adjuvant therapy. Brain metastasis that is RAI avid can be treated with RAI. Stereotactic EBRT and concomitant glucocorticoid therapy prior to ablation are recommended in this setting to prevent TSH-induced increase in tumor size and RAI-induced inflammatory response.

Empiric RAI for structurally identifiable disease that is not RAI avid is generally not recommended[77] but is considered by some experts when PET is also negative. Therapy is not recommended in stimulated thyroglobulin less than 10 ng/mL but may be considered in patients with rapidly rising thyroglobulin or anti-thyroglobulin levels with no evidence of active disease on anatomic or PET imaging. This may be repeated if there is evidence of thyroglobulin reduction.

While RAI is reasonably safe, side effects are not unknown. Salivary gland damage, dental caries, nasolacrimal duct obstruction, dysphasia in the long term, and secondary malignancies are reported. There is no direct evidence of increased risk in secondary malignancies after single administration of 30–100 mCi; it is clearly elevated with cumulative doses of more than 600 mCi. The risk of leukemia is increased, more in young individuals. Long-term rates of fertility in women do not appear to be affected; menopause appears to occur a year early. Temporary reduction in sperm counts and increase in follicle-stimulating hormone are seen in men. Single ablative doses do not appear to result in permanent infertility, risk of miscarriage, or congenital abnormalities. Avoidance by men for one sperm cycle (3 months) is recommended by some specialists. Sperm banking is recommended in men who may receive cumulative doses of more than 400 mCi.

Radioactive Iodine Refractory Differentiated Thyroid Cancer

Radioactive iodine refractory DTC occurs when the tumor/metastasis does not concentrate RAI primarily or loses the ability to do so over time. This can selectively involve some metastases. Sometimes, tumors may concentrate RAI but may be unresponsive. Choice of therapy depends on the extent, morbidity, and rapidity of progression. Presence of *BRAF* V600E may be a marker for progressive disease. Indolent tumors with low demonstrable morbidity and tumor progression may be followed clinically. Stereotactic radiation, radiofrequency, and cryoablation may be tried in individual distant metastasis. Radiotherapy is particularly effective in bone metastases. Radiofrequency ablation (RFA) may be used in lung lesions less than 3 cm. Radiofrequency ablation and cryoablation may be used for pain control in bone lesions. Cryoablation in association with cementoplasty may be used to stabilize bone lesions and can be used to treat larger lesions than RFA.

Systemic clinical therapy is beneficial in selected situations. Kinase inhibitors (sorafenib, sunitinib, lenvatinib, vandetanib, etc.) target the vascular endothelial growth factor (VEGF) receptor. Lenvatinib and sorafenib are approved for use in RAI-refractory DTC. Improvement in progression free survival but not overall survival or quality of life has been demonstrated. Kinase inhibitor therapy may be considered in RAI-refractory DTC with metastatic, rapidly progressive, symptomatic disease not amenable to other measures. While promising they are associated with numerous adverse effects including nausea, change in taste, diarrhea, weight loss, fatigue, hypertension, hepatotoxicity, and skin changes. These side effects are often debilitating and necessitate dosage reductions and discontinuation in up to 20% of patients. Rare but more serious risks include thrombosis, bleeding, heart failure, gastrointestinal fistula, and intestinal perforation. The risk of therapy-related death is up to 2%. Giving this therapy must be a carefully considered choice in which the patient is involved extensively in the decision-making.

Cytotoxic chemotherapy may be considered in selected patients unresponsive to kinase inhibitor therapy and in some patients with poorly differentiated cancer. Bisphosphonates or denosumab is preferred in patient with symptomatic bone metastasis.

Several agents have been tried in the past in an exercise to redifferentiate TC and make them RAI. Targeted blocking of the MAP kinase pathway appears to result in clinically relevant restoration of RAI avidity in RAI-refractory TC. The MEK inhibitor selumetinib and the BRAF inhibitor dabrafenib are promising in this respect. It is to be determined if these agents may be useful as an adjuvant to RAI.

RESOLUTION OF THE CASE

This patient has low risk for thyroid cancer. In the presence of low clinical risk and a Bethesda III cytology, the most appropriate steps would be to reevaluate the USG to ensure that there are no high risk features. This was done and the USG is consistent with a TIRADS score of 2. The next step would be to have the slide evaluated by a center with a high volume thyroid cytopathologist. This was done and the second reading reclassified the slide as Bethesda II. Molecular markers are of very little benefit in this setting. A GEC test may increase the negative predictive value but since the reading by the second cytologist was Bethesda II, this is unnecessary. Treatment options and risk of progression were discussed with this patient and the patient decided to continue clinical care without surgery.

CONCLUSION

The clinicians approach to thyroid nodule has changed over the years reflecting an increased understanding of the biologic pathways involved in tumorigenesis. This understanding has been augmented by the availability of improved imaging techniques and a concerted effort to standardize reporting of cytopathology. These have translated into reduction of unnecessary surgeries. Over the past few years, the development of panels of tumor markers have increased our ability to decrease uncertainty and provide targeted care to the high risk patient. The management of thyroid nodules and cancer epitomizes an example where multidisciplinary clinical, biochemical, molecular, and imaging expertise and wisdom come together in the care of the patient

REFERENCES

1. Haugen BR, Alexander EK, Bible KC, Doherty GM, Mandel SJ, Nikiforov YE, et al. 2015 American Thyroid Association Management Guidelines for Adult Patients with Thyroid Nodules and Differentiated Thyroid Cancer: The American Thyroid Association Guidelines Task Force on Thyroid Nodules and Differentiated Thyroid Cancer. Thyroid. 2015;26(1):1-133.
2. Guth S, Theune U, Aberle J, Galach A, Bamberger CM. Very high prevalence of thyroid nodules detected by high frequency (13 MHz) ultrasound examination. Eur J Clin Invest. 2009;39(8):699-706.

3. Mazzaferri EL. Management of a Solitary Thyroid Nodule. N Engl J Med. 1993;328(8):553-9.
4. Hedinger C, Williams ED, Sobin LH. The WHO histological classification of thyroid tumors. A commentary on the second edition. Cancer. 1989;63:908-11.
5. Thyroid Disease Manager. (2016). Thyroid nodules (DeGroot LJ, Pacini F). [online] Available from http://www.thyroidmanager.org/chapter/thyroid-nodules/. [Accessed February 2017]
6. Arturi F, Russo D, Schlumberger M, du Villard JA, Caillou B, Vigneri P, et al. Iodine symporter gene expression in human thyroid tumors. J Clin Endocrinol Metab. 1998;83:2493-6.
7. Demeester-Mirkine N, Van Sande J, Corvilain J, Dumont J. Benign thyroid nodule with normal iodide trap and defective organification. J Clin Endocrinol Metab 1975;41:1169-71.
8. Siegel RL, Miller KD, Jemal A. Cancer statistics, 2015. CA: A Cancer Journal for Clinicians. 2015;65(1):5-29.
9. Howlader N, Noone AM, Krapcho M, Garshell J, Miller D, Altekruse SF, et al. SEER Cancer Statistics Review, 1975-2012. Bethesda, MD: National Cancer Institute; 2015. Also available online http://seer.cancer.gov/csr/1975_2012/.
10. Kilfoy BA, Zheng T, Holford TR, Han X, Ward MH, Sjodin A, et al. International patterns and trends in thyroid cancer incidence, 1973-2002. Cancer Causes Control. 2009;20(5):525-31.
11. Aschebrook-Kilfoy B, Ward MH, Sabra MM, Devesa SS. Thyroid cancer incidence patterns in the United States by histologic type, 1992-2006. Thyroid. 2011;21(2):125-34.
12. Chia WK, Sharifah NA, Reena RMZ, Zubaidah Z, Clarence-Ko CH, Rohaizak M, et al. Fluorescence in situ hybridization analysis using PAX8- and PPARG-specific probes reveals the presence of PAX8-PPARG translocation and 3p25 aneusomy in follicular thyroid neoplasms. Cancer Genet Cytogenet. 2010;196(1):7-13.
13. Nikiforova MN, Lynch RA, Biddinger PW, Alexander EK, Dorn GW, Tallini G, et al. RAS Point Mutations and PAX8-PPAR Rearrangement in Thyroid Tumors: Evidence for Distinct Molecular Pathways in Thyroid Follicular Carcinoma. J Clin Endocrinol Metab. 2003;88(5):2318-26.
14. Basolo F, Giannini R, Monaco C, Melillo RM, Carlomagno F, Pancrazi M, et al. Potent Mitogenicity of the RET/PTC3 Oncogene Correlates with Its Prevalence in Tall-Cell Variant of Papillary Thyroid Carcinoma. Am J Pathol. 2002 Jan 1;160(1):247-54.
15. Battista S, Martelli ML, Fedele M, Chiappetta G, Trapasso F, De Vita G, et al. A mutated p53 gene alters thyroid cell differentiation. Oncogene. 1995;11(10):2029-37.
16. Franco AT, Malaguarnera R, Refetoff S, Liao X-H, Lundsmith E, Kimura S, et al. Thyrotrophin receptor signaling dependence of Braf-induced thyroid tumor initiation in mice. Proc Natl Acad Sci USA. 2011;108(4):1615-20.
17. Xing M. BRAF mutation in papillary thyroid cancer: pathogenic role, molecular bases, and clinical implications. Endocr Rev. 2006;28(7):742-62.
18. Elisei R, Ugolini C, Viola D, Lupi C, Biagini A, Giannini R, et al. BRAFV600E mutation and outcome of patients with papillary thyroid carcinoma: a 15-year median follow-up study. J Clin Endocrinol Metab. 2008;93(10):3943-9.
19. Guan H, Ji M, Bao R, Yu H, Wang Y, Hou P, et al. Association of High Iodine Intake with the T1799A BRAF Mutation in Papillary Thyroid Cancer. J Clin Endocrinol Metab. 2009 May 1;94(5):1612-7.
20. Pellegriti G, Vathaire FD, Scollo C, Attard M, Giordano C, Arena S, et al. Papillary thyroid cancer incidence in the volcanic area of sicily. J Natl Cancer Inst. 2009;101(22):1575-83.
21. Fagin JA, Matsuo K, Karmakar A, Chen DL, Tang SH, Koeffler HP. High prevalence of mutations of the p53 gene in poorly differentiated human thyroid carcinomas. J Clin Invest. 1993;91(1):179-84.
22. Choi JY, Lee KS, Kim HJ, Shim YM, Kwon OJ, Park K, et al. Focal thyroid lesions incidentally identified by integrated 18F-FDG PET/CT: clinical significance and improved characterization. J Nucl Med. 2006;47(4):609-15.
23. KwakJY, HanKH, YoonJH, MoonHJ, SonEJ, ParkSH, et al. Thyroid imaging reporting and data system for US features of nodules: a step in establishing better stratification of cancer risk. Radiology. 2011;260:892-9.
24. JehSK, JungSL, KimBS, LeeYS. Evaluating the degree of conformity of papillary carcinoma and follicular carcinoma to the reported ultrasonographic findings of malignant thyroid tumor. Korean J Radiol. 2007;8:192-7.
25. Kwak JY, Han KH, Yoon JH, Moon HJ, Son EJ, Park SH, et al. Thyroid imaging reporting and data system for US features of nodules: a step in establishing better stratification of cancer risk. Radiology. 2011;260(3):892-9.
26. Yoon JH, Lee HS, Kim E-K, Moon HJ, Kwak JY. Malignancy Risk Stratification of Thyroid Nodules: Comparison between the Thyroid Imaging Reporting and Data System and the 2014 American Thyroid Association Management Guidelines. Radiology. 2015;278(3):917-24.
27. Danese D, Sciacchitano S, Farsetti A, Andreoli M, Pontecorvi A. Diagnostic accuracy of conventional versus sonography-guided fine-needle aspiration biopsy of thyroid nodules. Thyroid. 1998;8(1):15-21.
28. Kim MJ, Kim E-K, Park SI, Kim BM, Kwak JY, Kim SJ, et al. US-guided fine-needle aspiration of thyroid nodules: indications, techniques, results. Radiographics. 2008;28(7):1869-86.
29. Lever EG, Refetoff S, Scherberg NH, Carr K. The influence of percutaneous fine needle aspiration on serum thyroglobulin. J Clin Endocrinol Metab. 1983;56(1):26-9.

30. Frates MC, Benson CB, Doubilet PM, Kunreuther E, Contreras M, Cibas ES, et al. Prevalence and distribution of carcinoma in patients with solitary and multiple thyroid nodules on sonography. J Clin Endocrinol Metab. 2006;91(9):3411-7.
31. Baloch ZW, LiVolsi VA, Asa SL, Rosai J, Merino MJ, Randolph G, et al. Diagnostic terminology and morphologic criteria for cytologic diagnosis of thyroid lesions: a synopsis of the National Cancer Institute Thyroid Fine-Needle Aspiration State of the Science Conference. Diagn Cytopathol. 2008;36(6):425-37.
32. Nayar R, Ivanovic M. The indeterminate thyroid fine-needle aspiration. Cancer Cytopathology. 2009;117(3):195-202.
33. Brauer VFH, Eder P, Miehle K, Wiesner TD, Hasenclever H, Paschke R. Interobserver variation for ultrasound determination of thyroid nodule volumes. Thyroid. 2005;15(10):1169-75.
34. Kwak JY, Koo H, Youk JH, Kim MJ, Moon HJ, Son EJ, et al. Value of US Correlation of a Thyroid Nodule with Initially Benign Cytologic Results. Radiology. 2009;254(1):292-300.
35. Faquin WC, Baloch ZW. Fine-needle aspiration of follicular patterned lesions of the thyroid: Diagnosis, management, and follow-up according to National Cancer Institute (NCI) recommendations. Diagn Cytopathol. 2010;38(10):731-9.
36. Banks ND, Kowalski J, Tsai H-L, Somervell H, Tufano R, Dackiw APB, et al. A diagnostic predictor model for indeterminate or suspicious thyroid FNA samples. Thyroid. 2008;18(9):933-41.
37. Rago T, Scutari M, Santini F, Loiacono V, Piaggi P, Coscio GD, et al. Real-time elastosonography: useful tool for refining the presurgical diagnosis in thyroid nodules with indeterminate or nondiagnostic cytology. J Clin Endocrinol Metab. 2010;95(12):5274-80.
38. Lippolis PV, Tognini S, Materazzi G, Polini A, Mancini R, Ambrosini CE, et al. Is elastography actually useful in the presurgical selection of thyroid nodules with indeterminate cytology? J Clin Endocrinol Metab. 2011;96(11):E1826-30.
39. Haymart MR, Greenblatt DY, Elson DF, Chen H. The role of intraoperative frozen section if suspicious for papillary thyroid cancer. Thyroid. 2008;18(4):419-23.
40. Moreno Egea A, Rodriguez Gonzalez JM, Sola Perez J, Soria Cogollos T, Parrilla Paricio P. Prognostic value of the tall cell variety of papillary cancer of the thyroid. Eur J Surg Oncol. 1993;19:517-21.
41. Xing M. BRAF mutation in thyroid cancer. Endocr Relat Cancer. 2005;12:245-62.
42. Chen JH, Faquin WC, Lloyd RV, Nose V. Clinicopathological and molecular characterization of nine cases of columnar cell variant of papillary thyroid carcinoma. Mod Pathol. 2011;24:739-49.
43. Asioli S, Erickson LA, Sebo TJ, Zhang J, Jin L, Thompson GB, et al. Papillary thyroid carcinoma with prominent hobnail features: a new aggressive variant of moderately differentiated papillary carcinoma. A clinicopathologic, immunohistochemical, and molecular study of eight cases. Am J Surg Pathol. 2010;34:44-52.
44. Nikiforov YE. Radiation-induced thyroid cancer: what we have learned from Chernobyl. Endocr Pathol. 2006;17:307-17.
45. Lam AK, Lo CY. Diffuse sclerosing variant of papillary carcinoma of the thyroid: a 35-year comparative study at a single institution. Ann Surg Oncol. 2006;13:176-81.
46. Rivera M, Ricarte-Filho J, Knauf J, Shaha A, Tuttle M, Fagin JA, et al. Molecular genotyping of papillary thyroid carcinoma follicular variant according to its histological subtypes (encapsulated vs infiltrative) reveals distinct BRAF and RAS mutation patterns. Mod Pathol. 2010;23:1191-200.
47. Proietti A, Giannini R, Ugolini C, Miccoli M, Fontanini G, Di Coscio G, et al. BRAF status of follicular variant of papillary thyroid carcinoma and its relationship to its clinical and cytological features. Thyroid. 2010;20:1263-70.
48. Vivero M, Kraft S, Barletta JA. Risk stratification of follicular variant of papillary thyroid carcinoma. Thyroid. 2013;23:273-9.
49. Cetta F, Montalto G, Gori M, Curia MC, Cama A, Olschwang S. Germline mutations of the APC gene in patients with familial adenomatous polyposis-associated thyroid carcinoma: results from a European cooperative study. J Clin Endocrinol Metab. 2000;85:286-92.
50. Nikiforov YE, Ohori NP. Follicular carcinoma. In: Nikiforov YE, Biddinger PW, Thompson LDR (Eds). Diagnostic Pathology and Molecular Genetics of the Thyroid, 1st edition. Philadelphia, PA: Lippincott; 2012. Pp. 152-82.
51. O'Neill CJ, Vaughan L, Learoyd DL, Sidhu SB, Delbridge LW, Sywak MS. Management of follicular thyroid carcinoma should be individualised based on degree of capsular and vascular invasion. Eur J Surg Oncol. 2011;37:181-5.
52. Laury AR, Bongiovanni M, Tille JC, Kozakewich H, Nose V. Thyroid pathology in PTEN-hamartoma tumor syndrome: characteristic findings of a distinct entity. Thyroid. 2011;21:135-44.
53. Vaisman F, Shaha A, Fish S, Michael TR. Initial therapy with either thyroid lobectomy or total thyroidectomy without radioactive iodine remnant ablation is associated with very low rates of structural disease recurrence in properly selected patients with differentiated thyroid cancer. Clin Endocrinol (Oxf). 2011;75:112-9.
54. Rosario PW, Xavier AC, Calsolari MR. Value of postoperative thyroglobulin and ultrasonography for the indication of ablation and 131I activity in patients with thyroid cancer and low risk of recurrence. Thyroid. 2011;21:49-53.
55. Tamilia M, Al-Kahtani N, Rochon L, Hier MP, Payne RJ, Holcroft CA, et al. Serum thyroglobulin predicts thyroid remnant ablation failure with 30 mCi iodine-131 treatment in patients with papillary thyroid carcinoma. Nucl Med Commun. 2011;32:212-20.

56. Schlumberger M, Lacroix L, Russo D, Filetti S, Bidart JM. Defects in iodide metabolism in thyroid cancer and implications for the follow-up and treatment of patients. Nat Clin Pract Endocrinol Metab. 2007;3(3):260-9.
57. Pacini F, Molinaro E, Castagna MG, Agate L, Elisei R, Ceccarelli C, et al. Recombinant human thyrotropin-stimulated serum thyroglobulin combined with neck ultrasonography has the highest sensitivity in monitoring differentiated thyroid carcinoma. J Clin Endocrinol Metab. 2003;88(8):3668-73.
58. Lee J, Yun MJ, Nam KH, Chung WY, Soh EY, Park CS. Quality of life and effectiveness comparisons of thyroxine withdrawal, triiodothyronine withdrawal, and recombinant thyroid-stimulating hormone administration for low-dose radioiodine remnant ablation of differentiated thyroid carcinoma. Thyroid. 2010;20:173-9.
59. Pacini F, Ladenson PW, Schlumberger M, Driedger A, Luster M, Kloos RT, et al. Radioiodine ablation of thyroid remnants after preparation with recombinant human thyrotropin in differentiated thyroid carcinoma: results of an international, randomized, controlled study. J Clin Endocrinol Metab. 2006;91(3):926-32.
60. Tala H, Robbins R, Fagin JA, Larson SM, Tuttle RM. Five-year survival is similar in thyroid cancer patients with distant metastases prepared for radioactive iodine therapy with either thyroid hormone withdrawal or recombinant human TSH. J Clin Endocrinol Metab. 2011;96:2105-11.
61. Van Nostrand D, Aiken M, Atkins F, Moreau S, Garcia C, Acio E, et al. The utility of radioiodine scans prior to iodine 131 ablation in patients with well-differentiated thyroid cancer. Thyroid. 2009;19(8):849-55.
62. Leger FA, Izembart M, Dagousset F, Barritault L, Baillet G, Chevalier A, et al. Decreased uptake of therapeutic doses of iodine-131 after 185-MBq iodine-131 diagnostic imaging for thyroid remnants in differentiated thyroid carcinoma. Eur J Nucl Med. 1998;25(3):242-6.
63. Carhill AA, Litofsky DR, Ross DS, Jonklaas J, Cooper DS, Brierley JD, et al. Long-term outcomes following therapy in differentiated thyroid carcinoma: NTCTCS Registry Analysis 1987-2012. J Clin Endocrinol Metab. 2015;100(9):3270-9.
64. Lamartine L, Durante C, Filet S, Cooper DS. Low-risk differentiated thyroid cancer and radioiodine remnant ablation: a systematic review of the literature. J Clin Endocrinol Metab. 2015;100:1748-61.
65. Kazaure HS, Roman SA, Sosa JA. Aggressive variants of papillary thyroid cancer: incidence, characteristics and predictors of survival among 43,738 patients. Ann Surg Oncol. 2012;19:1874-80.
66. Podnos YD, Smith DD, Wagman LD, Ellenhorn JD. Survival in patients with papillary thyroid cancer is not affected by the use of radioactive isotope. J Surg Oncol. 2007;96:3-7.
67. Cheng W, Ma C, Fu H, Li J, Chen S, Wu S, et al. Low- or high-dose radioiodine remnant ablation for differentiated thyroid carcinoma: a meta-analysis. J Clin Endocrinol Metab. 2013;98:1353-60.
68. Brabant G. Thyrotropin suppressive therapy in thyroid carcinoma: what are the targets? J Clin Endocrinol Metab. 2008;93:1167-9.
69. Pujo IP, Daures JP, Nsakala N, Baldet L, Bringer J, Jaffio IC. Degree of thyrotropin suppression as a prognostic determinant in differentiated thyroid cancer. J Clin Endocrinol Metab. 1996;81:4318-23.
70. Diess IS, Holzberger B, Mader U, Grelle I, Smit JW, Buck AK, et al. Impact of moderate vs stringent TSH suppression on survival in advanced differentiated thyroid carcinoma. Clin Endocrinol (Oxf). 2012;76:586-92.
71. Links TP, van Tol KM, Jager PL, Plukker JT, Piers DA, Boezen HM, et al. Life expectancy in differentiated thyroid cancer: a novel approach to survival analysis. Endocr Relat Cancer. 2005;12:273-80.
72. Gorges R, Maniecki M, Jentzen W, Sheu SN, Mann K, Bockisch A, et al. Development and clinical impact of thyroglobulin antibodies in patients with differentiated thyroid carcinoma during the first 3 years after thyroidectomy. Eur J Endocrinol. 2005;153:49-55.
73. Malandrino P, Latina A, Marescalco S, Spader A, Regalbuto C, Fulco RA, et al. Risk-adapted management of differentiated thyroid cancer assessed by a sensitive measurement of basal serum thyroglobulin. J Clin Endocrinol Metab. 2011;96:1703-9.
74. Bachelot A, Cailleux AF, Klain M, Baudin E, Ricard M, Bellon N, et al. Relationship between tumor burden and serum thyroglobulin level in patients with papillary and follicular thyroid carcinoma. Thyroid. 2002;12:707-11.
75. Leboulleux S, Rubino C, Baudin E, Caillou B, Hartl DM, Bidart JM, et al. Prognostic factors for persistent or recurrent disease of papillary thyroid carcinoma with neck lymph node metastases and/or tumor extension beyond the thyroid capsule at initial diagnosis. J Clin Endocrinol Metab. 2005;90:5723-9.
76. Grani G, Fumarola A. Thyroglobulin in lymph node fine-needle aspiration wash-out: a systematic review and meta-analysis of diagnostic accuracy. J Clin Endocrinol Metab. 2014;99:1970-82.
77. Sabra MM, Grewal RK, Tala H, Larson SM, Tuttle RM. Clinical outcomes following empiric radioiodine therapy in patients with structurally identifiable metastatic follicular cell-derived thyroid carcinoma with negative diagnostic but positive post-therapy 131I whole-body scans. Thyroid. 2012;22:877-83.
78. Amin MB, Edge S, Greene F, et al. AJCC Cancer Staging Manual, 7th Edition (1077). New York City: Springer Science and Business Media LLC; 2010.

CHAPTER 5

Thyroiditis

Pramila Kalra

INTRODUCTION

Thyroiditis is defined as inflammation of the thyroid gland. The types include acute suppurative thyroiditis, which is due to bacterial infection; subacute thyroiditis (SAT), which results from a viral infection of the gland; and chronic thyroiditis, which is usually autoimmune in nature. Secondary thyroiditis may be due to the administration of amiodarone to treat cardiac arrhythmias or the administration of interferon-α to treat viral diseases. Sometimes, there can be no evident inflammation of the gland when the illness is manifested primarily by thyroid dysfunction or goiter, e.g., painless thyroiditis and fibrous Riedel's thyroiditis.

Subacute thyroiditis is commonly called de Quervain's thyroiditis or nonsuppurative thyroiditis but other eponyms include granulomatous, pseudotuberculous, pseudogiant cell or giant cell thyroiditis, migratory or creeping thyroiditis, or struma granulomatosa, and is mostly a painful condition. It is also called painful subacute thyroiditis (PFSAT), but sometimes, it may be painless also.[1]

The other variety of SAT is called painless autoimmune subacute thyroiditis (PLSAT), which occurs spontaneously or following delivery when it is called postpartum thyroiditis. The pathophysiology is similar to Hashimoto's thyroiditis (HT) and is seen in 3.9–10% of pregnancies. The autoimmune origin is confirmed by the fact that these patients are mostly human leukocyte antigen (HLA)-Bw35 positive and they also frequently have thyroid peroxidase (TPO) or thyroglobulin (TG) antibody positivity.

Infectious thyroiditis is also called suppurative thyroiditis, and painless thyroiditis is also known as silent thyroiditis or lymphocytic thyroiditis with spontaneously resolving hyperthyroidism.

CASE 1

A 45-year-old female presented with anterior neck pain for 3 weeks with mild-to-moderate grade fever associated with chills but not rigors. She complained of 3 kg weight loss over past 1 month with complaints of palpitations and extreme malaise and fatigue. She complained of difficulty in swallowing and neck pain on lightly pressing over the neck. She did not complain of any change in the bowel habits and no difficulty in breathing or voice change.

She had been on combination of ibuprofen and paracetamol for past 2 weeks on advice of the family physician which gave her some symptomatic relief and she was also given a course of levofloxacin 500 mg for 7 days, but she did not get relief from her symptoms.

Disorders of Thyroid

On examination, her blood pressure was 140/86 mmHg and her pulse rate was 100/min. The thyroid examination showed enlargement of thyroid with an estimated weight of 40 g, was firm and tender on palpation with a nodular surface. She also had fine tremors with no eye signs of thyroid ophthalmopathy.

She said that she had become symptomatically better over the past 3 weeks.

Her laboratory evaluation revealed total thyroxine (T4) of 16 µg/dL and total triiodothyronine (T3) of 270 ng/dL and thyroid stimulating hormone (TSH) of 0.001 µIU/mL. Her erythrocyte sedimentation rate (ESR) was 60 mm/h. Her total leukocyte count was 7,000 cells/mm^3. Her C-reactive protein (CRP) level was 28.3 mg/L (normal 0.0–8.0 mg/L). Her technetium-99m (Tc-99m) pertechnetate scan showed a markedly reduced uptake in the thyroid gland. Her thyroid ultrasonography (USG) showed a small hypoechoic nodule in the thyroid about 6 mm size and the rest ultrasound examination was normal.

She was continued on anti-inflammatory and antipyretics for next 7 days and β-blockers were added. After 10 days, she was symptomatically better, and hence, was asked to continue on propranolol (β-blockers) 40 mg daily and was asked to follow-up after 6 weeks with repeat thyroid function tests. After 6 weeks, her TSH was 9 µIU/mL and she had regained 2 kg of weight and she also had reduction in the symptoms of fatigue and malaise. She was symptomatically better. She was told that this hypothyroidism could be transient and because the patient was largely asymptomatic, hence, she was advised to follow-up after 2 months and after 2 months she continued to be hypothyroid with a TSH value of 12 µIU/mL, and hence, was started on levothyroxine 50 µg/day and was told to follow-up. At 1 year follow-up, she has been maintaining a normal TSH with 50 µg of levothyroxine every day.

This case illustrates development of permanent primary hypothyroidism after recovery from SAT.

CASE 2

A 27-year-old female presented with a history of 6 days with severe neck pain and high grade fever.

She had symptoms of thyrotoxicosis and had lost 1 kg of weight over the past 1 week. She was taking anti-inflammatory and antipyretics for past 1 week, but it did not provide her any relief.

Her total T4 was 20 µg/dL, TSH was less than 0.001 µIU/mL and total T3 was 320 ng/dL. Her ESR was 66 mm/h and her CRP level was 31 mg/L (normal 0.0–8.0 mg/L). Her Tc-99m pertechnetate scan showed absent uptake in the thyroid gland.

She had severe neck tenderness and she was not allowing her neck to be touched. She also had high grade fever and symptoms suggestive of thyrotoxicosis, and hence, in view of the severe symptoms, she was started on prednisolone in a dose of 50 mg/day (in a dose of 1 mg/kg/day) which was tapered over 6 weeks with 5 mg tapering done every week. After starting steroids, she had a dramatic relief of her symptoms over the next 1 week and she continued to improve.

She became euthyroid after retesting after 6 weeks and at 3 months follow-up, her thyroid function tests continued to be normal and she is euthyroid now after 1 year of follow-up.

Thyroiditis can be classified as thyroiditis with pain and tenderness and thyroiditis without pain and tenderness.

THYROIDITIS WITH PAIN AND TENDERNESS

The common varieties include subacute, infectious, traumatic, and radiation thyroiditis. The SAT is the most common of these but other varieties are also seen.

What is de Quervain's Thyroiditis or Painful Subacute Thyroiditis?

It is called as painful (de Quervain's; granulomatous) thyroiditis. This was described by a Swiss surgeon, Fritz de Quervain who was an authority on thyroid disorders and he described the unique pathophysiology of the disease which comprises of granulomatous changes with giant cells in thyroid tissue as the pathological findings. The viral infection has been proposed in the pathogenesis of the disease, especially in genetically predisposed individuals.[2]

Epidemiology

It occurs more commonly in females and the age group mostly affected is above 40 years of age in both genders but, some studies have shown patients being affected a decade earlier than this.[3-6]

The prevalence is highest in the seasons of June to September which is superimposable on the higher incidence of *Enterovirus* infections like *Echovirus and Coxsackie A and B* viruses.[7,8]

Pathophysiology

Various viruses have been implicated in the etiology and virus-like particles have been seen in the follicular cells of thyroid in these patients.[9] The common viruses incriminated are influenza virus A, B, Adenovirus, cytomegalovirus (CMV), *Coxsackie A9, Bl, Echovirus 3, 7, 11, 12,* and *Epstein-Barr* virus.[10-12] High titers of mumps antibodies have been seen in patients with SAT and it can also be associated with orchitis or parotitis. It has also been found to be associated with measles, influenza, H1NI influenza, infectious mononucleosis, myocarditis, human immunodeficiency virus (HIV), and cat scratch fever.[13-17] *Erythrovirus B109* has been recently implicated in the pathophysiology of autoimmune thyroid disease and also for subacute thyroid disease.[18]

Subacute thyroiditis has been found to occur after usage of some drugs and vaccines. Etanercept has also been found to cause SAT.[19] Human chorionic gonadotropin has been implicated in the pathophysiology as it causes stimulation of the TSH receptor because it potentially stimulates thyroid follicular epithelium via cross-reactivity with the TSH receptor.[20] SAT can also be a possible outcome after influenza virus vaccination.[21] The patients on immunosuppressive treatment for kidney transplant have been shown to develop SAT.[22]

Drug-induced hypersensitivity syndrome can manifest as severe multiorgan system and adverse drug reaction with reactivation of human Herpesviruses (HHVs) such as HHV-6, HHV-7, CMV, and Epstein-Barr virus. SAT has also been reported approximately 2 months after the onset of drug-induced hypersensitivity syndrome.[23]

Sometimes, attacks have been shown to occur in small clusters in school children could be attributed to some unidentified viruses.[24]

Correlation with Thyroid Peroxidase Antibodies

Autoimmunity does not appear to be the primary event in the pathogenesis of painful SAT though a transient autoimmune phenomenon may happen as a secondary response.[25] The patients have been shown to mount a transient autoimmune response during the course of illness.

About 4% of the cases showed overlap of chronic lymphocytic thyroiditis (CLT) or HT and SAT showed combined clinico-cytomorphological features of both lesions.[26]

Diagnosis

Clinical Features

The diagnosis is mostly clinical. Most of the patients present with complaints of anterior neck pain preceded by an upper respiratory tract infection mostly 2 weeks prior to the onset of thyroiditis. The patient's differential diagnosis in such scenario can be acute (suppurative, thyroid abscess) thyroiditis which is usually a painful nodular enlargement of the thyroid, or unusual presentations of Graves' or nodular thyroid disease with pain generated by capsular stretching. The patients mostly present with neck pain which is aggravated by swallowing and radiates behind the ears.

Malaise, myalgias, fatigue, and arthralgias are common presentation. It is called creeping thyroiditis as patient may have pain in one lobe. The patients mostly have mild-to-moderate degree of fever but some may have high grade fever up to 104°F and may also present sometimes as pyrexia of unknown origin.[27] The disease reaches a peak in 4 days and subsides in about a month but, in some patients, it may take longer period also and may continue with a fluctuating course for 3–6 weeks. Sometimes, the course is more protracted to about 3–4 months.

The disease mostly has four phases. The destructive inflammation results temporarily in thyrotoxic phase followed by euthyroidism. After a transient hypothyroidism, the disease becomes inactive and the thyroid function is normalized but some patients become permanently hypothyroid on recovery.[28,29]

Fever may be seen in about 54%, prior upper respiratory illness in 17%, symptoms of thyrotoxicosis in 47%, sore throat in 36%, and painful thyroid swelling in 77%. The less common presentations include vocal cord paresis or paralysis and hard thyroid mass.[30,31]

Some patients can present with psychotic symptoms and especially if they are abrupt and unusual associated with onset of SAT, they can be attributed to it and may resolve with treatment of SAT.[32]

Laboratory Parameters

Sometimes, a time lag exists between the onset of clinical symptoms and the laboratory parameters and even a normal thyroid function tests in the setting of high clinical suspicion of SAT should be kept in mind and this disease should not be excluded from the differential diagnosis.[33]

The laboratory parameters show high T4 and T3 levels and suppressed TSH suggesting thyrotoxicosis. The patients usually have a high ESR, elevated ESR and CRP.

The ratio of T3 (ng/dL) to T4 (µg/dL) is less than 20 in all forms of SAT. Erythrocyte sedimentation rate is almost always greater than 50 mm/h, white blood cell (WBC) counts and CRP levels are usually elevated in PFSAT.

Elevated WBC count is seen in 25–50% and elevated ESR can be seen in 85% of patients, Abnormal thyroid function documented in 60%, rise of alkaline phosphatase, alanine transaminase (ALT) and aspartate transaminase (AST) is common.

The PFSAT mostly have absent or low titers of anti-TPO and thyroglobulin antibodies (TPOAb and TGAb). These antibodies either one or both are typically positive in PLSAT and postpartum thyroiditis (PPT). The thyrotropin receptor antibodies (TRAb) are usually absent or in very low titer in patients with PFSAT as well as PPT.

Rarely, these patients can also have hypercalcemia as one of the presenting laboratory abnormality (Table 1).[30]

TABLE 1: Differential diagnosis of a thyrotoxic patient

	Painful subacute thyroiditis	Painless autoimmune subacute thyroiditis	Postpartum thyroiditis	Graves' disease
History of preceding URI	Yes	No	No	No
Neck pain	Mostly yes	No	No	No
Systemic symptoms	Yes	No	No	No
Recent pregnancy	No	No	Yes	No
Symptoms of thyrotoxicosis	Yes	Yes	Yes	Yes
ESR	Elevated	Normal	Normal	Normal
CRP	Elevated	Normal	Normal	Normal
Total T4 or Free T4	Normal or elevated	Normal or elevated	Normal or elevated	Normal or elevated
Total T3	Normal or elevated	Normal or elevated	Normal or elevated	Normal or elevated
T3 (ng/dL) or T4 (µg/dL)	<20	<20	<20	>20
TSH	Mostly suppressed or sometimes normal	Mostly suppressed or sometimes normal	Mostly suppressed or sometimes normal	Suppressed
Thyroglobulin	Elevated	Elevated	Elevated	Elevated
TPOAb	Mostly negative	Mostly positive	Mostly positive	Mostly positive
TgAb	Mostly negative	Mostly positive	Mostly positive	Mostly positive
TSHrAb	Negative	Negative	Negative	Positive
Tc-99m scan	Reduced uptake. During recovery phase can be rarely increased	Reduced uptake	Reduced uptake	Increased uptake
Echogenicity of thyroid on ultrasound	Hypoechoic	Hypoechoic	Hypoechoic	Hypoechoic
Vascularity	Decreased	Decreased	Decreased	Increased

CRP, C-reactive protein; ESR, erythrocyte sedimentation rate; PPT, postpartum thyroiditis; T3, triiodothyronine; T4, thyroxine; Tc, technetium; TPOAb, thyroid peroxidase antibody; TgAb, thyroglobulin antibody; TSH, thyroid stimulating hormone; TSHrAb, TSH-receptor antibody; URI, upper respiratory illness.

Imaging

Most of the cases do not need imaging but in atypical cases, imaging may be of help in ruling out other pathologies.

Ultrasonography is the most common imaging modality. The commonest finding is hypoechoic and heterogeneous areas with irregular margin but painless and painful hypoechoic nodules are commonly seen. The finding of nodules in cases with SAT is very common and many of these nodules resolve after the resolution of SAT.

A characteristic observation on USG is the lava flow which consists of diffuse, hypoechoic, and confluent areas with typical negative margins. The color Doppler mostly does not show any increase in the vascularity.[34] Color Doppler may be a noninvasive, useful, and rapid modality to differentiate it from Graves' disease (GD) and also for monitoring and follow, of lesions in cases with SAT.[35]

Nuclear Imaging

Technetium-99m pertechnetate mostly reveals homogeneously reduced or no activity in the thyroid gland. The imaging studies have shown diffuse increased uptake of Tc-99m sestamibi and Tc-99m tetrofosmin in the thyroid region of patients in the acute phase (thyrotoxic) of SAT reflecting the inflammatory process. Thus, both these agents have the ability to detect the inflammatory process associated with the disease.[36-38]

Fine Needle Aspiration Cytology

It may give accurate results and mostly clinches the diagnosis, especially in the situation when there is a doubt about the diagnosis.

The most remarkable characteristic in fine needle aspiration cytology (FNAC) is the presence of mononuclear giant cells with cytoplasm, a dirty background consisting of cellular debris, blood elements, and pink amorphous acellular material, with mild-to-moderate cellularity, degenerated proliferated follicular epithelium cells, rare epithelioid granulomas, and mixed type inflammatory cells can also be seen. Multinuclear giant cell is an invariable characteristic in all the cases. Fine needle aspiration cytology typically shows lymphocytes, macrophages, polymorphonuclear leukocytes, giant cells which are seen in 100% of cases.[39] It is mostly not needed but only when the diagnosis is in doubt, it needs to be done.

Treatment

Analgesic therapy with nonsteroidal anti-inflammatory drugs (NSAIDs) provides relief in most cases.

Beta blockers can be used in the initial stages for relief of symptoms of SAT but there is no role of antithyroid drugs because the high levels result from the release of preformed T4 and T3 from the inflamed thyroid gland.[39]

Though mostly not required but rarely thyroidectomy may be indicated in cases of recurrent thyroiditis or those cases who are not responding to steroids and the pain is severe and debilitating.

Steroid Therapy

If the NSAIDS do not provide symptomatic relief and the symptoms are severe, then prednisolone can be used in a dose of 40-60 mg or the dose can be calculated as 1 mg/kg/day to be tapered over 6 weeks period. The indications of steroid therapy include severe neck pain, severe symptoms not responding to conventional NSAIDS, and rare presentations like vocal cord paresis and paralysis and hypercalcemia.[40]

In one study, steroid replacement with prednisolone was administered in a dose of 15 mg/day and 51.6% achieved remission within 6 weeks, while 27.9% went into remission within 7-8 weeks,[19] and none experienced recurrence. It has been shown that 6 weeks period is required before tapering steroid therapy to prevent recurrence.[41,42]

After 1–2 weeks of treatment, the dose is tapered over a period of 6 weeks. Most of the patients do not have a recrudescence of symptoms but if it happens rarely, the dose of steroid needs to be increased. The recurrence rate of painful thyroiditis is about 20–22% after stopping steroids and has not been shown to be dependent on the baseline parameters.[43]

A novel treatment using a mixture of lidocaine and dexamethasone using an insulin pen has also been tried for the treatment of SAT.[44]

Sequelae

Permanent hypothyroidism can be a sequelae of SAT. In about 85% of patients, there is recovery of normal thyroid function after recovery from SAT and thyroid may show scarring post recovery with islands of normal functioning thyroid tissue. The rate of permanent hypothyroidism has been reported to range from 11 to 20% after recovery.[45,46]

Recurrence

Recurrence of thyroiditis is rare and occurs mostly after 12 months of thyroiditis. The recurrences in up to 2% of cases have been reported after the first episode and the clinical manifestations are mostly milder in the second episode.[47]

ATYPICAL PRESENTATIONS OF SUBACUTE THYROIDITIS

Many times, the presentation may not be typically with thyroid pain, swelling, or fever or thyroid function tests abnormalities and on USG, these cases may present with painless and hard thyroid nodules in the thyroid which may be a diagnostic dilemma. The reported incidence of atypical presentation is up to 36% of the cases.[48]

The development of GD after SAT is very rare, and only a limited number of cases of GD occurring after SAT have been reported. The GD can occur after many years of occurrence of SAT.[49] Rarely, SAT has been reported to precipitate thyroid crisis also.[50]

One case of granulomatosis with polyangiitis accompanied by SAT during immunosuppressive therapy has also been reported in literature.[51]

Even though it is a rare event, most associations of thyroid carcinoma with SAT described in the literature are related to granulomatous form (de Quervain's thyroiditis). The presence of features suggestive of malignancy like hard painless thyroid nodule with USG evidence of a suspicious thyroid nodule, microcalcification focus in the heterogeneous thyroid parenchyma, and cervical lymphadenopathy warrant further investigations for confirmation of diagnosis. A further cytological examination needs to be done in cases presenting with suspicious thyroid nodule and/or non-nodular hypoechoic (>1 cm) or heterogeneous areas with microcalcification focus.[52] Some typical features of thyroid nodules in patients with SAT which have been documented include a poorly defined margin and also grayscale feature of centripetal reduction in echogenicity which is specific for atypical SAT, and the color Doppler feature of internal vascularity rules out SAT. These features may help in ruling out malignancy and doing unnecessary FNAC, biopsies, and surgeries in these cases.[53]

Disorders of Thyroid

> **CASE 3**
>
> A 19-year-old boy presented with gradually increasing swelling in the neck for past 1 year which was not painful. He had no systemic symptoms.
>
> The patient had come for the treatment of the swelling. He did not have any features suggestive of hyperthyroidism or hypothyroidism. He also had cervical lymphadenopathy.
>
> The thyroid gland on examination was hard with bosselations and no nodule was discernable. The gland was enlarged to 2.5 times the size and it was hard to touch and nontender. The patient also had cervical lymph nodes enlargement which were matted.
>
> The thyroid function tests showed euthyroid status with TSH of 3 µIU/mL, T4 of 10 µg/dL, T3 of 120 ng/dL, and anti-TPO was negative (3 IU/mL).
>
> The USG examination of the thyroid showed an enlarged thyroid with bosselations. The cervical lymph nodes were also enlarged and matted.
>
> The patient was subjected to thyroid FNAC which showed acid-fast bacilli suggestive of tubercular pathology. He was then subjected to cervical lymph node biopsy which also showed caseation and granuloma suggestive of tubercular pathology. The tuberculin test was performed which showed an induration of 15 mm at 72 hours.
>
> A chest X-ray to rule out pulmonary pathology was done which showed no infective focus and no pleural thickening.
>
> He was started on antitubercular treatment and was followed up in the outpatient department which showed reduction in the size of the thyroid gland.
>
> The thyroid swelling and cervical lymphadenopathy resolved after 6 months of treatment with antitubercular therapy.

INFECTIOUS THYROIDITIS

Infectious thyroiditis can be acute or chronic. The acute infection may present with abscess formation which may be caused by Gram-positive or Gram-negative organisms. These organisms may reach the thyroid by hematogenous route and is especially seen in patients who are immunocompromised or via fistula from the pyriform sinus adjacent to the larynx which is the commonest cause of suppurative thyroiditis. The common organisms are *Staphylococcus* and *Streptococcus*, but many other rare pathogens like *Nocardia asteroides* have also been reported. The chronic infections include mycobacterial-like tuberculosis, fungal and pneumocystis infections mostly occurring in immunocompromised patients.[54-58]

Acute infectious thyroiditis is characterized by sudden onset of neck pain with high grade fever and chills and signs and symptoms of infection. Patients may present with unilateral neck mass which may fluctuate in size but, sometimes hemorrhage into the thyroid gland and acute stage of SAT may also mimic this.[59]

The diagnosis is made on the basis of clinical presentation and imaging by USG to look for presence of single or multiple abscesses. The ultrasound may help in differentiating it from SAT and also FNAC may help in differentiation as SAT shows multinucleated giant cell granulomas versus fluid collection with microbes on bacteriologic examination and culture in infectious thyroiditis.

An adequate intravenous antibiotic therapy needs to be given as per the culture sensitivity report of the pus or blood culture reports. The drainage of the pus may be required if patient is not responding to antibiotic therapy and conservative management.

The laboratory evaluation may show normal thyroid function or thyrotoxicosis in few cases.

Patients with chronic thyroid infection mostly present with bilateral disease and less pain and tenderness on examination. Fine needle aspiration cytology helps in making the diagnosis and confirming the microorganism.

Radiological studies may be required to confirm the fistula or the tract causing the infection.

The presence of tubercular thyroiditis though rare should be suspected in our country where extrapulmonary tuberculosis could rarely manifest as thyroiditis.[60] The thyroid gland is normally resistant to tubercular infection because of antibacterial action of colloid material, high vascularity of the gland, excess of iodine content, and enhanced phagocytic activity in hyperthyroid states.

In cases of tubercular thyroiditis, the thyroid function is usually well-preserved with only rare case reports documenting hypothyroidism or hyperthyroidism.

RADIATION THYROIDITIS

The patients with GD who receive radioiodine for ablation may develop neck pain and tenderness after 5-10 days of radioiodine therapy. The cause may be due to radiation-induced injury and necrosis of the thyroid follicular cells. The symptoms are mostly mild and resolve over a period of few days with symptomatic therapy. Sometimes, these patients may have transient exacerbation of hyperthyroidism and may even present as thyroid crisis.[61]

Painless thyrotoxic thyroiditis has also been reported after radiation is given to the neck for any other malignancy.[62]

TRAUMA INDUCED THYROIDITIS

Sometimes, the patients may present with thyroid pain and tenderness and thyrotoxic state after rigorous palpation of the thyroid gland or manipulation during biopsy and surgery for parathyroid gland. This resolves mostly with spontaneous treatment.

PAINLESS CAUSES OF THYROIDITIS

Thyroiditis can also present as painless condition which includes postpartum, drug-induced, and fibrous thyroiditis.

Painless or Silent Thyroiditis

It is characterized by transient hyperthyroidism, followed by temporary or rarely permanent hypothyroidism. It is also called as silent thyroiditis, subacute lymphocytic thyroiditis, and lymphocytic thyroiditis with spontaneously resolving thyrotoxicosis. It constitutes about 0.5-5% of the cases of thyrotoxicosis. It excludes women who have painless thyroiditis within 1 year of delivery or miscarriage when it is labelled as PPT.[63,64]

Pathogenesis

This is considered as a variant of Hashimoto's thyroiditis. Many patients with painless thyroiditis can have very high levels of TPOAb and anti-thyroglobulin antibodies and may manifest chronic autoimmune thyroiditis (AIT) after several years. It is found to be more common in women. It has been found to be associated with specific HLA haplotypes, most often HLA-DR3. The other predisposing factors for painless thyroiditis include excess iodine intake and various cytokines. A similar syndrome can occur in patients treated with lithium, interferon-α, interleukin-2, and tyrosine kinase inhibitors, etc. The cytokines released in response to some (subclinical) injury or infections are thought to initiate the disorder.

Clinical Features

An approximately 5-20% of patients with painless thyroiditis have the characteristic sequence of thyrotoxicosis, followed by hypothyroidism, and then recovery. The thyrotoxic phase develops over a period of 1-2 weeks and usually lasts up to 8 weeks before subsiding. The symptoms are usually mild. The thyroid gland is not painful or tender, but is usually minimally diffusely enlarged and sometimes firm in texture.

This may be followed by recovery or hypothyroidism which is usually clinically mild or even asymptomatic for 2-8 weeks, followed by recovery. Approximately 10% of patients may have additional episodes of painless thyroiditis, typically occurring years apart. About 50% of patients develop chronic AIT with permanent hypothyroidism, goiter, or both.

Investigations

The laboratory evaluation in the thyrotoxic phase will be normal or high total T4, normal or high total T3, and supressed TSH.

The Tc-99m pertechnetate can help to confirm the diagnosis which shows a reduced uptake in the thyroid gland. The scan typically shows a markedly reduced uptake in the gland. Any of the incriminating drugs described earlier if included in the treatment should point towards a diagnosis of painless thyroiditis.

Ultrasound may not provide much diagnostic information. It may show a heterogeneous, hypoechogenic, normal-sized or slightly enlarged thyroid gland, and a normal or decreased Doppler flow.

Treatment

The treatment include β-blockers if the symptoms and signs of thyrotoxicosis are present and in the hypothyroid phase, levothyroxine supplementation may be required if hypothyroidism is not recovering.

RIEDEL'S THYROIDITIS

Riedel's thyroiditis is an extremely rare form of thyroiditis. Women are mostly affected with a female to male ratio of 4:1 and peak age incidence is the fifth decade.[65] It is characterized by extensive fibrosis involving the thyroid and contiguous neck structures. It has been found to be associated with idiopathic fibrosis in other sites of the body, such as the retroperitoneum. A rare complication of the disease is entrapment of the recurrent laryngeal nerve which can lead to vocal cord paralysis.[66]

POSTPARTUM THYROIDITIS

The prevalence ranges from 1 to 17%. It is found to be more common in women with type 1 diabetes mellitus and a previous history of postpartum thyroiditis.

Clinical Course

The clinical course of thyroid dysfunction is similar to SAT but with no anterior neck pain or tenderness of the thyroid. The prevalence of PPT ranges from 3 to 8% of all pregnancies.

It occurs within 6 months (typically, 2–4 months) after delivery and runs a clinical course identical to that of painless thyroiditis occurring rarely without relation to pregnancy. The clinical course is almost similar to SAT but is not associated with any neck pain or fever. It starts with destructive thyroiditis which is painless and resolves over few months leading to hypothyroidism 3–6 months after delivery which is mostly temporary.

Pathogenesis

Postpartum thyroiditis is known to occur because of an immune rebound phenomenon.[67-71]

Most women with subclinical AIT and antithyroid microsomal antibodies of more than 1:5,120 before pregnancy develop PPT. After delivery, other forms of autoimmune thyroid dysfunction may also occur, including GD, transient hypothyroidism without preceding destructive thyrotoxicosis and persistent hypothyroidism. The risk of PPT in women with AIT before pregnancy has been found to be higher among women with preserved thyroid functional capacity.

Investigations

The investigations show mostly suppressed TSH and high total T4, FT4, FT3, T3, or FT4, T4, FT3, T3 can be normal. The second phase may show TSH levels high with low or normal total T4, FT4, T3, and FT3. The Tc-99m scan is not indicated in patients as most of them are breastfeeding. The patients may need to go for ultrasound examination if clinically indicated.

The TSH-receptor antibody levels may help to differentiate if there is a doubt about the diagnosis in a postpartum woman and GD is strongly suspected as Tc-99m scan may not be advisable if the woman is breastfeeding, but in case it is done, then breastfeeding has to be suspended for 24 hours.

RECENT ADVANCES IN DIAGNOSIS OF POSTPARTUM THYROIDITIS

Spectral Doppler sonography has been recently shown to be a useful and accurate method for thyroid dysfunction evaluation during the postpartum period. The peak systolic velocity in hyperthyroid PPT was found to significantly lower than in hypothyroid PPT and GD. The anti-C1q levels were higher in the TPOAb positive women than in controls. The anti-C1q positive pregnant women screened positive for autoimmune thyroid disease were shown to have higher TSH levels than anti-C1q negative ones.[72]

Treatment

The treatment remains same as for SAT. In the thyrotoxic phase, symptomatic treatment with β-blockers is indicated, and in the hypothyroid phase, treatment with levothyroxine supplementation is indicated which may be temporary or sometimes permanent.

CONCLUSION

The diagnosis of thyroiditis is mostly clinical and laboratory investigations and imaging help in confirming it. The treatment of SAT is mostly symptomatic with nonsteroidal anti-inflammatory agents and in few cases, steroids for up to 6 weeks. The atypical presentations may pose a diagnostic dilemma and laboratory diagnosis and imaging and follow-up will help in making a correct diagnosis. The acute infectious thyroiditis presents with systemic symptoms and antibiotics as per the organism sensitivity are indicated. The tubercular thyroiditis though uncommon is seen in our country because of the wide prevalence of tuberculosis.

The painless thyroiditis presents like SAT but there is no pain associated with it. The PPT is recognized by its presentation in the postpartum period. The follow-up for development of primary hypothyroidism is important as some of these cases may continue to be hypothyroid permanently and may require levothyroxine supplementation for the same.

REFERENCES

1. Hennessey JV. Subacute Thyroiditis. In: De Groot LJ, Chrousos G, Dungan K, Feingold KR, Grossman A, Hershman JM, Koch C, Korbonits M, McLachlan R, New M, Purnell J, Rebar R, Singer F, Vinik A (Eds). Endotext [Internet]. South Dartmouth (MA): MDText.com, Inc.; 2000-2015.
2. Engkakul P, Mahachoklertwattana P, Poomthavorn P. Eponym: de Quervain thyroiditis. Eur J Pediatr. 2011;170(4):427-31.
3. Shrestha RT, Hennessey J. Acute and Subacute, and Riedel's Thyroiditis. In: De Groot LJ, Chrousos G, Dungan K, Feingold KR, Grossman A, Hershman JM, Koch C, Korbonits M, McLachlan R, New M, Purnell J, Rebar R, Singer F, Vinik A (Eds). Endotext [Internet]. South Dartmouth (MA): MDText.com, Inc.; 2000-2015.
4. Sweeney LB, Stewart C, Gaitonde DY. Thyroiditis: an integrated approach. Am Fam Physician. 2014;90(6):389-96.
5. Erdem N, Erdogan M, Ozbek M, Karadeniz M, Cetinkalp S, Ozgen AG, et al. Demographic and clinical features of patients with subacute thyroiditis: results of 169 patients from a single university center in Turkey. J Endocrinol Invest. 2007;30(7):546-50.
6. Kalra P, Kumar KM, Kallur KG, Vadyanathan V, Nadig M, Shankar M. Demographic data of thyroiditis from a south Indian city. Indian J Endocrinol Metab. 2015;19(2):300-2.
7. Martino E, Buratti L, Bartalena L, Mariotti S, Cupini C, Aghini-Lombardi F, et al. High prevalence of subacute thyroiditis during summer season in Italy. J Endocrinol Invest. 1987;10(3):321-3.
8. Kitaoka H, Sakurada T, Fukazawa H, Suzuki M, Kaise N, Kaise K, et al. An epidemiological study of subacute thyroiditis in northern Japan. Nihon Naibunpi Gakkai Zasshi. 1985;61(5):554-70.
9. Sato M. Virus-like particles in the follicular epithelium of the thyroid from a patient with subacute thyroiditis (De Quervain). Acta Pathol Jpn. 1975;25(4):499-501.
10. Volta C, Carano N, Street ME, Bernasconi S. Atypical subacute thyroiditis caused by Epstein-Barr virus infection in a three-year-old girl. Thyroid. 2005;15(10):1189-91.
11. Luotola K, Hyöty H, Salmi J, Miettinen A, Helin H, Pasternack A. Evaluation of infectious etiology in subacute thyroiditis--lack of association with coxsackievirus infection. APMIS. 1998;106(4):500-4.
12. Mori K, Yoshida K, Funato T, Ishii T, Nomura T, Fukuzawa H, et al. Failure in detection of Epstein-Barr virus and cytomegalovirus in specimen obtained by fine needle aspiration biopsy of thyroid in patients with subacute thyroiditis. Tohoku J Exp Med. 1998;186(1):13-7.
13. Kimura M, Amino N, Takada K, Miyai K. Subacute thyroiditis associated with systemic multi-organ disorders. Endocrinol Jpn. 1989;36(6):859-64.
14. Bouillet B, Petit JM, Piroth L, Duong M, Bourg JB. A case of subacute thyroiditis associated with primary HIV infection. Am J Med. 2009;122(4):e5-6.
15. Engkakul P, Mahachoklertwattana P, Poomthavorn P. de Quervain thyroiditis in a young boy following hand-foot-mouth disease. Eur J Pediatr. 2011;170(4):527-9.
16. Ogawa E, Katsushima Y, Fujiwara I, Iinuma K. Subacute thyroiditis in children: patient report and review of the literature. J Pediatr Endocrinol Metab. 2003;16(6):897-900.

17. Dimos G, Pappas G, Akritidis N. Subacute thyroiditis in the course of novel H1N1 influenza infection. Endocrine. 2010;37(3):440-1.
18. Page C, Duverlie G, Sevestre H, Desailloud R. Erythrovirus B19 and autoimmune thyroid diseases. Review of the literature and pathophysiological hypotheses. J Med Virol. 2015;87(1):162-9.
19. Yasuji I. Subacute thyroiditis in a patient with juvenile idiopathic arthritis undergoing etanercept treatment: a case report and review of the literature. Mod Rheumatol. 2013;23(2):397-400.
20. Lamos EM, Munir KM. Thyroid swelling and thyroiditis in the setting of recent hCG injections and fine needle aspiration. Case Rep Endocrinol. 2016;2016.
21. Altay FA, Güz G, Altay M. Subacute thyroiditis following seasonal influenza vaccination. Hum Vaccin Immunother. 2016;12(4):1033-4.
22. D'Amico G, Di Crescenzo V, Caleo A, Garzi A, Vitale M. Sub-acute thyroiditis in a patient on immunosuppressive treatment. Recenti Prog Med. 2013;104(7-8):459-61.
23. Sato M, Mizuno Y, Matsuyama K, Shu E, Kanoh H, Suwa T, et al. Drug-induced hypersensitivity syndrome followed by subacute thyroiditis. Case Rep Dermatol. 2015;7(2):161-5.
24. Ogura T, Hirakawa S, Suzuki S, Ota Z, Togawa T, Nogami I. Five patients with painless thyroiditis simultaneously developed in a nursery school. Endocrinol Jpn. 1988;35(2):225-30.
25. Volpé R. Thyroiditis: current views of pathogenesis. Med Clin North Am. 1975;59(5):1163-75.
26. Kalita A, Baruah R. Thyroiditis: a clinico-cytomorphological study with a reference to the ethnic groups of northeast regions of India. Indian J Otolaryngol Head Neck Surg. 2015;67(4):403-6.
27. Sardesai V. Pyrexia of unknown origin--an uncommon presentation of subacute thyroiditis. J Indian Med Assoc. 2013;111(2):135.
28. Oláh R, Hajós P, Soós Z, Winkler G. De Quervain thyroiditis. Corner points of the diagnosis. Orv Hetil. 2014;155(17):676-80.
29. Fatourechi V, Aniszewski JP, Fatourechi GZ, Atkinson EJ, Jacobsen SJ. Clinical features and outcome of subacute thyroiditis in an incidence cohort: Olmsted County, Minnesota, study. J Clin Endocrinol Metab. 2003;88(5):2100-5.
30. Huang C, Wang X. Subacute thyroiditis manifesting as a thyroid mass, vocal cord paralysis, and hypercalcemia. Endocr Pract. 2012;18(2):e17-20.
31. Chang M, Khoo JB, Tan HK. Reversible recurrent laryngeal nerve palsy in acute thyroiditis. Singapore Med J. 2012;53(5):e101-3.
32. Lee KA, Park KT, Yu HM, Jin HY, Baek HS, Park TS. Subacute thyroiditis presenting as acute psychosis: a case report and literature review. Korean J Intern Med. 2013;28(2):242-6.
33. Tachibana T, Orita Y, Ogawara Y, Matsuyama Y, Abe I, Nakada M, et al. Time-lag between symptom onset and laboratory findings in patients with subacute thyroiditis. Auris Nasus Larynx. 2014;41(4):369-72.
34. Cappelli C, Pirola I, Gandossi E, Formenti AM, Agosti B, Castellano M. Ultrasound findings of subacute thyroiditis: a single institution retrospective review. Acta Radiol. 2014;55(4):429-33.
35. Hiromatsu Y, Ishibashi M, Miyake I, Soyejima E, Yamashita K, Koike N, et al. Color Doppler ultrasonography in patients with subacute thyroiditis. Thyroid. 1999;9(12):1189-93.
36. Hiromatsu Y, Ishibashi M, Nishida H, Kawamura S, Kaku H, Baba K, et al. Technetium-99 m sestamibi imaging in patients with subacute thyroiditis. Endocr J. 2003;50(3):239-44.
37. Hiromatsu Y, Ishibashi M, Miyake I, Nonaka K. Technetium-99m tetrofosmin imaging in patients with subacute thyroiditis. Eur J Nucl Med. 1998;25(10):1448-52.
38. Bahn Chair RS, Burch HB, Cooper DS, Garber JR, Greenlee MC, Klein I, et al. Hyperthyroidism and other causes of thyrotoxicosis: management guidelines of the American Thyroid Association and American Association of Clinical Endocrinologists. Thyroid. 2011;21(6):593-646.
39. Vural Ç, Paksoy N, Gök ND, Yazal K. Subacute granulomatous (De Quervain's) thyroiditis: Fine-needle aspiration cytology and ultrasonographic characteristics of 21 cases. Cytojournal. 2015;12:9.
40. Koirala KP, Sharma V. Treatment of acute painful thyroiditis with low dose prednisolone: a study on patients from western Nepal. J Clin Diagn Res. 2015;9(9):MC01-3.
41. Kubota S, Nishihara E, Kudo T, Ito M, Amino N, Miyauchi A. Initial treatment with 15 mg of prednisolone daily is sufficient for most patients with subacute thyroiditis in Japan. Thyroid. 2013;23(3):269-72.
42. Arao T, Okada Y, Torimoto K, Kurozumi A, Narisawa M, Yamamoto S, et al. Prednisolone dosing regimen for treatment of subacute thyroiditis. J UOEH. 2015;37(2):103-10.
43. Mizukoshi T, Noguchi S, Murakami T, Futata T, Yamashita H. Evaluation of recurrence in 36 subacute thyroiditis patients managed with prednisolone. Intern Med. 2001;40(4):292-5.

44. Ma SG, Bai F, Cheng L. A novel treatment for subacute thyroiditis: administration of a mixture of lidocaine and dexamethasone using an insulin pen. Mayo Clin Proc. 2014;89(6):861-2.
45. Stagnaro-Green A, Schwartz A, Gismondi R, Tinelli A, Mangieri T, Negro R. High rate of persistent hypothyroidism in a large-scale prospective study of postpartum thyroiditis in southern Italy. J Clin Endocrinol Metab. 2011;96(3):652-7.
46. Kitchener MI, Chapman IM. Subacute thyroiditis: a review of 105 cases. Clin Nucl Med. 1989;14(6):439-42.
47. Iitaka M, Momotani N, Ishii J, Ito K. Incidence of subacute thyroiditis recurrences after a prolonged latency: 24-year survey. J Clin Endocrinol Metab. 1996;81(2):466-9.
48. Stein AA, Hernandez I, McClintock JC. Subacute granulomatous thyroiditis: a clinicopathologic review. Ann Surg. 1961;153(1):149-56.
49. Hoang TD, Mai VQ, Clyde PW, Shakir MK. Simultaneous occurrence of subacute thyroiditis and Graves' disease. Thyroid. 2011;21(12):1397-400.
50. Sherman SI, Ladenson PW. Subacute thyroiditis causing thyroid storm. Thyroid. 2007;17(3):283.
51. Mukae H, Furusyo N, Murata M, Ogawa E, Kainuma M, Shimizu M, et al. A case of granulomatosis with polyangiitis preceded by subacute thyroiditis. Clin Case Rep. 2015;3(3):139-44.
52. Valentini RB, Macedo BM, Izquierdo RF, Meyer EL. Painless thyroiditis associated to thyroid carcinoma: role of initial ultrasonography evaluation. Arch Endocrinol Metab. 2016;60(2):178-82.
53. Pan FS, Wang W, Wang Y, Xu M, Liang JY, Zheng YL, et al. Sonographic features of thyroid nodules that may help distinguish clinically atypical subacute thyroiditis from thyroid malignancy. J Ultrasound Med. 2015;34(4):689-96.
54. Paes JE, Burman KD, Cohen J, Franklyn J, McHenry CR, Shoham S, et al. Acute bacterial suppurative thyroiditis: a clinical review and expert opinion. Thyroid. 2010;20(3):247-55.
55. Raman L, Murray J, Banka R. Primary tuberculosis of the thyroid gland: an unexpected cause of thyrotoxicosis. BMJ Case Rep. 2014;2014.
56. Guttler R, Singer PA, Axline SG, Greaves TS, McGill JJ. Pneumocystis carinii thyroiditis. Report of three cases and review of the literature. Arch Intern Med. 1993;153(3):393-6.
57. Aamir S, Rizvi AA. Visual vignette. Suppurative thyroiditis due to Nocardia asteroides. Endocr Pract. 2012;18(3):426.
58. Abe K, Fujita H, Matsuura N, Minami H, Sato T. A fistula from pyriform sinus in recurrent acute suppurative thyroiditis. Am J Dis Child. 1981;135(2):178.
59. Adesola AO. Acute suppurative thyroiditis (with a report of 3 cases). West Afr Med J. 1962;11:248-54.
60. Chaurasia JK, Garg C, Agarwal A, Naim M. Tubercular thyroiditis with multinodular goitre with adenomatous hyperplasia: a rare coexistence. BMJ Case Rep. 2013;2013.
61. Aizawa T, Hashizume K. Radiation thyroiditis. Ryoikibetsu Shokogun Shirizu. 1993;1:349-51.
62. Aizawa T, Watanabe T, Suzuki N, Suzuki S, Miyamoto T, Ichikawa K, et al. Radiation-induced painless thyrotoxic thyroiditis followed by hypothyroidism: a case report and literature review. Thyroid. 1998;8(3):273-5.
63. Meng Z, Zhang G, Sun H, Tan J, Yu C, Tian W, et al. Differentiation between Graves' disease and painless thyroiditis by diffusion-weighted imaging, thyroid iodine uptake, thyroid scintigraphy and serum parameters. Exp Ther Med. 2015;9(6):2165-72.
64. Akamizu T, Amino N, DeGroot LJ. Hashimoto's Thyroiditis. In: De Groot LJ, Chrousos G, Dungan K, Feingold KR, Grossman A, Hershman JM, Koch C, Korbonits M, McLachlan R, New M, Purnell J, Rebar R, Singer F, Vinik A (Eds). Endotext [Internet]. South Dartmouth (MA): MDText.com, Inc.; 2000-2013.
65. Arowolo OA, Ige FS, Odujoko O, Agbakwuru EA. Riedel's thyroiditis in a black African: A case report and review of literature. Niger J Clin Pract. 2016;19(4):549-55.
66. Ng SA, Corcuera-Solano I, Gurudutt VV, Som PM. A rare case of Reidel thyroiditis with associated vocal cord paralysis: CT and MR imaging features. AJNR Am J Neuroradiol. 2011;32(11):E201-2.
67. Azizi F. Treatment of post-partum thyrotoxicosis. J Endocrinol Invest. 2006;29(3):244-7.
68. Postpartum thyroiditis. Lancet. 1987;1(8539):962.
69. Akamizu T. Postpartum Thyroiditis. In: De Groot LJ, Chrousos G, Dungan K, Feingold KR, Grossman A, Hershman JM, Koch C, Korbonits M, McLachlan R, New M, Purnell J, Rebar R, Singer F, Vinik A (Eds). Endotext [Internet]. South Dartmouth (MA): MDText.com, Inc.; 2000-2015.
70. Gaberšček S, Osolnik J, Zaletel K, Pirnat E, Hojker S. An advantageous role of spectral Doppler Sonography in the evaluation of thyroid dysfunction during the postpartum period. J Ultrasound Med. 2016;35(7):1429-36.
71. Vitkova H, Jiskra J, Springer D, Limanova Z, Telicka Z, Bartakova J, et al. Anti-C1q autoantibodies are linked to autoimmune thyroid disorders in pregnant women. Clin Exp Immunol. 2016;186(1):10-7.
72. Argatska A, Nonchev B, Orbetzova M, Pehlivanov B. Postpartum thyroid dysfunction in women with autoimmune thyroiditis. Gynecol Endocrinol. 2016;32(5):379-82.

CHAPTER 6

Depression and Hypothyroidism

Gumpeny R Sridhar, Gumpeny Lakshmi

> **CASE 1**
>
> A 26-year-old woman presented with clinical and biochemical features of hypothyroidism. She had anorexia, weakness, shortness of breath, body pains, excessive daytime sleepiness, irregular bowel movement, and slowness of mental activity. Her menstrual cycles were regular. She had no family history of thyroid disease.
>
> Her last childbirth occurred 6 years ago. She has been under the care of a psychiatrist for management of depression, which was diagnosed earlier, and was prescribed Fluvac.
>
> On physical examination, she had a goiter (grade 2), with, hypokinesis, and dry skin.
>
> Concerned by the suboptimal response to antidepressant medication and suspicious clinical features, thyroid function was evaluated, which confirmed the diagnosis of hypothyroidism, with an elevated level of thyrotropin (19.4 µIU/mL).
>
> She was then started on thyroxine (T4) replacement (100 µg/day) which led to improvement of hypothyroid features, as well as a better response to the antidepressant drug.

> **CASE 2**
>
> A 27-year-old woman, diagnosed to have primary hypothyroidism 3 years ago was on thyroxine 100 µg/day. She did not have any symptoms of thyroid dysfunction and was clinically euthyroid (no goiter, normal skin, brisk deep tendon reflexes).
>
> During the course, she developed behavioral abnormalities and was referred to a psychiatrist, who diagnosed she had paranoid schizophrenia.
>
> At the time of her psychiatric abnormality, she stopped using thyroxine without medical advice and developed hypothyroidism [thyroid-stimulating hormone (TSH) 33 µIU/mL]. She is under follow up after restarting thyroxine replacement (125 µg/day).

BACKGROUND

Thyroid hormones are well-recognized to have critical roles in the development of the central nervous system. Neonatal deficiency leads to cognitive and growth dysfunction. Thyroxine passes to the brain via hormone transporters where it is converted to its active form [triiodothyronine (T3)] which acts on specific thyroid hormone receptors in the brain. It is conceivable that lack of thyroid hormones in adulthood can result in cognitive dysfunction short of gross intellectual deficit of neonatal hypothyroidism.

In hypothyroidism, a reported ranging of psychiatric abnormalities were reported from agitation to schizophrenia (paranoid and affective). Poor memory and depression are also reported. These defects were attributed to reduced cerebral blood flow and metabolism.[1] Among other conditions, epidemiological studies linked hypothyroidism with Alzheimer's disease, although the cause-effect was not definitely established.[2]

A variety of pathways exist between the action of thyroid hormone and neuro-psychiatric dysfunction involving brain uptake of the hormone, activation and influence on neurotransmitter generation.[3] In addition, genetic variations and mutation of proteins affect the action of thyroid hormone. An understanding of the polymorphisms of thyroid hormone receptors in the brain offers newer avenues for diagnosis and treatment.[4]

However, in adults, hypothyroidism is most often associated with depression and dementia, via dysregulation of specific target transcription.[5] In a prospective cohort study of 2,269 adult men (range: 45–59 years), a positive association was weakly associated between total T4 level and chronic psychiatric morbidity. However, pooling data from other studies, the meta-analysis showed a positive association between depression and T4 level. This intriguing result suggested that high normal T4 levels were associated with increased risk of depression.[6] Nevertheless, hypothyroidism affects cognitive functioning and mood the more. It leads to slowing of information processing, reduced efficiency in functions related to executive function, as well as increased susceptibility to depression.[7]

Such uncertainty was expressed even in 2004, when Bahls stated that mild abnormalities of thyroid function predisposes to developing depression.[8] There has been a recent suggestion that a bidirectional relation may exist between psychiatric diseases and dysfunction of the thyroid.[9]

CLINICAL FEATURES

Subclinical hypothyroidism is more common than overt hypothyroidism; the former refers to a "compensated state" where the level of free T4 is normal, but TSH is elevated, suggesting that thyronormalcy is achieved at the cost of increased stimulation by the hypothalamic-pituitary signals on the thyroid. There is evidence for depression and cognitive impairment in subclinical hypothyroidism, although there are conflicting reports.[10] A review on the relation between hypothyroidism and depression showed that people on thyroxine had poorer psychological well-being even when biochemically euthyroid.[11] The authors suggested that misdiagnosis may be due to "initial misdiagnosis and misattribution of symptoms". Box 1 shows the features common to both depression and hypothyroidism.[12] Gender differences in the prevalence of thyroid diseases, with women being more affected, could also be contributing to the expression of mood disorders.[13] Difficulties may arise in the diagnosis of depression if undetected depression coexists.

Box 1: Features common to both depression and hypothyroidism	
• Depressed mood • Apathy • Emotional lability • Poor appetite • Excessive sleep • Weight gain	• Fatigue • Poor concentrations • Memory loss • Suicidal ideation • Delusions
Source: Bathla M, Singh M, Relan P. Prevalence of anxiety and depressive symptoms among patients with hypothyroidism. Indian J Endocrinol Metab. 2016;20:468-74.	

Giving support to the gender differences, both hypothyroidism and disorders of mood are common in pregnancy and the postpartum period. Changes in brain function could underlie as the cause for both, which has only been suggested, not yet studied.[14]

Although depression often occurs with hypothyroidism and mania with hyperthyroidism, contrariwise associations were reported. There were 13 subjects of hypothyroidism who presented with acute maniac episode (Diagnostic and Statistical Manual of Mental Disorders, 4th Edition, Text Revision criteria). Of the three who were followed up, all improved with thyroxine replacement along with drugs for mania.[15] Similarly, depression and psychotic behavior was reported in a young man with thyrotoxicosis due to subacute thyroiditis, which normalized with achievement of euthyroid state.[16]

A recent study from India reported the prevalence of depressive symptoms and anxiety in subjects with hypothyroidism. The sample comprised mostly in the age group of 26–35 years (n:41), with nearly twice as many women (n:33) as men (n:18). In the total sample, 60% had some degree of depression: 37% mild, 14% moderate, and 9% severe. There were no gender differences. In the anxiety score, 29% had mild, 14% had moderate, and 9% had severe anxiety, without any gender difference.[12] Depressive symptoms were the most common among men, whereas in women they formed the third commonest symptoms (following gastrointestinal somatic symptoms and hypochondriasis).

Subclinical Hypothyroidism

It is established that subclinical hypothyroidism does not present with widespread and severe dysfunctions in cognition, which are mild and limited; thyroxine replacement does not markedly improve clinical improvement. Therefore, mild symptoms may be common, but are not significantly reversed by thyroxine therapy.[1] Correction of biochemical hypothyroidism may still result in residual cognitive symptoms, which may need to be managed independent of thyroxine replacement, though a potential role of antithyroid antibodies has been postulated.

PATHOGENESIS

Thyroid hormones are critical for the development and function of both neuronal and glial cells; abnormalities lead to changes in the architecture and function of the brain. Disturbances in the transport and metabolism in astrocytes lead to abnormalities of microglia and oligodendrocytes and may, thus, contribute to cognitive dysfunction. This has been named as the glioendocrine system.[17]

Daylight regulates the suprachiasmatic nucleus and melatonin secretion. Melatonin secretion affects the production of TSH and T3 in the hypothalamus. It has been postulated that irregular circadian sleep timing and thyroid hormone homeostasis can lead to depression.[18] Iodothyronine deiodinases are well-recognized selenoproteins that influence thyroid hormone action. A recent meta-analysis has shown that deiodinase type 1 (D1) polymorphisms have a moderate to strong relation with thyroid hormone levels, insulin, bipolar mood disorder, as well as well-being.[19] Thus, variants of deiodinase may be involved in cognitive pathological conditions. The deiodinase type 2 (D2) variant was shown to be associated with well-being, independent of serum levels of thyroid hormone levels, suggesting an independent regulation of these hormones at the tissue level.[20]

There is emerging evidence for the role of autoantibodies in the pathogenesis of cognitive dysfunction and depression. Considering the existence of autoimmunity in the pathogenesis of hypothyroidism, Iseme et al. postulated that autoantibodies may account for symptoms similar to depression.[21] To support evidence for such an association, thyroid peroxidase antibodies were associated for "trait markers of depression".[22] Subjects with depression had altered function of hypothalamic-pituitary-thyroid axis, leading to elevated T4 level, lack of nocturnal rise of TSH and a blunted response of TSH to thyrotropin-releasing hormone, along with predisposition to autoimmune thyroiditis. This led to the postulation of "brain hypothyroidism" as a pathway to the pathogenesis of depression.[23] Depression was suggested to be a condition of tissue hypothyroidism in the brain, even though the peripheral levels of the hormone are normal. Brain type 2 deiodinase inhibition is believed to inhibit transfer of T4 across the blood-brain barrier.

While overt hypothyroidism is uncommon among subjects with depression, altered thyroid function has been reported. The mediation may occur through autoimmune processes.[24] This might be associated with abnormal hypothalamic-pituitary-adrenal axis as well as involvement of other mediators such as leptin and dehydroepiandrosterone.[25]

Finally, changes in the brain cellular high-energy phosphate metabolism have also been studied in subjects with major depression. Thyroid hormones were postulated to affect its metabolism, and correction by thyroxine replacement could be a therapeutic option,[26] particularly in the treatment of resistant depression.

In addition to measurement of thyroid hormones and thyroid autoantibodies in the peripheral blood, imaging methods of the brain using single photon emission computed tomography and positron emission tomography were employed in investigating psychiatric disorders in thyroid dysfunction. Particularly in hypothyroid dementia, decrease in cerebral metabolism and blood flow occurs in brain regions mediating attention, motor speed, and visuospatial processing.[27]

TREATMENT

Overt or even subclinical hypothyroidism is managed by thyroxine replacement, the latter based on a case-by-case basis.

There have been reports of thyroxine being used as a supplement to conventional drugs for treatment of depression. This has been particularly tried when there is a delay in the onset of effect of antidepressant agents, or when the response is poor. Triiodothyronine has been employed in an effort to hasten or augment the response to antidepressant drugs, especially tricyclic antidepressants.[28] Such intervention may be necessary only in a subgroup of depressed subjects with specific demographic, clinical, and genetic characteristics, although the recommendation is based on theoretical grounds rather than clinical evidence-base. In an analysis on the use of thyroxine supplementation in subclinical hypothyroidism associated with depression, there was no clinical benefit.[29] Further clinical studies are required before a clear answer can be obtained about the concomitant use of thyroxine in the treatment of depression.

In the 5–10% cases where symptoms of anxiety or depression persist despite achieving normal TSH levels with thyroxine replacement, there is evidence for combining it with T3 in selected patients having genetic polymorphisms of thyroid hormone transporters and deiodinases that result in hypothyroidism at the level of the brain cells.[30] A recent review on the subject relating to improving quality of life with combined T3 and T4 replacement suggested the need for prospective randomized controlled trials that can mimic physiological profile of thyroid hormone levels.[31]

Thyroxine Treatment in Resistant Depression and Other Conditions

Literature in the field of psychiatry provides evidence for the role of thyroxine as an adjuvant in the treatment of resistant depression. When bipolar disorder responds unsatisfactorily to conventional pharmacotherapy, T3 supplementation was also employed as an adjuvant; however, most studies were small and had competing treatment regimens, which mandates conduct of properly designed trials with controls and adequate follow-up.[32] In an earlier study that the addition of thyroxine did not improve the outcome of depression, it was concluded that "maintaining a good quality relationship between patient and doctor may be more important".[33] Resistant depression being a fairly common recalcitrant condition, augmenting agents such as thyroid hormones and lithium were employed, although uncommonly.[34] The authors cautioned that despite the various adjunct treatments attempted, it "represents an area of unmet medical need".[34]

Menstrual psychosis is an uncommon condition, with 80 reported cases with substantial evidence. It presents features with maniac depressive disorder. Unconventional treatments such as thyroid hormones and clomiphene were suggested to be effective by action at the hypothalamus, interfering with the interaction between bipolar diathesis and menstruation.[35]

Another intriguing report reviewed the role of preventive pharmacotherapy in postpartum depression with agents including thyroid, but concluded that evidence for its efficacy was equivocal.[36] It raises interesting questions, but answers must await further evidence.

A more provocative suggestion was made by Malhotra that T4 in high doses may help in augmenting the effect of mood stabilizers in the treatment of disorders of mood.[37]

CONCLUSION

Both overt and subclinical hypothyroidism may be associated with changes in mood, particularly depression. They share some common clinical features, and the contribution of each must be carefully dissected. Common pathogenic factors may be responsible such as autoimmunity, abnormalities of hypothalamic-pituitary-adrenal axis, changes in energy metabolism, and blood flow. Frank hypothyroidism must be corrected with thyroxine; evidence exists for addition of thyroxine to treat recalcitrant or poorly responsive resistant depression

REFERENCES

1. Schuff KG, Samuels MH, Whybrow PC, Bauer M. Psychiatric and cognitive effects of hypothyroidism. In: Braverman LE, Cooper DS (Eds). Werner and Ingbar's The Thyroid. New Delhi: Wolters Kluwer; 2013. pp. 596-600.
2. Brent GA, Weetman AP. Hypothyroidism and thyroiditis. In: Melmed S, Polonsky KS, Larsen PR, Kronenberg HM (Eds). Williams Textbook of Endocrinology. Philadelphia: Elsevier; 2016. pp. 416-48.
3. Feldman AZ, Shreshta RT, Hennessey JV. Neuropsychiatric manifestations of thyroid disease. Endocrinol Metab Clin North Am. 2013;42:453-76.
4. Bunevicius R. Thyroid disorders in mental patients. Curr Opin Psychiatry. 2009;22:391-5.
5. Aszalos Z. Some neurologic and psychiatric complications in endocrine disorders: the thyroid gland. Orv Hetil. 2007;148:303-10.
6. Williams MD, Harris R, Dayan CM, Evans J, Gallacher J, Ben-Shlomo Y. Thyroid function and the natural history of depression: findings from the Caerphilly Prospective Study (CaPS) and a meta-analysis. Clin Endocrinol (Oxf) 2009;70:484-92.
7. Davis JD, Tremont G. Neuropsychiatric aspects of hypothyroidism and treatment reversibility. Minerva Endocrinol. 2007;32:49-65.

8. Bahls SC, de Carvalho GA. The relation between thyroid function and depression: a review. Rev Bras Psiquiatr. 2004;26:41-9.
9. Kalra S, Balhara YP. Euthyroid depression: the role of thyroid hormone. Recent Pat Endocr Metab Immune Drug Discov. 2014;8:38-41.
10. Baumgartner C, Blum MR, Rodondi N. Subclinical hypothyroidism: summary of evidence in 2014. Swiss Med Wkly. 2014;144:w14058.
11. Dayan CM, Panicker V. Hypothyroidism and depression. Eur Thyroid J. 2013;2:168-79.
12. Bathla M, Singh M, Relan P. Prevalence of anxiety and depressive symptoms among patients with hypothyroidism. Indian J Endocrinol Metab. 2016;20:468-74.
13. Bauer M, Glenn T, Pilhatsch M, Pfennig A, Whybrow PC. Gender differences in thyroid system function: relevance to bipolar disorder and its treatment. Bipolar Disord. 2014;16:58-71.
14. Basraon S, Constantine MM. Mood disorders in pregnant women with thyroid dysfunction. Clin Obstet Gynecol. 2011;54:506-14.
15. Khemka D, Ali JA, Koch CA. Primary hypothyroidism associated with acute mania: case series and literature review. Exp Clin Endocrinol Diabetes. 2011;119:513-7.
16. Rizvi AA. "Thyrotoxic psychosis" associated with subacute thyroiditis. South Med J. 2007;100:837-40.
17. Noda M. Possible role of glial cells in the relationship between thyroid dysfunction and mental disorders. Front Cell Neurosci. 2015;9:194.
18. Kripke DF, Elliott JA, Welsh DK, Youngstedt SD. Photoperiodic and circadian bifurcation theories of depression and mania. F1000Res. 2015;4:107.
19. Verloop H, Dekkers OM, Peetters RP, Schoones JW, Smit JW. Genetics in endocrinology: genetic variation in deiodinases: a systematic review of potential clinical effects in humans. Eur J Endocrinol. 2014;171:R123-35.
20. Dayan CM, Panicker V. Novel insights into thyroid hormones from the study of common genetic variations. Nat Rev Endocrinol. 2009;5:211-8.
21. Isema RA, McEvoy M, Kelly B, Agnew L, Attia J, Walker FR. Autoantibodies and depression: evidence for a causal link? Neurosci Biobehav Rev. 2014;40:62-79.
22. Duntas LH, Mallis A. Hypothyroidism and depression: salient aspects of pathogenesis and management. Minerva Endocrinol. 2013;8:365-77.
23. Foltyn W, Nowakowska-Zajdel E, Danikiewica A, Brodziak A. Hypothalamic-pituitary-thyroid axis in depression. Psychiatr Pol. 2002;36:281-92.
24. Fountoulakis KN, Kantartzis S, Siamouli M, Panagiotidis P, Kaprinis S, Iacovides A, et al. Peripheral thyroid dysfunction in depression. World J Biol Psychiatry. 2006;7:131-7.
25. Tichomirowa MA, Kech ME, Schneider HJ, Paez-Pereda M, Renner U, Holsboer F, et al. Endocrine disturbances in depression. J Endocrinol Invest. 2005;28:89-99.
26. Iosifescu DV, Renshaw PE. 31P-magnetic resonance spectroscopy and thyroid hormones in major depressive disorder: toward a bioenergetic mechanism in depression? Harv Rev Psychiatry. 2003;11:51-63.
27. Lass P, Slawek J, Derejko D, Rubello D. Neurological and psychiatric disorders in thyroid dysfunctions. The role of nuclear medicine: SPECT and PET imaging. Minerva Endocrinol. 2008;33:75-84.
28. Cooper R, Lerer B. The use of thyroid hormones in the treatment of depression. Harefuah. 2010;149:529-34.
29. van Harten AC, Leue C, Verhey FR. Should depressive symptoms in patients with subclinical hypothyroidism be treated with thyroid hormone? Tijdschr Psychiatr. 2008;50:539-43.
30. Wiersinga WM. Paradigm shifts in thyroid hormone replacement therapies for hypothyroidism. Nat Rev Endocrinol. 2014;10:164-74.
31. Biondi B, Wartofsky L. Combination treatment with T4 and T3: toward personalized replacement therapy in hypothyroidism? J Clin Endocrinol Metab. 2012;97:2256-71.
32. Poon SH, Sim K, Sum MY, Kuswanto CN, Baldessarini RJ. Evidence-based options for treatment-resistant adult bipolar disorder patients. Bipolar Disord. 2012;14:573-84.
33. Treatment-resistant depression: no panacea, many uncertainties. Adverse effects are a major factor in treatment choice. Prescrire Int. 2011;20:128-33.
34. Shelton RC, Osuntokun O, Heinloth AN, Corya SA. Therapeutic options for treatment-resistant depression. CNS Drugs. 2010;24:131-61.
35. Brockington IF. Menstrual psychosis: a bipolar disorder with a link to the hypothalamus. Curr Psychiatry Rep. 2011;13:193-7.
36. Dennis CL. Preventing postpartum depression part 1: a review of biological interventions. Can J Psychiatry. 2004;49:467-75.
37. Chakrabarti S, Malhotra. Thyroid hormones in treatment of mood disorders. Indian J Med Sci. 2001;55:501-7.

CHAPTER 7

Subclinical Hyperthyroidism

Rana Bhattacharjee, Sujoy Ghosh

INTRODUCTION

Subclinical hyperthyroidism is characterized by low thyroid-stimulating hormone (TSH) with normal free thyroxine (T4) and triiodothyronine (T3) values. Etiology is similar to overt hyperthyroidism. They are often discovered incidentally or during workup of thyroid nodule.

At the end of this chapter, the reader should be able to formulate a diagnostic plan and make treatment decision for an individual patient with subclinical hyperthyroidism. This chapter will start with a case vignette.

> **CASE 1**
> A 67-year-old lady was referred by her primary care physician for goiter. The patient noticed swelling in front of her neck 2 years back. Since then it had not increased in size much, but she visited the physician on her relative's insistence. She had her last menstrual period 17 years back. She was healthy and does not take any medication. Her thyroid function report done 2 months back was as follows—TSH 0.03 mU/mL (normal 0.5–4), free T4 1.6 ng/dL (normal 0.8–1.9), and T3–173 ng/dL (80–190).
>
> On examination, she was found to have multinodular goiter, which was nontender. There was no lymphadenopathy. Her pulse rate was 90 per minute, regular. Repeat thyroid function test showed persistence of hyperthyroidism. Technetium-99m (Tc-99m) pertechnetate scan was consistent with toxic multinodular goiter (TMNG). Bone mineral density (BMD) dual energy X-ray absorptiometry (DEXA) T-score was −2.6 at hip.
>
> **Management**
> Considering her age, comorbidity, and pathogenesis of subclinical hyperthyroidism, decision was made to treat the patient and treatment options were discussed with her. Radioiodine ablation was done with 20 mCi of I^{131}. Calcium and vitamin D supplementation were also given. She became hypothyroid and started with levothyroxine replacement. After 28 months, repeat BMD DEXA T-score and mineral density improved (T −2.2). Her thyroid function test continued to be normal with replacement and she is being followed up.

DEFINITION

Subclinical hyperthyroidism is a biochemical entity. It is said to be present when serum TSH level is below the lower limit of normal but T4 or free T4 level is within the age-specific normal range. Although, the term thyrotoxicosis classically denotes excessive amount of circulating thyroid hormone level and hyperthyroidism implies that thyrotoxicosis is due to hyperfunction of thyroid gland, in this chapter both the terms will be used interchangeably.

EPIDEMIOLOGY

It is estimated that around 1.27% of Indian urban adult population suffer from subclinical hyperthyroidism.[1] In third National Health and Nutrition Examination Survey (NHANES III), subclinical hyperthyroidism was found to be commoner in females, older persons, smokers, and persons living in areas with mild-moderate iodine deficiency.[2]

ETIOLOGY

Causes of subclinical hyperthyroidism are similar to overt hyperthyroidism. Common causes are listed in table 1.

- Overtreatment of overt or subclinical hyperthyroidism: 11% of urban adult population in India suffers from overt hypothyroidism, whereas 8% suffers from subclinical hyperthyroidism.[1] They are at risk of overtreatment and consequent development of subclinical hyperthyroidism
- Thyroid hormone suppressive therapy: TSH suppression therapy is employed in many patients with differentiated thyroid carcinoma. Sometimes, it is used to reduce the size of benign thyroid nodule
- Destruction of thyroid gland architecture: In subacute and silent thyroiditis, excessive amount of thyroid hormone is released into circulation due to destruction of follicular structure. In mild cases, subclinical hyperthyroidism may occur
- Overproduction from thyroid gland: Patients with Graves' disease can have subclinical hyperthyroidism in early stages of disease. Subclinical hyperthyroidism like thyroid function test can also occur in patients who are well controlled with medical therapy, but TSH level is yet to recover. Many patients of TMNG and toxic adenoma (TA) have subclinical hyperthyroidism and it is often discovered during evaluation of nodule
- Human chorionic gonadotropin (HCG)-related: High level of HCG can stimulate TSH receptor due to its cross-reactivity with TSH. Late first trimester pregnancy and hydatidiform mole can lead to biochemical change consistent with subclinical hyperthyroidism by this mechanism.

TABLE 1: Common causes of subclinical hyperthyroidism

Exogenous	1. Unintentional	Over-replacement
	2. Intentional	Suppressive therapy
Endogenous	1. Graves' disease 2. Toxic multinodular goiter 3. Toxic adenoma 4. Subacute thyroiditis or silent thyroiditis (thyrotoxicosis without hypothyroidism) 5. HCG-induced—late first trimester pregnancy, molar pregnancy	–

HCG, human chorionic gonadotropin.

NATURAL HISTORY

Many persons with mild decrease in TSH have spontaneous reversion whereas very low TSH levels tend to persist. Few patients may progress to overt hyperthyroidism. In a follow-up study on subjects more than 60 years of age with low but detectable TSH, 76% (38 out of 50) showed spontaneous reversion at the end of 12 months. On the contrary, 14 out of 16 subjects with undetectable TSH had persistence of low TSH level at 12 months. Only one of them developed overt hyperthyroidism.[3] In another study, 52% subjects with TSH less than 0.35 μU/mL became biochemically euthyroid without any treatment.[4]

SYSTEMIC EFFECTS

Cardiovascular System

Patients with subclinical hyperthyroidism have increased risk for atrial fibrillation (AF), sinus tachycardia, and left ventricular hypertrophy, coronary artery disease, and heart failure. atrial fibrillation is commoner in elderly persons. Tachyarrhythmias can lead to palpitation and exercise intolerance. The risk of AF is higher in patients with TSH of less than 0.1 μU/mL than in patients with TSH between 0.1 and 0.44 μU/mL.[5-7]

Bone and Mineral Metabolism

Effect of subclinical hyperthyroidism on bone density and fracture risk is controversial as results from various studies are conflicting. In postmenopausal women, exogenous subclinical hyperthyroidism leads to increased bone turnover and mineral loss. The degree of these changes depends on extent of TSH suppression and calcium intake. In men and premenopausal women, BMD is not affected significantly. In endogenous subclinical hyperthyroidism, the effect on bone is difficult to interpret, as disease duration is variable. Overall, cortical bone is more affected than trabecular bone. The association of fracture with subclinical hyperthyroidism is unclear.[5]

Central Nervous System

Various studies showed increased incidence of dementia in subclinical hyperthyroidism.[8-10] But causality is doubtful as dementia itself leads to low TSH level. Moreover, autoimmunity may be a common link between many cases of subclinical hyperthyroidism and dementia.[5]

Quality of Life

Quality of life seems to be impaired in both the endogenous and endogenous subclinical hyperthyroidism.[5] Sleep disturbance, palpitation, effort intolerance, and mood changes are likely contributing factor in some of the patients.

APPROACH TO A PATIENT WITH SUBCLINICAL HYPERTHYROIDISM

Algorithm stating the approach to a patient with subclinical hyperthyroidism is depicted in flowchart 1.

Disorders of Thyroid

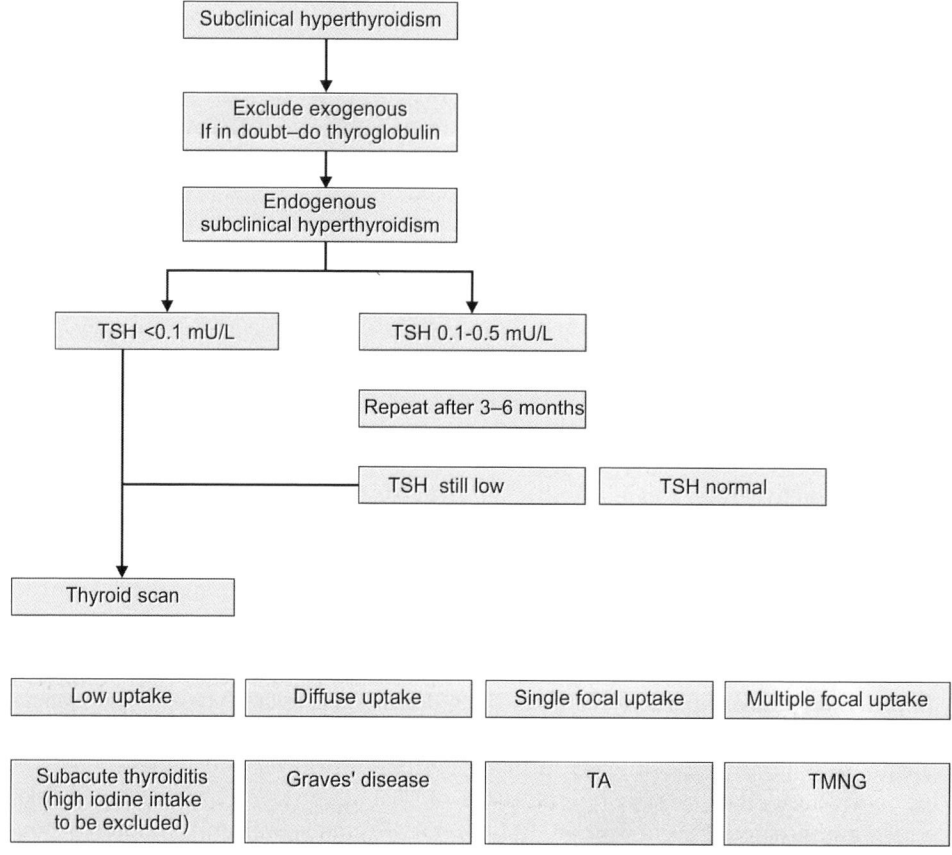

FLOWCHART 1: Diagnostic algorithm

TA, toxic adenoma; TMNG, toxic multinodular goiter; TSH, thyroid-stimulating hormone.

- Exclusion of other conditions: Although low TSH and normal T4 or free T4 and T3 define subclinical hyperthyroidism, few other conditions can present with similar biochemical picture
    - Recovery from Graves' disease: Serum TSH level may take months to years to recover after normalization of T4 and T3 levels
    - Central hypothyroidism: A small subset of patient of central hypothyroidism may have low TSH with low normal TSH (c/f high normal TSH in subclinical hyperthyroidism)
    - "Sick euthyroid" syndrome: Some patients with serious non-thyroidal illness can have low TSH with normal T4 and low normal T3 (though low T3 is commoner). TSH suppression is more common in a patient receiving high dose glucocorticoid and/or dopamine
- Searching for etiology: Thorough history taking and physical examination often leads to diagnosis. History of sore throat and fever suggest subacute thyroiditis, whereas presence of orbitopathy suggests Graves' disease. Presence of diffuse goiter or nodule should be noted. Sometimes patient "forgets" to tell about levothyroxine he or she is taking unless specifically asked for. History of missed period may point toward early pregnancy.

In endogenous subclinical hyperthyroidism, Tc-99m pertechnetate scan may be employed to confirm the etiology. Alternatively, radioactive iodine uptake study can differentiate between subacute thyroiditis and over-activity of thyroid gland. Low uptake value point toward the former, whereas high or "normal" (which is inappropriately high for low TSH) uptake suggests the latter. Patients with surreptitious intake of levothyroxine will have low thyroglobulin level (however, antibody interference should be excluded by doing a simultaneous anti-thyroglobulin level).

- Search for comorbidities: One should search for associated conditions, which would influence the management of subclinical hyperthyroidism. History of fragility fracture and presence of risk factors for osteoporosis should be sought. Presence of underlying cardiac disease, particularly tachyarrhythmias should be noted. These conditions put the patient in higher risk of complication from subclinical hyperthyroidism.

MANAGEMENT

Adequate calcium and vitamin D intake should be ensured in all patients with subclinical hyperthyroidism.[11]

Exogenous Subclinical Hyperthyroidism

Patients who are taking levothyroxine for primary hyperthyroidism, TSH should be monitored regularly to keep it in the normal range to avoid subclinical hyperthyroidism. This is particularly true in elderly men, postmenopausal women, and patients with high-risk features.

Patients who are on suppressive dose of levothyroxine, lowest possible dose necessary to achieve TSH target for that particular patient should be employed.

Endogenous Subclincial Hyperthyroidism

Randomized controlled trial looking at "hard" clinical endpoints following treatment of subclinical hyperthyroidism is not available. First and foremost, thyroid function test needs to be repeated over a period of 3-6 months to exclude transient subclinical hyperthyroidism.[12] Subsequent management depends on degree of TSH suppression, age, and presence of high risk features.

Patients with high risk of cardiac and skeletal complication (age >65 years, with or at risk of cardiac arrhythmia, postmenopausal women with or at risk of osteoporosis): If TSH is less than 0.1 µIU/mL, underlying cause of subclinical hyperthyroidism should be treated. If TSH is between 0.1 and 0.5 µIU/mL, treatment is usually considered in patients with established cardiac disease or osteoporosis. Treatment threshold is also lower when TMNA or TA causes subclinical hyperthyroidism because chance of progression to overt hyperthyroidism is more in these patients. Treatment options are similar to overt hyperthyroidism. Target of therapy is normalization of TSH. Patient with Graves' disease in this TSH range without high risk of complication may be followed up with thyroid function test every 3 months. Beta blocker may also be used in patients with AF.[12]

Patients with low risk of cardiac and skeletal complication: If TSH is less than 0.1 µIU/mL, treatment is usually considered. Patients are followed up without treatment if TSH is between 0.1 and 0.5 mu/L (Table 2).

TABLE 2: **Treatment guidelines for subclinical hyperthyroidism**[12]

Factor	TSH (<0.1 mU/L)	TSH (0.1–0.5 mU/L)[a]
Age >65	Yes	Consider treating
Age <65 with comorbidities		
Heart disease	Yes	Consider treating
Osteoporosis	Yes	No
Menopausal	Consider treating	Consider treating
Hyperthyroid symptoms	Yes	Consider treating
Age <65, asymptomatic	Consider treating	No

[a]Where 0.5 mU/L is the lower limit of the normal range.

CONCLUSION

Despite lack of randomized controlled trial, subclinical hyperthyroidism can be treated depending on underlying cause, risk factors, and TSH level.

REFERENCES

1. Unnikrishnan AG, Kalra S, Sahay RK, Bantwal G, John M, Tewari N. Prevalence of hypothyroidism in adults : An epidemiological study in eight cities of India. Indian J Endocrinol Metab. 2013;17(4):647-52.
2. Belin RM, Astor BC, Powe NR, Ladenson PW. Smoke exposure is associated with a lower prevalence of serum thyroid autoantibodies and thyrotropin concentration elevation and a higher prevalence of mild thyrotropin concentration suppression in the third National Health and Nutrition Examination Survey (NHANES III). J Clin Endocrinol Metab. 2004;89(12):6077-86.
3. Parle JV, Franklyn JA, Cross KW, Jones SC, Sheppard MC. Prevalence and follow-up of abnormal thyrotrophin (TSH) concentrations in the elderly in the United Kingdom. Clin Endocrinol (Oxf). 1991;34(1):77-83.
4. Meyerovitch J, Rotman-Pikielny P, Sherf M, Battat E, Levy Y, Surks MI. Serum thyrotropin measurements in the community: five-year follow-up in a large network of primary care physicians. Arch Intern Med. 2007;167(14):1533-8.
5. Biondi B, Cooper DS. The clinical significance of subclinical thyroid dysfunction. Endocr Rev. 2008;29(1):76-131.
6. Collet TH, Gussekloo J, Bauer DC, den Elzen WP, Cappola AR, Balmer P, et al. Subclinical hyperthyroidism and the risk of coronary heart disease and mortality. Arch Intern Med. 2012;172(10):799-809.
7. Nanchen D, Gussekloo J, Westendorp RG, Stott DJ, Jukema JW, Trompet S, et al. Subclinical thyroid dysfunction and the risk of heart failure in older persons at high cardiovascular risk. J Clin Endocrinol Metab. 2012;97(3):852-61.
8. Ceresini G, Lauretani F, Maggio M, Ceda GP, Morganti S, Usberti E, et al. Thyroid function abnormalities and cognitive impairment in elderly people: results of the Invecchiare in Chianti study. J Am Geriatr Soc. 2009;57(1):89-93.
9. Kalmijn S, Mehta KM, Pols HA, Hofman A, Drexhage HA, Breteler MM. Subclinical hyperthyroidism and the risk of dementia. The Rotterdam study. Clin Endocrinol (Oxf). 2000;53(6):733-7.
10. Vadiveloo T, Donnan PT, Cochrane L, Leese GP. The Thyroid Epidemiology, Audit, and Research Study (TEARS): morbidity in patients with endogenous subclinical hyperthyroidism. J Clin Endocrinol Metab. 2011;96(5):1344-51.
11. Bone metabolism during anti-thyroid drug treatment of endogenous subclinical hyperthyroidism. Mudde AH, Houben AJ, Nieuwenhuijzen Kruseman AC .Clin Endocrinol (Oxf). 1994;41(4):421.
12. Bahn Chair RS, Burch HB, Cooper DS, Garber JR, Greenlee MC, Klein I, et al. Hyperthyroidism and other causes of thyrotoxicosis: management guidelines of the American Thyroid Association and American Association of Clinical Endocrinologists. Thyroid. 2011;21(6):593-646.

CHAPTER 8

Subclinical Hypothyroidism

Vedavati B Purandare, Unnikrishnan AG

> **CASE 1**
>
> A 25-year-old unmarried lady presented for routine annual health checkup. Physical examination suggested grade 1 thyromegaly which on enquiry was nonprogressive. Her biochemical parameters suggested impaired fasting glucose and thyroid-stimulating hormone (TSH) levels of 7.1 µIU/mL. She was advised lifestyle modification in the form of healthy diet and regular exercise. In view of raised TSH, she was advised to review with total triiodothyronine (T3), total thyroxine (T4), and thyroid peroxidase (TPO) antibody test. She was noncompliant with this advice and presented after 3 years with complaints of menstrual irregularity and change in voice.
>
> **On examination**
> - Her weight: 76 kg
> - Body mass index (BMI): 29
> - Blood pressure (BP): 130/90 mmHg
> - Skin was dry.
>
> **Investigations**
> - Serum TSH: 35 µIU/mL (reference range 0.25–5 µIU/mL)
> - Serum T3: 26.2 ng/dL (reference range 60–175 ng/dL)
> - Serum T4: 1.3 µg/dL (reference range 5.5–12.3 µg/dL)
> - Thyroid peroxidase antibody: Positive.
>
> **Management**
>
> Levothyroxine 100 µg orally once a day in the morning on empty stomach was prescribed. She was asked to follow up after 6 weeks for repeat thyroid profile.
>
> **Impression**
>
> Subclinical hypothyroidism (SCH) (autoimmune etiology) progressed to overt hypothyroidism over a period of time.
>
> **Discussion**
>
> Subclinical hypothyroidism is known to progress to overt hypothyroidism. Especially in subjects with autoimmune thyroid disease, this may occur more frequently. This issue is discussed in detail in this chapter.

> **CASE 2**
>
> A 68-year-old gentleman known to have type 2 diabetes mellitus and hypertension visited his physician with complaints of constipation and inability to lose weight. He is worried about abnormal thyroid profile report.
>
> He read about the symptoms of hypothyroidism on the internet and wants to know whether his symptoms will improve after thyroxine replacement.
>
> On examination:
> - Weight: 96 kg
> - Body mass index: 32 kg/m^2
> - Blood pressure: 130/90 mmHg.
>
> Investigations:
> - Thyroid stimulating hormone: 6.2 µIU/mL (reference range 0.25–5 µIU/mL)
> - Serum T3 levels: 72.6 ng/dL (reference range 60–175 ng/dL)
> - Serum T4 levels: 6.1 µg/dL (reference range 5.5–12.3 µg/dL).
>
> Impression
> Subclinical hypothyroidism.
>
> Discussion
> This gentleman was explained about the age-related rise in TSH. He was further explained that current evidence does not suggest benefit from replacement of thyroxine in his scenario; in fact it may have harmful effects on his bone and cardiovascular health, as discussed in the chapter.

INTRODUCTION

Contrary to its nomenclature, "subclinical hypothyroidism" is a term which is defined biochemically and not clinically. Irrespective of the clinical presentation, a normal serum thyroid hormone concentration in the presence of an elevated serum TSH concentration is termed as "subclinical hypothyroidism" making it mandatory to have a thyroid function test report for the diagnosis.[1] It is observed that most of the subjects diagnosed to have SCH are indeed clinically asymptomatic.[2] What makes SCH an important disease to consider is its prevalence. It is one of the most common problems encountered by general physicians as well as endocrinologists. This makes it necessary to have clear recommendations about SCH in terms of predicting clinical impact of SCH, knowing who should be screened for SCH, determining the subgroup of people who have a high clinical risk arising from the condition and selecting who will benefit most from the treatment. The evidence has travelled a long way from the earlier descriptions of SCH to the present day understanding of its clinical impact and therapeutic decision-making. Most of the evidence is generated from observational studies instead of randomized control trials and the cost-effectiveness of the treatment is unclear.

DEFINING SUBCLINICAL HYPOTHYROIDISM—WHAT IS THE NORMAL RANGE OF THYROID STIMULATING HORMONE?

Referring back to the biochemical definition of SCH stating requirement of thyroid hormones to be in normal range and TSH above the upper limit of normal range, it becomes important to have a reliable reference range of serum TSH from respective laboratories. Generally, reference ranges of a parameter for a given population are derived by obtaining values from individuals without evidence of the disorder in question. There has been an ongoing controversy about the upper limit of normal serum TSH which is specific to age, time and method of determination of TSH. There are fewer controversies about determining the lower limit.[3,4] In consideration to TSH, the controversies relate to the definition of normal population, consideration about iodine sufficiency as well as supplementation and the status of the antithyroid antibodies in the population. It has been observed that patients with TSH values above 2.5 µIU/L have a higher rate of positive antithyroid antibodies representing early stage of autoimmune thyroid illness and are at higher risk of progression to clinical hypothyroidism. Does this translate to 2.5 µIU/L being the upper limit of normal TSH? The answer is no, because this doubles or sometimes triples the number of people getting classified as hypothyroid, and studies have shown that they do not get benefit of therapy.[5] Currently, upper limit of normal level of TSH between 4 and 5 µIU/L depending on assay system is acceptable for general population.[6] There are exceptions to this rule in certain subgroups in which evidence has clearly shown benefits of lowering the upper limit of normal for therapeutic decision-making. This is discussed in further details in the later chapter Clinicians commonly encounter subjects with slightly elevated TSH which may fall into normal range on repeat testing. In this scenario, especially when there are no clinical features or compelling indications for treatment, it is considered prudent to repeat TSH testing after 6-12 weeks to observe the trend of serial values. Few explanations for a transiently high TSH include recovery from thyroiditis, a nonthyroidal illness or a laboratory error.[7]

EPIDEMIOLOGY

The prevalence of SCH is dependent of age, gender, iodine sufficiency status, status of positive thyroid antibody, and the considered reference range of TSH. Population studies show the prevalence of SCH to be 4–15%.[8-12] In the United States National Health and Nutrition Examination Survey III (NHANES III), which surveyed 16,533 people, prevalence of SCH was 4.3%.[13] The prevalence was higher in elderly females than males, and Whites compared to Blacks. There is a physiological rise in TSH with age; hence, the higher estimates of SCH in elderly population may be an overestimation of the actual prevalence.

Subclinical hypothyroidism is more prevalent in areas of iodine sufficiency ranging from 4.2% in iodine-deficient areas to 23.9% in iodine-sufficient areas irrespective of antithyroid peroxidase (anti-TPO) antibodies positivity.[14] In India, the prevalence of SCH is estimated to be 8% and is higher in women and elderly.[15]

ETIOLOGY

The first step to classify the patients with SCH is to make a distinction of patients with known thyroid disease. The etiologies of SCH and overt hypothyroidism are essentially same and are summarized in table 1. The most common cause of SCH in people without prior history of thyroid illness is autoimmune thyroiditis or Hashimoto's thyroiditis.

TABLE 1: Etiological classification of subclinical hypothyroidism

Previous history of thyroid illness	Without known thyroid illness	Conditions with raised TSH but not classified as SCH
• Inadequate therapeutic thyroid hormone (for overt hypothyroidism) supplementation due to poor adherence, drug interactions, or inadequate monitoring of treatment • Therapy for treatment of hyperthyroidism (radioactive iodine, medications or surgery) • Partial thyroidectomy	• Chronic autoimmune thyroiditis • Persistent TSH increase after an episode of subacute thyroiditis, postpartum thyroiditis, or painless thyroiditis • External radiotherapy of head and neck • Drugs impairing thyroid function (iodine, amiodarone) • Infiltrative disorders of the thyroid gland (amyloidosis, sarcoidosis, hemochromatosis, or Riedel's thyroiditis) • Iodine deficiency • Transient SCH after subacute, painless, or postpartum thyroiditis	• Laboratory errors • TSH-secreting pituitary adenoma • Recovery from critical illness • TSH with reduced biological activity • Impaired renal function • Untreated adrenal insufficiency

TSH, thyroid-stimulating hormone; SCH, subclinical hypothyroidism.

CLINICAL IMPACT OF SUBCLINICAL HYPOTHYROIDISM

Subclinical Hypothyroidism and Clinical Symptoms

Clinical symptoms of hypothyroidism, whether it is overt or subclinical, are neither sensitive nor specific. In other words, it is difficult to differentiate euthyroidism, SCH, and overt hypothyroidism from clinical examination. Additionally, severity of symptoms and signs does not relate to biochemical thyroid dysfunction neither does it affect the treatment of overt hypothyroidism. However, it does have impact on decision-making for treatment of SCH. The trials on patients with SCH have included patients with varied range of TSH. However, subgroup analysis of subjects with serum TSH between 4.5 and 10 µIU/L does not show any improvement in clinical parameters with thyroxine therapy in this group.[16]

Progression to Overt Hypothyroidism

The chance of progression of SCH to overt symptomatic hypothyroidism is dependent on the initial serum TSH concentration, which is the underlying cause of the disease with most important being presence of anti-TPO antibodies.[17-19] The rate of conversion of SCH to overt hypothyroidism in women with raised TSH and positive thyroid antibody is reported to be 4.3% per year.[20] Patients with past history of radioiodine therapy or high-dose external radiotherapy are also more likely to progress to overt hypothyroidism. Spontaneous recovery is observed in up to 62% of patients with normalization more likely in patients with negative antithyroid antibodies and serum TSH levels less than 10 µIU/L, and within the first 2 years after diagnosis.[21]

Cardiovascular Disease

Raised TSH has been shown to be associated with multiple cardiovascular effects like slowing of heart rate, slowing of left ventricular relaxation, increased oxygen consumption at rest, poor left ventricle function, impaired endothelial function, impairment in coronary reserve, and reduced global myocardial function.[22-24] The magnitude of effect varies according to the level of TSH with significant association TSH more than or equal to 10 μIU/L. Cardiovascular effects do not seem to be affected by age, gender, or past history of cardiovascular disease. However, treatment of SCH has not been shown to benefit cardiovascular outcomes.

Dyslipidemia

Effect of overt hypothyroidism on dyslipidemia in the form of raised total and low-density lipoprotein cholesterol is clear and has been documented to reverse after thyroxine replacement therapy. Patients with SCH too have been seen to have higher levels of apolipoprotein B. The effect of thyroxine replacement in SCH on lipid profile is unclear but is probably favorable.[25]

Metabolic Syndrome

In addition to dyslipidemia, SCH has been found to coexist with other atherosclerotic cardiovascular risk factors or surrogate markers like insulin resistance, inflammatory markers, obesity, and diabetes. There are multiple confounding factors to doubt a causal relationship between SCH and metabolic derangement. However, observational trials have suggested that raised TSH may be a part and parcel of metabolic syndrome as the mean TSH in people with metabolic syndrome is significantly higher than the controls.[26,27] In fact, it is observed that even in the euthyroid state, raised TSH seems to predispose to higher cholesterol, glucose, insulin levels, and insulin resistance. Thyroid stimulating hormone and free thyroxine concentrations are associated with differing metabolic markers in euthyroid subjects.[28] However, currently, no evidence suggests that the outcome of the risk can be modified by therapy of SCH.

Neurological and Psychiatric Symptoms

Preclinical studies estimate an association between neuromuscular dysfunction which can be reversed upon normalization of thyroid function[29] but recent clinical studies have negated the usefulness of thyroxine replacement for management of peripheral neuropathy.[30] Evidence exists on the either side of association between SCH and depression, decrements in mood, and memory. However, the most recent meta-analysis showed a weak but definitely positive relationship between depression and serum thyroxine, and an inverse association with serum TSH.[31] Until any conclusive answer from a large randomized control trial is derived, it is prudent to have low threshold for a therapeutic trial of levothyroxine for patients with SCH in patients with neuropsychiatric symptoms except for minimal cognitive and memory disturbances in elderly patients.

Subclinical Hypothyroidism and Old Age

The upper limit of normal level of TSH increases with age. Accordingly, it can be as high as 7.0 μIU/L for people with more than 70 years of age (Fig. 1). This increase in TSH with age has been linked to survival benefit in very old. Additionally, significance of association

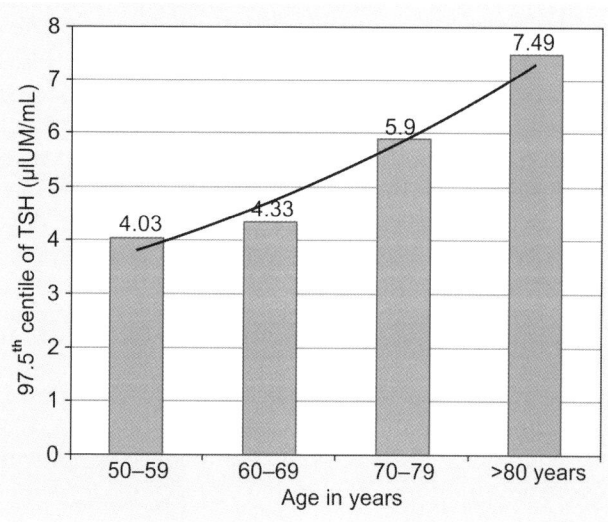

TSH, thyroid-stimulating hormone.
FIG. 1: Age-related rise in serum thyroid stimulating hormone[32]

between SCH and cardiovascular risk from almost all the observational trials is very weak in subgroup of people other than age 65. Same holds true for benefit of thyroxine therapy for SCH on improvement of cognitive dysfunction and memory in older patients. In conclusion, the threshold for decision-making of thyroxine replacement for SCH in elderly should be high. Overtreatment of hypothyroidism in the elderly may increase the risk of osteoporosis and cardiac arrhythmias. In general, conservative management is advisable in the elderly.

Pregnancy

Fetal thyroid gland does not function significantly prior to 20 weeks of gestation.[33] Many studies have shown that pregnant women with SCH (TSH >2.5 µIU/mL) have increased incidences of miscarriage, preterm delivery, placenta abruption,[34-37] and neuropsychiatric maldevelopment of the offsprings.[38,39] The risk of recurrent miscarriage has also been found to be more in women with positive antithyroid antibodies even with normal serum TSH levels. Yet, the evidence to support thyroxine therapy in antibody-positive euthyroid women is not convincing.[40] Most guidelines recommend to treat SCH in pregnancy with target level of TSH as 2.5 and 3 µIU/mL in first and later trimesters, respectively.

Screening for Subclinical Thyroid Dysfunction

There is no widespread agreement on screening parameters for thyroid dysfunction in population. However, the American Association of Clinical Endocrinologists and the American Thyroid Association suggest case finding for thyroid dysfunction in high-risk conditions (Box 1).

Subclinical Hypothyroidism

> **Box 1: Indications of screening for subclinical thyroid dysfunction**
> - Presence of other autoimmune disease, e.g., type 1 diabetes, pernicious anemia, alopecia
> - History of first-degree relative with autoimmune thyroid disease
> - History of neck radiation for treatment of hyperthyroidism and neck malignancies
> - History of thyroid surgery
> - Presence of goiter on examination
> - Psychiatric disorders
> - Patients taking amiodarone or lithium
> - Patients with International Classification of Diseases-Ninth Revision (ICD-9) diagnoses like adrenal insufficiency, unclassified anemia or cardiac dysrhythmia, changes in skin texture, congestive heart failure, constipation, dementia, unexplained hypercholesterolemia, malaise and fatigue, and unexplained weight gain.

MANAGEMENT OF SUBCLINICAL HYPOTHYROIDISM

Decision to Treat

Most guidelines agree on the decision to treat patients of SCH with TSH more than 10 μIU/mL. Another subgroup where a clear evidence of benefit from treatment of SCH is available is pregnancy where the threshold for stating treatment is TSH level of 2.5 μIU/mL. Individualized approach is required for other patients depending on the level TSH, status of anti-TPO antibodies, presence of certain clinical features and coexisting conditions. Proposed algorithm[1] for deciding thyroxine replacement in SCH is depicted in flowchart 1.

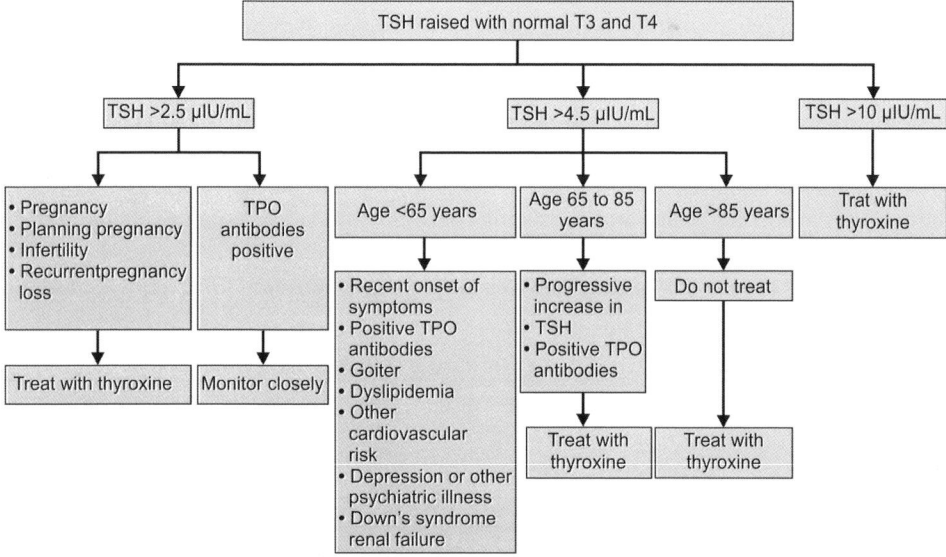

TSH, thyroid-stimulating hormone; TPO, thyroid peroxidase; T3, triiodothyronine; T4, thyroxine.

FLOWCHART 1: Algorithm for deciding thyroxine replacement in subclinical hypothyroidism (in adults)

Thyroxine therapy in younger patients with TSH more than 10 µIU/mL has been shown to improve:
- Symptoms of hypothyroidism, specifically tiredness
- Mood and cognition
- Improvement in cardiovascular function and reversal of preexisting dysfunction, if any, including systolic and diastolic dysfunction, endothelial function, and carotid intima-media thickness
- All-cause mortality
- Rate of miscarriage
- Rate of premature delivery.

Conflicting results about improvement in lipid abnormalities are present suggesting significant improvement in subjects with high baseline cholesterol.

Though different guidelines differ in recommending selection of patients who will benefit from thyroxine therapy, general consensus exists that thyroxine therapy is not indicated for lone purpose of weight loss in obese people with SCH.

How to Treat

The only evidence-based treatment for SCH is levothyroxine. The starting dose is generally lower than that of over hypothyroidism. Depending on the age and weight of the patient, it is recommended to start with 25–75 µg levothyroxine per day in nonpregnant subjects. The starting dose of thyroxine is lower in older people and patients with coexisting cardiovascular disorder. Pregnant women require higher dose and the starting dose may be 75 µg.

How to Follow Up

Goal of the therapy of SCH is normalization of TSH value. Thyroid stimulating hormone levels should be rechecked after 4–6 weeks of initiation of thyroxine therapy or change in the dose till stabilization of TSH. After that TSH should be followed every 6–12 months. During pregnancy, monitoring should be done every 4–6 weeks till the TSH is stabilized and at least once in each trimester thereafter. Anti-TPO antibody testing is a one-time investigation and should not be used for monitoring the disease response. The TSH targets vary according to age and coexisting condition and are summarized in table 2.

TABLE 2: Target thyroid-stimulating hormone for patients with subclinical hypothyroidism on thyroxine replacement

Condition	Target thyroid-stimulating hormone (µIU/mL)
• Pregnancy	
○ First trimester	<2.5
○ Second trimester	<3
○ Third trimester	<3–3.5
• Planning pregnancy	<2.5
• Nonpregnant adults aged <65 years	<4.5
• Nonpregnant adults aged <65 to 85 years	<7
• Nonpregnant adults aged >85 years	<8

CONCLUSION

Subclinical hypothyroidism is a common disorder with overall prevalence of around 10%. Thyroid stimulating hormone levels rise with age, apparently increasing prevalence of subclinical hypothyroidism in elderly. Three out of four patients with subclinical hypothyroidism have TSH below 10 µIU/mL. Some patients with mildly elevated serum TSH may normalize spontaneously on repeat testing. Observational data suggests increased risk of cardiovascular disorders in younger individuals with subclinical hypothyroidism. However, randomized controlled studies are needed to confirm this observation. Clinical impact and benefit of thyroxine replacement therapy are most marked in patients with persistent serum TSH above 10 µIU/mL. All pregnant women and women planning pregnancy with subclinical hypothyroidism should receive thyroxine therapy. In nonpregnant subjects with subclinical hypothyroidism and serum TSH below 10 µIU/L, an individualized and selective rather than uniform approach is recommended.

REFERENCES

1. Cooper DS, Biondi B. Subclinical thyroid disease. Lancet. 2012;379:1142-54.
2. Bensenor IM, Olmos RD, Lotufo PA. Hypothyroidism in the elderly: diagnosis and management. Clin Interv Aging. 2012;7:97-111; Waring AC, Arnold AM, Newman AB, et al. Longitudinal changes in thyroid function testing in the oldest old and survival: the cardiovascular health study all-stars study. Thyroid. 2011;21:A48-9.
3. Fatourechi V. Subclinical hypothyroidism and subclinical hyperthyroidism. Expert Rev Endocrinol Metab. 2010;5:359-73.
4. Surks MI, Goswami G, Daniels GH. The thyrotropin reference range should remain unchanged. J Clin Endocrinol Metab. 2005;90:5489-96.
5. Fatourechi V, Klee GG, Grebe SK, Bahn RS, Brennan MD, Hay ID, et al. Effects of reducing the upper limit of normal TSH values. JAMA. 2003;290:3195-6.
6. Boucai L, Hollowell JG, Surks MI. An approach for development of age-, gender-, and ethnicity-specific thyrotropin reference limits. Thyroid. 2011;21:5-11.
7. Unnikrishnan AG. Thyrotropin and the ever-narrowing reference ranges. Thyroid Research and Practice. 2006;3:50-5.
8. Tunbridge WM, Evered DC, Hall R, Appleton D, Brewis M, Clark F, et al. The spectrum of thyroid disease in a community: the Whickham survey. Clin Endocrinol (Oxf). 1977;7:481-93.
9. Bagchi N, Brown TR, Parish RF. Thyroid dysfunction in adults over age 55 years. A study in an urban US community. Arch Intern Med. 1990;150:785-7.
10. Kanaya AM, Harris F, Volpato S, Pérez-Stable EJ, Harris T, Bauer DC. Association between thyroid dysfunction and total cholesterol level in an older biracial population: the health, aging and body composition study. Arch Intern Med. 2002;162:773-9.
11. Canaris GJ, Manowitz NR, Mayor G, Ridgway EC. The Colorado thyroid disease prevalence study. Arch Intern Med. 2000;160:526-34.
12. Parle JV, Franklyn JA, Cross KW, Jones SC, Sheppard MC. Prevalence and follow-up of abnormal thyrotrophin (TSH) concentrations in the elderly in the United Kingdom. Clin Endocrinol (Oxf). 1991;34:77-83.
13. Hollowell JG, Staehling NW, Flanders WD, Hannon WH, Gunter EW, Spencer CA, et al. Serum TSH, T(4), and thyroid antibodies in the United States population (1988 to 1994): National Health and Nutrition Examination Survey (NHANES III). J Clin Endocrinol Metab. 2002;87:489-99.
14. Szabolcs I, Podoba J, Feldkamp J, Dohan O, Farkas I, Sajgó M, et al. Comparative screening for thyroid disorders in old age in areas of iodine deficiency, long-term iodine prophylaxis and abundant iodine intake. Clin Endocrinol (Oxf). 1997;47:87-92.
15. Unnikrishnan AG, Kalra S, Sahay RK, Bantwal G, John M, Tewari N. Prevalence of hypothyroidism in adults: An epidemiological study in eight cities of India. Indian J Endocrinol Metab. 2013;17:647-52.
16. Villar HC, Saconato H, Valente O, Atallah AN. Thyroid hormone replacement for subclinical hypothyroidism. Cochrane Database Syst Rev. 2007;3:CD003419.
17. Huber G, Staub JJ, Meier C, et al. Prospective study of the spontaneous course of subclinical hypothyroidism: prognostic value of thyrotropin, thyroid reserve, and thyroid antibodies. J Clin Endocrinol Metab. 2002;87:3221-6.

18. Rosenthal MJ, Hunt WC, Garry PJ, Goodwin JS. Thyroid failure in the elderly. Microsomal antibodies as discriminant for therapy. JAMA. 1987;258:209.
19. Díez JJ, Iglesias P. Spontaneous subclinical hypothyroidism in patients older than 55 years: an analysis of natural course and risk factors for the development of overt thyroid failure. J Clin Endocrinol Metab. 2004;89:4890-7.
20. Vanderpump MP, Tunbridge WM, French JM, Appleton D, Bates D, Clark F, et al. The incidence of thyroid disorders in the community: a twenty-year follow-up of the Whickham Survey. Clin Endocrinol (Oxf). 1995;43:55-68.
21. Díez JJ, Iglesias P, Burman KD. Spontaneous normalization of thyrotropin concentrations in patients with subclinical hypothyroidism. J Clin Endocrinol Metab. 2005;90:4124-7.
22. Duntas LH, Biondi B. New insights into subclinical hypothyroidism and cardiovascular risk. Semin Thromb Hemost. 2011;37:27-34.
23. Biondi B, Galderisi M, Pagano L, Sidiropulos M, Pulcrano M, D' Errico A, et al. Endothelial-mediated coronary flow reserve in patients with mild thyroid hormone deficiency. Eur J Endocrinol. 2009;161:323-9.
24. Biondi B, Palmieri EA, Lombardi G, Fazio S. Subclinical hypothyroidism and cardiac function. Thyroid. 2002;12:505-10.
25. Meier C, Staub JJ, Roth CB, Guglielmetti M, Kunz M, Miserez AR, et al. TSH-controlled L-thyroxine therapy reduces cholesterol levels and clinical symptoms in subclinical hypothyroidism: a double blind, placebo-controlled trial (Basel Thyroid Study). J Clin Endocrinol Metab. 2001;86:4860-6.
26. Chugh K, Goyal S, Shankar V, Chugh SN. Thyroid function tests in metabolic syndrome. Indian J Endocrinol Metab. 2002;16:958-61.
27. Meher LK, Raveendranathan SK, Kota SK, Sarangi J, Jali SN. Prevalence of hypothyroidism in patients with metabolic syndrome. Thyroid Res Pract. 2013;10:60-4.
28. Garduño-Garcia Jde J, Alvirde-Garcia U, López-Carrasco G, Padilla Mendoza ME, Mehta R, Arellano-Campos O, et al. TSH and free thyroxine concentrations are associated with differing metabolic markers in euthyroid subjects. Eur J Endocrinol. 2010;163:273-8.
29. Monzani F, Caraccio N, Del Guerra P, Casolaro A, Ferrannini E. Neuromuscular symptoms and dysfunction in subclinical hypothyroid patients: beneficial effect of L-T-4 replacement therapy. Clin Endocrinol (Oxf). 1999;51:237-42.
30. Misiunas A, Niepomniszcze H, Ravera B, Faraj G, Faure E. Peripheral neuropathy in subclinical hypothyroidism. Thyroid. 1995;5:283-6.
31. Williams MD, Harris R, Dayan CM, Evans J, Gallacher J, Ben-Shlomo Y. Thyroid function and the natural history of depression: findings from the Caerphilly Prospective Study (CaPS) and a meta-analysis. Clin Endocrinol (Oxf). 2009;70:484-92.
32. Surks MI, Hollowell JG. Age-specific distribution of serum thyrotropin and antithyroid antibodies in the US population: implications for the prevalence of subclinical hypothyroidism. J Clin Endocrinol Metab. 2007;92:4575-82.
33. Glinoer D. Potential repercussions for the progeny of maternal hypothyroxinemia during pregnancy. Thyroid. 2000;10:59-62.
34. Haddow JE. Preventing, identifying and managing thyroid deficiency in prenatal practice. Expert Rev Obstetr Gynecol. 2013;8:213-22.
35. Goel P, Kaur J, Saha PK, Tandon R, Devi L. Prevalence, associated risk factors and effects of hypothyroidism in pregnancy: a study from north India. Gynecol Obstet Invest. 2012;74:89-94.
36. Su PY, Huang K, Hao JH, Xu YQ, Yan SQ, Li T, et al. Maternal thyroid function in the first twenty weeks of pregnancy and subsequent fetal and infant development: a prospective population-based cohort study in China. J Clin Endocrinol Metab. 2011;96:3234-41.
37. Rosario PW, Purisch S. Thyroid dysfunction in pregnancy: definition of TSH cut-off should precede the decision of screening in low-risk pregnant women. Gynecol Endocrinol. 2011;27:205-8.
38. LaFranchi SH, Haddow JE, Hollowell JG. Is thyroid inadequacy during gestation a risk factor for adverse pregnancy and developmental outcomes? Thyroid. 2005;15:60-71.
39. Hollowell JG, LaFranchi S, Smallridge RC, Spong CY, Haddow JE, Boyle CA. Where do we go from here? – Summary of working group discussions on thyroid function and gestational outcomes. Thyroid. 2005;15:72-6.
40. Negro R, Mestman JH. Thyroid disease in pregnancy. Best Pract Res Clin Endocrinol Metab. 2011;25:927-43.

CHAPTER 9

Thyroid Imaging: From an Endocrinologist's Point of View

Mythri Shankar, Shrivalli Nandikoor

INTRODUCTION

Thyroid is a bilobed endocrine gland in front of larynx and the first tracheal ring. The right and left lobes are connected in front of trachea through the isthmus, which is the narrowest part of the gland. Normal gland is about 4 × 1.5 × 2 cm (volume: 18 g).[1] Occasionally, a small triangular pyramidal lobe is seen at superior margin of isthmus.[2] The gland is surrounded by a pencil-thin echogenic capsule on ultrasound.

RELATIONS

The thyroid bed is confined by strap muscles anteriorly; sternocleidomastoid muscles anterolaterally; carotid and jugular vessels laterally; and trachea, esophagus, and longus coli muscles posteriorly.

Thyroid imaging has gained importance because it is the most common endocrine gland to go for malignancy[3] and only 5% of malignancies are clinically palpable. Incidental thyroid nodules are detected in about 40–50% of the older, general populations,[4] though majority of them are benign on histopathology.

The common thyroid diseases demanding imaging include wide spectrum of congenital and acquired conditions. Developmental abnormalities like ectopic thyroid, thyroglossal cyst, and hypoplasia needs imaging assistance to confirm the normal gland in thyroid bed and to search for ectopic location. Thyroid is one of the commonest endocrine gland to go for inflammatory involvement or immune-mediated damage. Incidental imaging findings may be the earliest clue for clinician to suspect the inflammation. It helps to assess the chronicity of inflammation in conditions such as Graves' disease, Hashimoto's thyroiditis. Though infection of thyroid is very rare, suppurative thyroiditis is known and can progress to form an abscess. Thyroid neoplasms are the most common conditions demanding wide spectrum of imaging to localize and to show the extent of the lesion. It also helps to characterize cystic versus solid masses and to narrow down the diagnosis of benignity versus malignancy. Imaging also assists in interventions like fine needle aspiration (FNA) cytology, biopsy, and chemical ablation. Patient may be referred for imaging even after treatment to look for recurrent or residual disease.

IMAGING MODALITIES

Although a wide array of imaging modalities are available to evaluate thyroid disease, it is important for the clinician to refer the most appropriate test for the particular condition.

Disorders of Thyroid

Radiographs

Radiograph is rarely performed nowadays to detect thyroid disease. Most often, it incidentally detects thyroid-related problems when cervical spine or chest radiographs are performed.

Plain radiograph may show tracheal compression, retrosternal extension, calcification, cartilage or bone destruction, and mediastinal or lung involvement (Fig. 1).

Ultrasound

Ultrasound of thyroid is recommended in extended neck with high frequency probe of 12–15 MHz.[4] It is the commonest recommended radiological investigation for thyroid imaging,[1] since it can detect lesions of 2–3 mm size. It can localize the lesion to thyroid lobes or to an extrathyroidal location. It characterizes the lesion as probably benign or malignant, describes the extent of lesion, presence of extracapsular extension, and lymph nodal extension (Fig. 2).

The other advantages of this modality are that it is freely available, technically easy, cost-effective, radiation-free, and painless. This modality does not require patient preparation such as stopping of medication and can be performed in patients of any age group as well as in pregnant and lactating mothers.

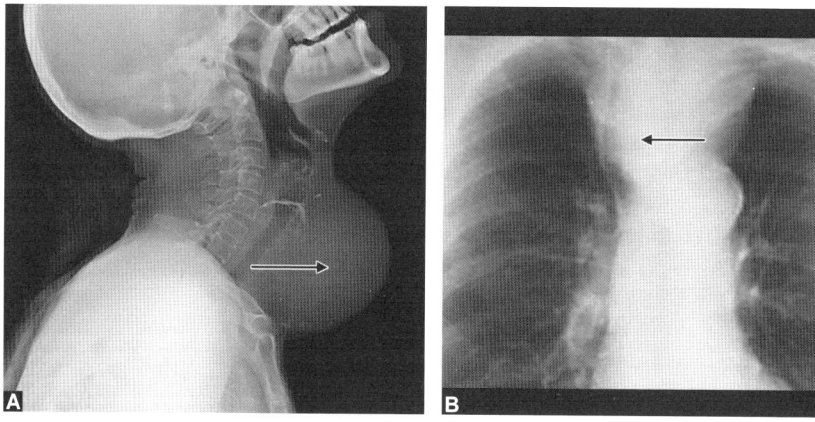

FIG. 1: A, Lateral neck radiograph; soft tissue mass with punctuate calcifications compressing trachea; **B,** Frontal chest radiograph; widened superior mediastinum, displacement and narrowing of the trachea

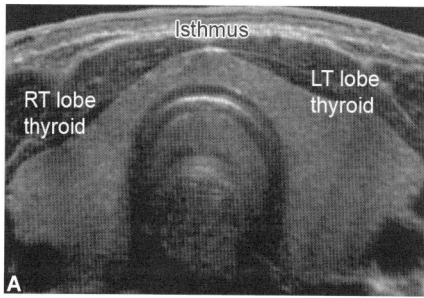 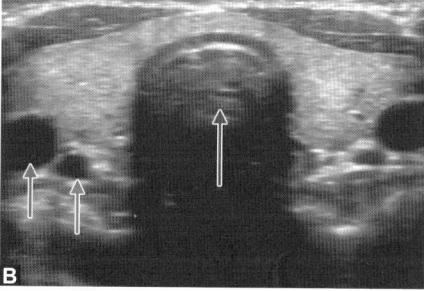

FIG. 2: Gray scale ultrasound of normal thyroid gland (white arrow: internal carotid artery, thin black arrow: internal jugular vein, thick black arrow: trachea)

Imaging Appearance

Normal gland has characteristic homogeneous, medium to high level echogenicity and a speckled pattern. The gland is darker than the surrounding hyperechoic adipose tissue and brighter than adjacent hypoechoic neck muscles.

Diffuse thyroid diseases have a wide spectrum of sonographic characteristics, with respect to size and internal echotexture and have overlapping ultrasonographic, and Doppler features. Most of the acutely inflamed glands are hypoechoic, enlarged, and hypervascular. Whereas in chronic and resolving inflammation, the gland appears heterogeneously hyperechoic and returns to normal size and vascularity or shrinks in size.[1] In cases of focal thyroid masses, color Doppler shows neovascularity of the lesion, rest of the thyroid gland, adjacent vascular invasion, vascular encasement, and tumor thrombosis.

Some of the important sonographic characteristics that help to narrow down the diagnosis of benign versus malignancy is tabulated below[4,5] (Table 1) (Figs 3 and 4).

Ultrasound can also help in detecting metastatic neck lymph nodes in cases of thyroid malignancies. Common features of metastatic lymph nodes include rounded shape instead of normal oval nodes, absent hyperechoic hilar fat, and vessels entering along the periphery unlike normal hilar vessel.[2,6] These nodes also show replacement of normal homogenous, smooth hypoechoic cortex by heterogeneous cystic areas or microcalcifications or simply focal cortical thickening, breach in the smooth nodal capsule with perinodal extension.

Newer advances in ultrasound techniques include microbubble contrast and shear or strain wave elastography. They help to further narrow down the diagnosis. Strain tissue elastography (SE) evaluates the tumor strain on compression or pressure over mass and gives the value as an absolute number with color coding in comparison with the normal gland. It is based on the principle that benign lesions are softer and have less strain whereas malignancies have higher strain or stiffness. Higher the absolute strain value, more is the probability of malignancy (absolute stain value >66 kilopascal) with sensitivity of 80% and specificity of 90.5%[7] (Fig. 5).

TABLE 1: Differentiating features between malignant and benign lesions[4,5]

High risk for thyroid cancer	Low risk for thyroid cancer
Hypoechoic	Hyperechoic (colloid or Hashimoto's)
Microcalcification	Large, coarse calcifications (except medullary cancer)
Central vascularity	Peripheral vascularity
Irregular margins	Looks like Napoleon or puff pastry
Incomplete/absent halo/refractive margins	Comet-tail shadowing (condensed inspissated colloid)
Nodule is taller than wide	Purely/Predominantly (>50%) cystic lesion
Documented interval enlargement of a nodule	Less than 10 mm size
Associated rounded adenopathy (especially with cystic spaces)	Colloid plug—honeycomb or spongiform nodule
Homogenously oval mass with thin capsule	–
Extraglandular extension	–
Size >10 mm or interval increase in size	–

Disorders of Thyroid

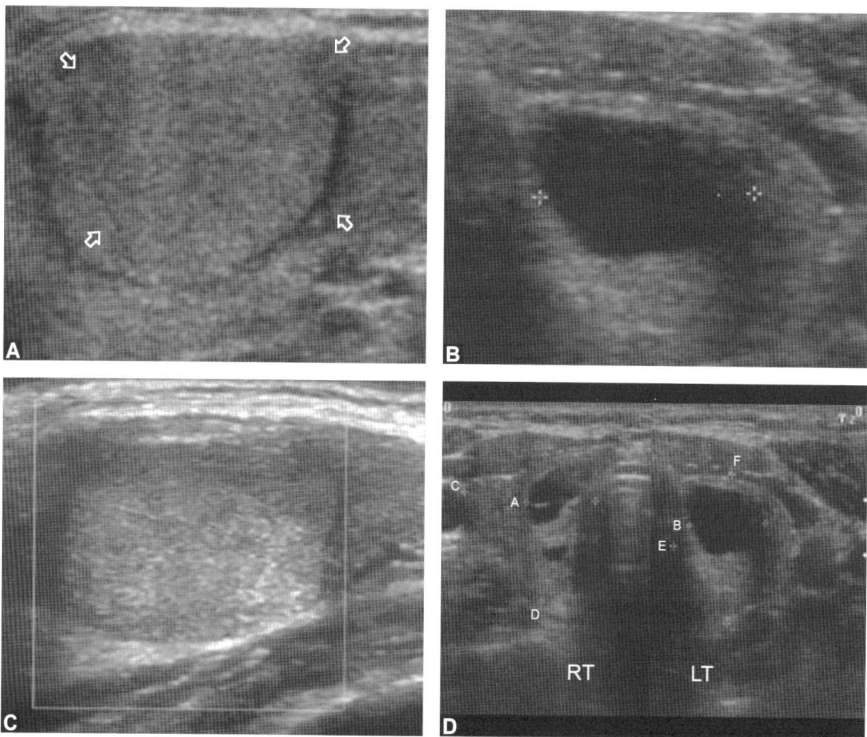

FIG. 3: Ultrasonographic features of benign thyroid lesions. **A,** Solid nodule complete hypoechoic hal; **B,** predominantly cystic; **C,** echogenic nodule with avascularity; **D,** enlarged thyroid with multiple nodule

Thyroid Image Reporting and Data System Classification

With the success of Breast Imaging Reporting and Data System (BIRADS) classification for breast masses, efforts were made to implement the same for thyroid masses. Thus, Thyroid Image Reporting and Data System (TIRADS) classification was introduced by Horvath initially[8] and later by few other authors. But, it is still not implemented widely.
- TIRADS 1: Normal thyroid gland
- TIRADS 2: Benign conditions (0% malignancy)
- TIRADS 3: Probably benign nodules (5% malignancy)
- TIRADS 4: Suspicious nodules (5–80% malignancy rate)
  - 4a: Malignancy between 5 and 10%
  - 4b: Malignancy between 10 and 80%
- TIRADS 5: Probably malignant nodules (malignancy 80%)
- TIRADS 6: Category included biopsy proven malignant nodules.

Ultrasound-guided Procedures

Ultrasound is of great value in diagnostic as well as therapeutic management of the thyroid nodules.

It assists in sampling nonpalpable/tiny nodules, helps to choose the most malignant appearing nodule in patients with multiple nodules for sampling, helps to choose solid/hypervascular components in a complex nodule for sampling and simultaneously helps to get cytology from lymph nodes. It also guides the radiologist for ablative procedures using alcohol or for tetracycline sclerotherapy.[2]

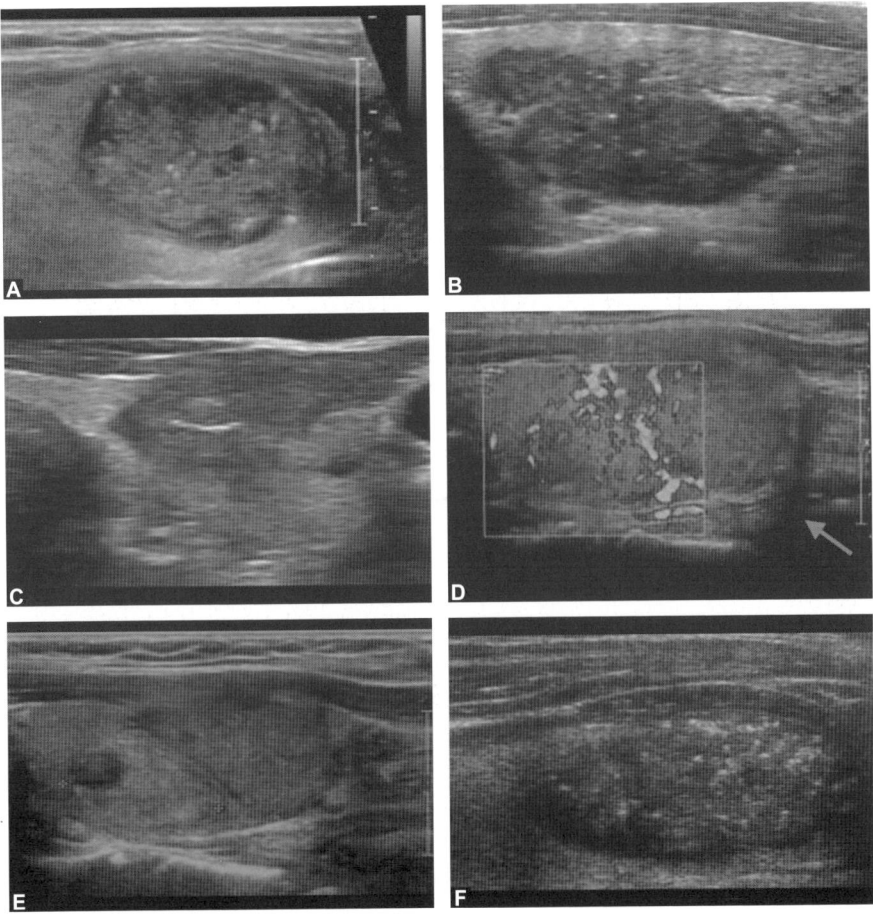

FIG. 4: Ultrasonographic features suggestive of malignancy. **A,** Microcalcifications; **B,** ill defined margins; **C,** extension beyond thyroid margin; **D,** increased central vascularity + reverberation halo; **E,** absent peripheral halo; **F,** cervical lymph node metastsis *(For color version, see Plate 1)*

Criteria for Ultrasound-guided Aspiration Cytology (Fig. 6)

Fine needle aspiration cytology is considered as primary method of evaluating thyroid nodules before surgery. Ultrasound-guided FNA allows a more precise and adequate sampling of thyroid nodular lesions and is associated with a lower rate of false-negatives, thus improving global diagnostic accuracy in the preoperative selection of thyroid cancer.[9] It is observed that on FNA about 60–70% of nodules are found to be benign, and therefore require only follow-up, another 3–7% of nodules are malignant and remaining nodules are indeterminate.[10] Hence, to get the best results on FNA, it is advisable to follow American Thyroid Association[11] or Society of Radiologists in Ultrasound[12] criteria to choose patients appropriately (Table 2). Testing of FNA specimens for the thyroid cancer molecular mutations has recently become a useful adjunct tool.[3]

Thyroid Scintigraphy

It is an integral part of diagnostics while evaluating the largest endocrine gland in the body. The thyroid gland includes the following:[13]

Disorders of Thyroid

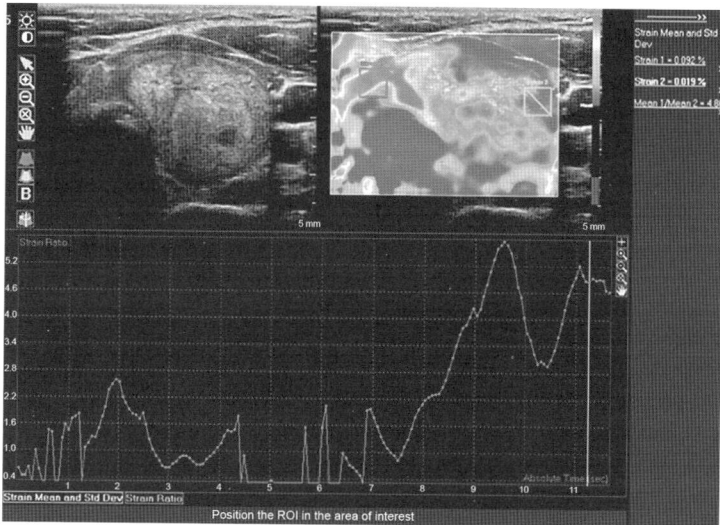

FIG. 5: Strain tissue elastography image showing varying grades of tissue stiffness *(For color version, see Plate 2)*

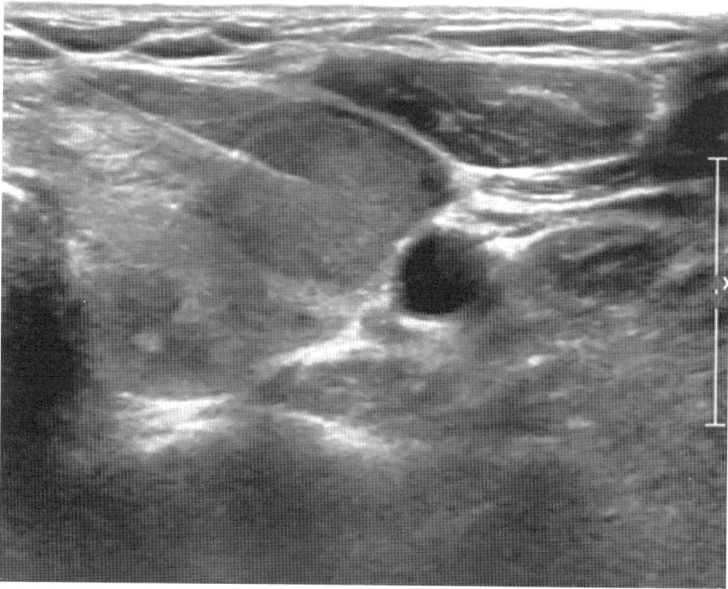

FIG. 6: Ultrasonographic image showing needle tract for fine needle aspiration cytology

- Technetium-99m (Tc-99m) uptake and scan: Tc-99m pertechnetate has a half-life of about 6 hours and is a γ-emitter. It is transported into the follicular cells of the thyroid and trapped but not organified within the thyroid tissue. It is a 140 keV photon, with a half-life of 6 hours. The administered dose ranges from 1–5 mCi given intravenously. The imaging is done 10–30 minutes later for about 20–40 minutes. It is commonly used in diagnosis of thyroiditis, Graves' and nodules

TABLE 2: American Thyroid Association and Society of Radiologists in Ultrasound criteria to choose appropriate patients for fine needle aspiration

Size of nodule (mm)	American Thyroid Association guidelines[11]	Society of Radiologists in Ultrasound guidelines[12]
5–10	FNA if clinical risk factors and suspicious ultrasonographic features	No recommendation
10–15	FNA if nodule contains microcalcification or is solid	Strongly consider FNA if nodule contains microcalcifications
15–20	FNA if nodule contains microcalcification, is solid, or is both solid and cystic with suspicious features	Strongly consider FNA if nodules contain microcalcifications, or is solid with coarse calcifications
>20	FNA for all nodules except the purely cystic ones	Strongly consider FNA if nodule contains microcalcifications, is solid with coarse calcifications, is both solid and cystic, or is cystic with mural nodules or substantial growth

FNA, fine needle aspiration.

- Iodine-123 scan: I-123 with a half-life of 13 hours is a γ-emitter with 159 keV. Its dose in the range of 100–300 uCi is given orally in form of liquid or capsule on an empty stomach. Uptake values calculated at 4 hours and 24 hours
- Iodine-131 scan and uptake: Iodine-131 being a β- and γ-emitting radioisotope may be used for both imaging and therapy. It predominantly emits a γ-photon of 364 keV and has a half-life of 8.04 days. It is exclusive to the thyroid tissue which is organified. Administered dose can vary depending upon the technique used; for uptake purposes, it is 3–5 uCi; for scanning purposes, it is 50–100 uCi[14] and for cancer imaging, higher doses are used

  Normal scan would show homogenous uptake of the tracer with distinct margins, common variations like pyramidal or cephalad lobe. Physiologic uptake in the salivary glands and lacrimal glands and artefacts in the esophagus or gut can be easily identified.

  Non- or faint visualization or low uptake is seen in cases of increased iodine pool in the body [recent computed tomography (CT) contrast, ingestion of certain foods (sea weeds, kelp, goitrogenic foods like turnips, and cabbages, medications (betadine, antipertusives, propylthiouracil, methimazole)] and in conditions like thyroiditis (acute, subacute/De Quervain's, chronic, Hashimoto's and Riedel's), hypothyroidism (primary, secondary or tertiary), and ectopic thyroid tissue.

  Nodules can be single, multiple, cold (nonfunctioning), or hot (functioning). Solitary cold nodules are of significance and need to be evaluated further to distinguish between an adenoma, cyst, primary thyroid carcinoma, hematoma, focal thyroiditis, etc. Multiple cold nodules are commonly seen in multinodular goiter (Fig. 7) and rarely in post radiation neoplasms
- Iodine-131 therapy: Treatment doses are much higher than diagnostic doses and call for radiation precautions in the patient post administration. This is rather a controversial topic. Administered doses can vary from 5 to 30 mCi given on an outpatient basis for

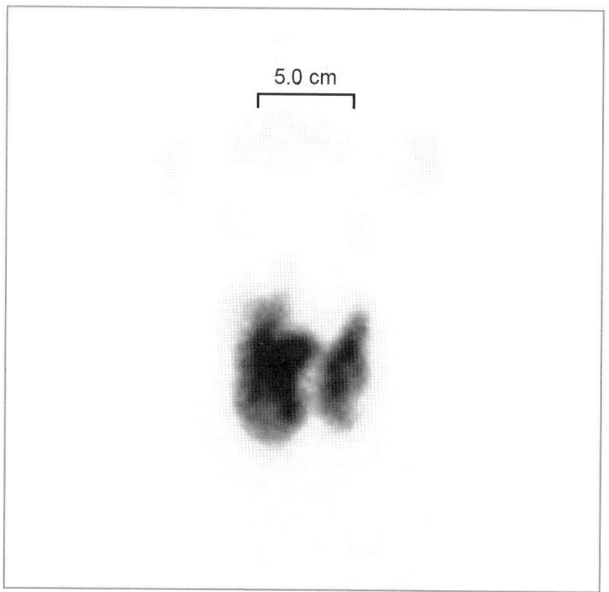

FIG. 7: Multiple nodules with heterogeneous uptake (multinodular goiter) *(For color version, see Plate 2)*

Graves', autonomous nodule and remnant ablation. Much higher doses (30–200 mCi) are used for treatment of thyroid cancer which requires an inpatient facility. Typically, a posttreatment scan is done after 2–3 days of administration. Since most patients die from local invasion, it is very important to adequately treat these patients. Survival with distant metastasis is also significantly decreased, particularly in patients with lung and bone metastasis.[15] Common post-treatment complications would include nausea, vomiting, and sialoadenitis. Rare complications include leukemia, breast cancer, bladder cancer, bone marrow depression.[16]

Most common clinical scenarios: Which test to order and when?
- Trapping function thyroid gland/nodule: Tc-99m scans should suffice in most patients when being evaluated for uptake and nodules. Patient with hyperthyroidism can be diagnosed further depending in the uptake scan. Increased uptake is seen in Graves' disease and toxic nodular goiter whereas low iodine uptake is seen in thyroiditis, factitious hyperthyroidism and struma ovary. It can help the physician plan the management better, since it can be totally different in both case scenarios[17] (Figs 8–10)
- Evaluation of functional status of a nodule: Nodules can be visualized as areas of increased (hot) functioning or decreased (cold) tracer activity. Hot nodules (which are typically adenomas) are more often benign than cold lesions (Fig. 11)
- Differentiate between multinodular goiter and toxic adenoma: Thyroid scans can distinguish between toxic nodular goiter or toxic adenoma/toxic nodule. It is important to identify a toxic adenoma, since it requires higher doses of radioiodine ablation (Fig. 12)
- Evaluation of additional functioning status of thyroid tissue: Iodine scans are preferred for diagnosis of discordant nodules and retrosternal or substernal goiter. Additional tests like the perchlorate washout test and triiodothyronine (T3) suppression test can add value in the diagnosis of organification defects (peroxidase deficiency) and borderline hyperthyroidism respectively

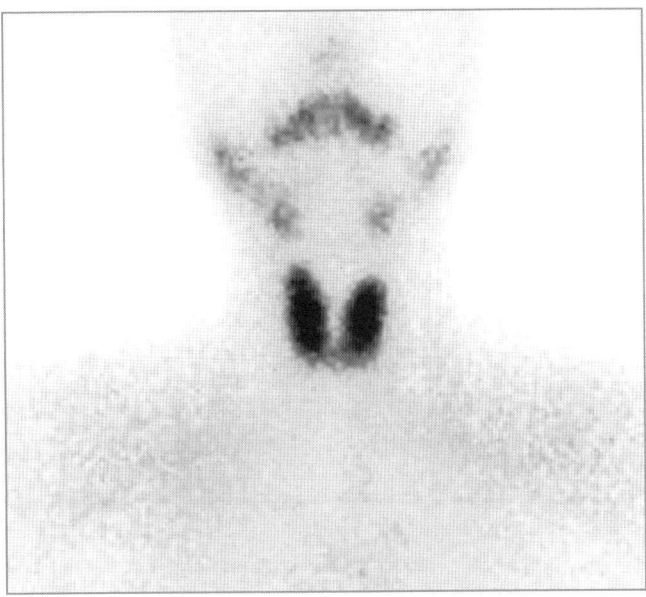

FIG. 8: Normal thyroid gland with normal uptake values *(For color version, see Plate 3)*

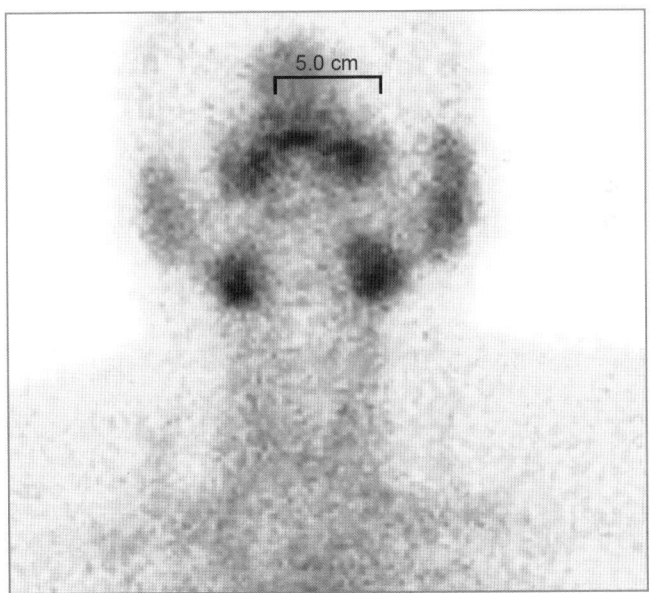

FIG. 9: Low uptake or decreased trapping function (thyroiditis) *(For color version, see Plate 3)*

- Identification of ectopic thyroid tissue: In a rare case of suspected struma ovary, additional images can detect iodine avid tissue in the pelvis. A larger field of view is required when evaluating a newborn for hypothyroidism (sublingual thyroid and agenesis) (Fig. 13)
- Postsurgical thyroid status: Any remnant or residual thyroid tissue after surgery/post total thyroidectomy (Fig. 14)

Disorders of Thyroid

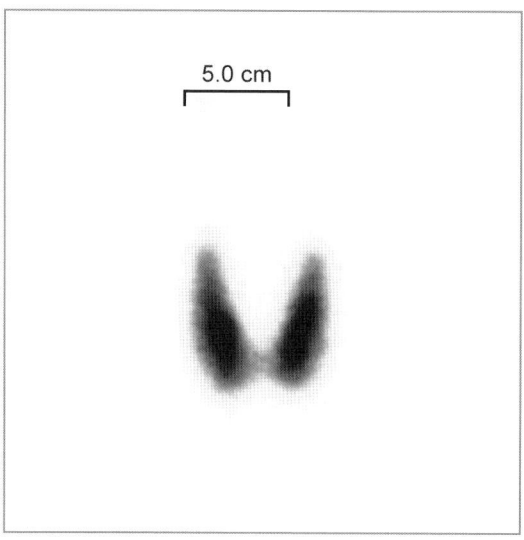

FIG. 10: High uptake (Graves' disease) *(For color version, see Plate 4)*

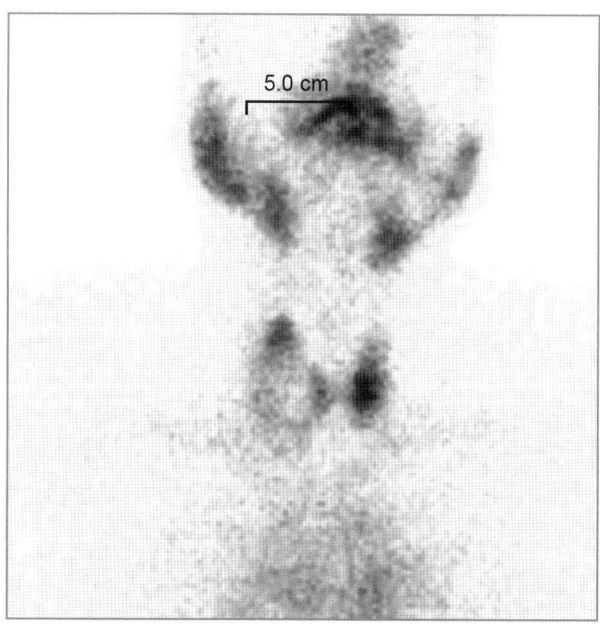

FIG. 11: Solitary nodule with low uptake (Cold nodule) *(For color version, see Plate 4)*

- Routine whole body iodine scans for staging of thyroid cancer: Iodine avid cancers like papillary and follicular. can show metastasis to locoregional lymph nodes, bone, and lungs. Treatment is based on as to how extensive the cancer has spread (Figs 15 and 16).

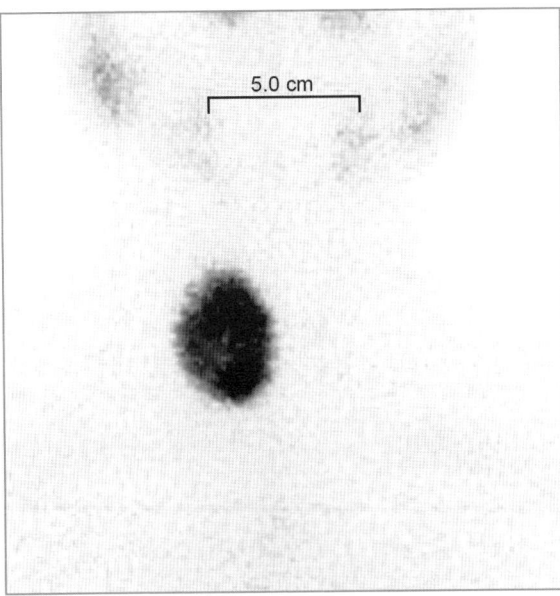

FIG. 12: Solitary nodule with high uptake and suppression of contralateral gland (toxic or autonomous nodule) *(For color version, see Plate 5)*

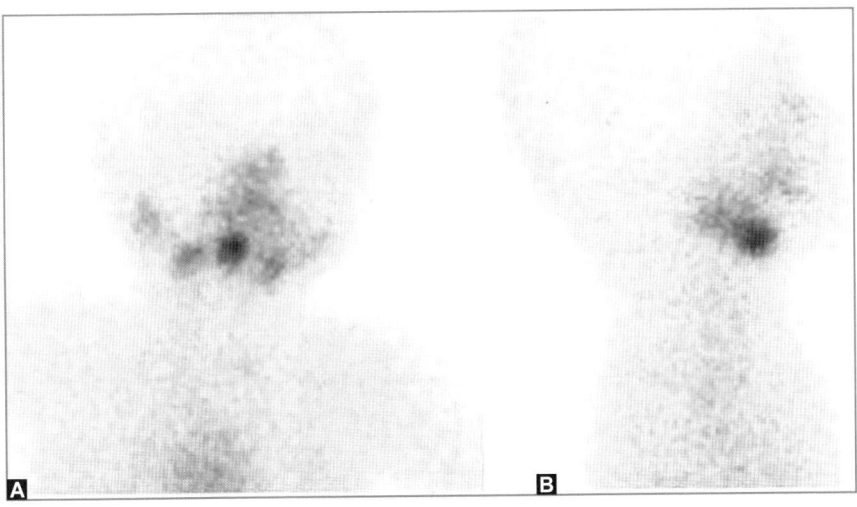

FIG. 13: Lingual thyroid in a pediatric patient (Better appreciated in lateral views). **A,** Anterior; **B,** right lateral *(For color version, see Plate 5)*

- Stimulated thyroid scan: In post total thyroidectomy state, patients are stimulated with thyroid-stimulating hormone (TSH) either exogenously (recombinant TSH) or endogenously (off thyroid medications) to optimally stimulate the thyroid gland and elevate TSH levels (>30 units). A whole body iodine scan done in this state will detect residual/recurrent or metastatic disease (Fig. 17).

Disorders of Thyroid

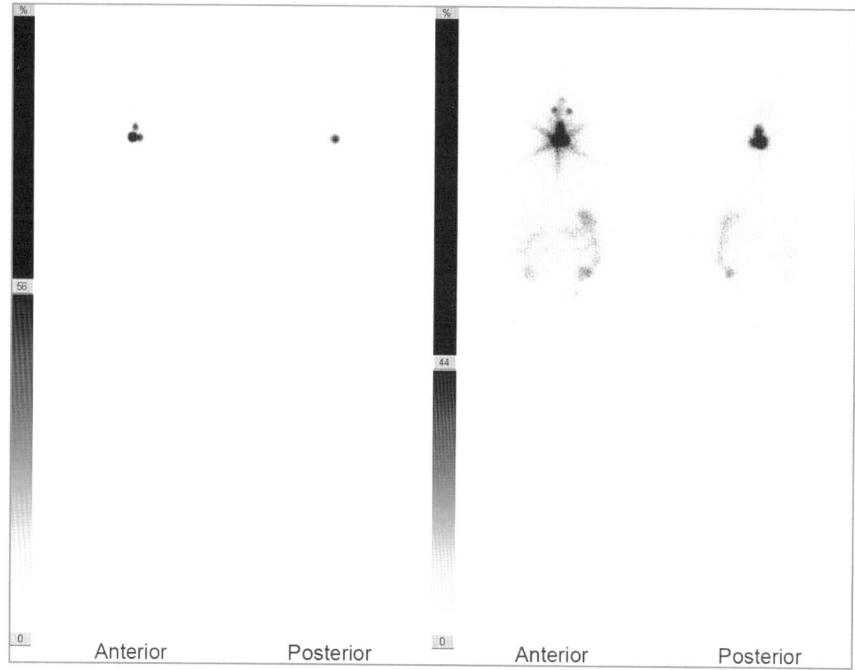

FIG. 14: Positive whole body iodine scan showing iodine avid tissue in the thyroid bed suggestive of residual thyroid tissue *(For color version, see Plate 6)*

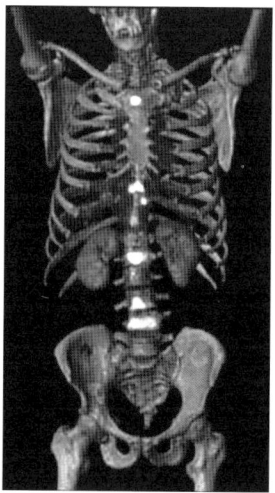

FIG. 15: Fluorodeoxyglucose positron emission tomography computed tomography showing multiple skeletal metastasis *(For color version, see Plate 6)*

Patient Preparation

Low iodine diet is recommended. Medications which interfere with thyroid uptake need to be discontinued (for e.g., thyroid hormones-T3 for 2–3 weeks and thyroxine (T4) for 6 weeks, antithyroid drugs, amiodarone, etc.). Patients should refrain from using

Thyroid Imaging: From an Endocrinologist's Point of View

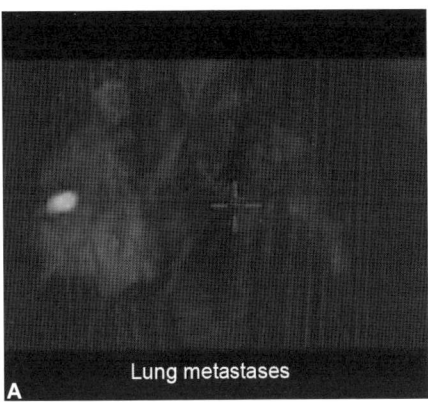
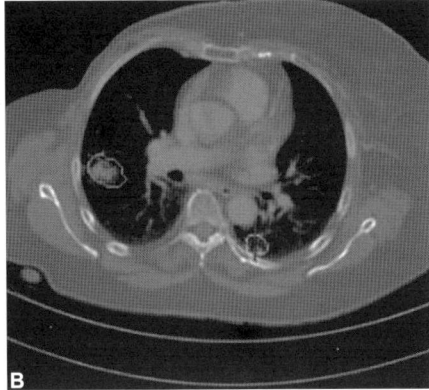

FIG. 16: Fluorodeoxyglucose positron emission tomography computed tomography showing pulmonary metastasis *(For color version, see Plate 7)*

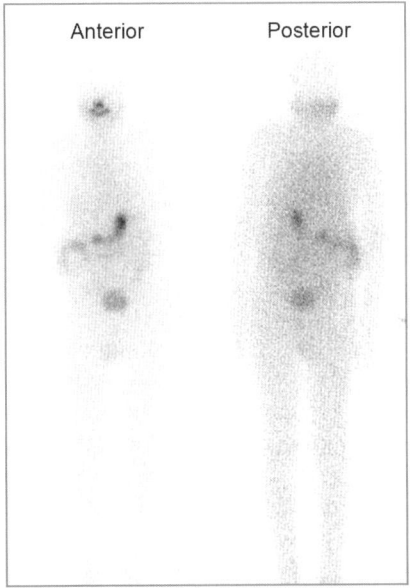

FIG. 17: Negative whole body iodine scan status post thyroidectomy (no iodine avid tissue suggestive of residual tissue or recurrent or metastatic disease)

antibacterial soaps and multivitamins or food supplements which may contain iodine. Patients who have undergone CT scans with iodinated contrast need to be scheduled accordingly, since it may take over 3 months to clear completely from the body.

Radiation Safety Precautions

Application of the ALARA (As Low As Reasonably Achievable) principle is of key importance, keeping in mind the three parameters to reduce radiation burden—time, distance, and shielding.

Women who are pregnant and likely to be pregnant should inform the nuclear medicine physician. Pregnancy is an absolute contraindication for iodine administration.

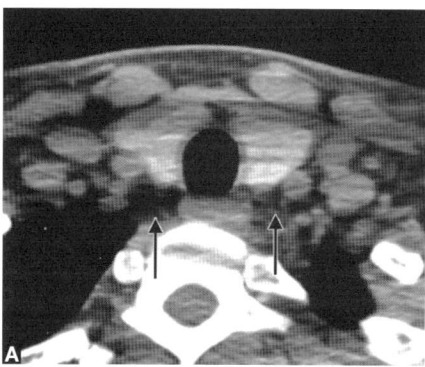 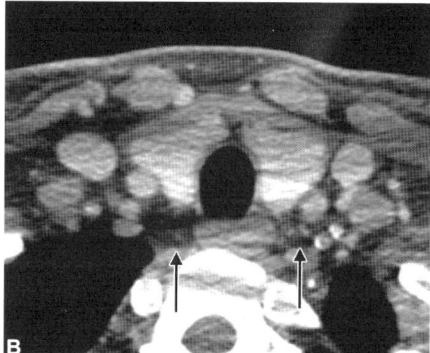

FIG. 18: Nonenhanced and contrast enhanced computed tomography images show normal thyroid gland

Special instructions for nursing and pregnant women is given. Lactating mothers may resume nursing in 24 hours when undergoing Tc-99m scans. However, significant amount of iodine is excreted in breast milk, and therefore, nursing needs to be discontinued for 6-8 weeks. In cases of high dose therapy, pregnancy should be avoided for 1 year after administration of treatment dose.

Usage of radioisotopes falls under the purview of Atomic Energy Regulatory Board and requires extensive infrastructure and manpower in the nuclear medicine department. Special licenses are required to import or procure these time-sensitive radiopharmaceuticals.

COMPUTED TOMOGRAPHY SCAN

Normal thyroid gland on CT[5] appears more radiopaque than the rest of the soft tissues of the neck because of its high iodine content (Fig. 18). It is homogeneous, except for regions of abnormal enhancement that correspond to nodules, cysts, hemorrhage, and calcification. Characterization of small intrathyroid lesions is poor. Computed tomography is rarely advised nowadays due to its limitations and due to the presence of better imaging modalities like sonography. It is less sensitive than ultrasonography in detecting millimeter-sized intrathyroid nodules. Since intravenous contrast agents used in CT are iodine based, it is known to interfere with radioisotope studies and iodine therapy. In addition, excessive iodine may cause hyperthyroidism, cardiac arrhythmias and hypothyroidism, depending on the underlying precontrast thyroid status. Computed tomography also involves the use of radiation and must be avoided in children and lactating mothers. However, it scores over sonography for the locoregional staging of thyroid malignancies.

MAGNETIC RESONANCE IMAGING

Magnetic resonance imaging (MRI) is rarely indicated for benign pathologies as it is time consuming, not cost-effective, provides nonspecific imaging features. Normal thyroid is slightly more intense than muscle on a T1-weighted image, and thyroid tumor usually hyperintense (brighter). It is poor in delineation of malignant versus benign thyroid tissue.[5] MRI is useful for locoregional staging and extra capsular extension (Fig. 19).

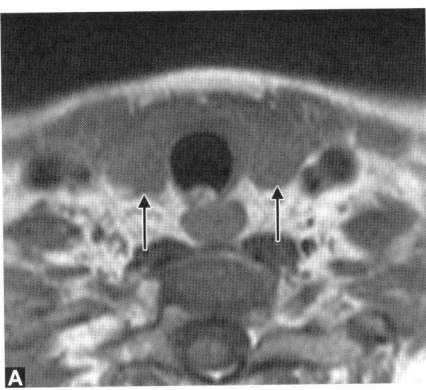 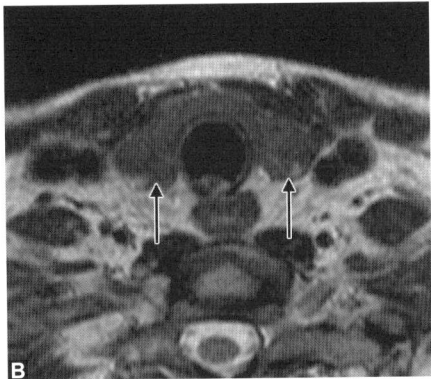

FIG. 19: T1-weighted and T2-weighted magnetic resonance images show the appearance of normal thyroid gland

FLUORODEOXYGLUCOSE POSITRON EMISSION TOMOGRAPHY SCAN

Fluorine-18 fludeoxyglucose (FDG) is a glucose analog and a positron emitter with a half-life of 120 minutes.[18] Dosage is in the range of 10–15 mCi given intravenously. It gets trapped and accumulates in cancer cells at a higher concentration than normal tissue. It is used in diagnosis and staging of thyroid cancer, particularly in the setting of thyroglobulin elevated negative iodine scan patients.[19] Though I-131 scanning is the mainstay for the evaluation of recurrent thyroid carcinoma, not all recurrences are iodine avid due to progressive tumor dedifferentiation. Patients with elevated human thyroglobulin levels (post-TSH stimulation value greater than 10 ug/L), but negative I-131 scans pose a diagnostic and therapeutic dilemma.

Fluorodeoxyglucose positron emission tomography (FDG PET) imaging can help in the detection of metastatic disease in these patients. Unlike conventional imaging, FDG PET imaging can detect metastatic disease to normal sized lymph nodes and complement an I-131 scan. Tumor uptake is also related to the degree of tumor differentiation and is expressed in terms of an SUV value (standardized uptake value) which is essentially quantification of the level of metabolic activity in the cancer tissue. These values are particularly useful in following up treatment response and have a favorable prognosis when they show a downward trend. In general, well-differentiated thyroid carcinoma will be I-131 positive and FDG PET negative, while less differentiated cancers will show the reverse, i.e., FDG PET positive and I-131 negative. This has been linked to decrease in sodium-iodide symporter expression and an increase in glucose transporter-1 expression. This has not been proven to be used as an indicator for worse prognosis. It can certainly help in identification of unsuspected secondary malignancies as well. One of the benefits of FDG PET imaging is that patients do not necessarily need to discontinue hormonal replacement therapy prior to imaging.

Iodine-124 (half-life 4.18 days) is a new positron emitting agent which may hold promise for imaging differentiated thyroid cancer.

Disorders of Thyroid

CASE STUDIES

CASE 1 (FIG. 9)

A 45-year-old homemaker presented with symptoms of thyrotoxicosis for the last 1 week. She presented with weight loss of 1 kg, tremors in both hands and increased sweating.

On examination she had a mildly enlarged diffuse thyroid gland. On examination, the gland was tender. There were no enlarged lymph nodes in the neck. Clinical diagnosis of thyrotoxicosis due to thyroidites or Graves' disease was made.

Investigations revealed elevated serum T3, serum T4, and suppressed TSH. Confirming the diagnosis of thyrotoxicosis, technitium scan with Tc-99m was performed. The nuclear scan of the thyroid showed faintly visualized thyroid gland. There were no nodules in the thyroid. Homogenous low uptake of the technitium was observed.

Clinically, it is difficult to differentiate Graves' thyrotoxicosis from thyroidites unless features like ophthalmopathy and dermopathy are present, which confirms Graves' disease. Presence of tenderness of the thyroid is a feature of thyroidites, but painless thyroidites will not have tenderness of thyroid on palpation. Technitium scan or radio iodine scan will help in differentiating Graves' disease from thyroidites as in this case.

CASE 2 (FIG. 15)

A 25-year-old postgraduate university student was referred to nuclear medicine department with a past history of total thyroidectomy 3 weeks back. The histopathological examination of the surgical specimen was confirmed as papillary carcinoma of the thyroid. The size of the tumor surgically removed was less than 4 mm and the staging of the tumor was T1, N0, M0. The TSH was 45 mIU/mL 3 weeks after total thyroidectomy. Serum thyroglobulin was negative. Antithyroglobulin antibody was negative. 3-week postoperative scan showed presence of residual thyroid disease. Radioiodine ablation was given to the patient and followed in the thyroid clinic regularly.

CASE 3 (FIGS 16–18)

A 56-year-old lady, who underwent thyroidectomy for follicular carcinoma 5 years back, was referred to nuclear medicine department. Initial iodine scan was negative. However, thyroglobulin levels were elevated at 5 years post operation. Positron emission tomography CT scan shows skeletal and pulmonary metastatic lesions.

CONCLUSION

With a wide variety of imaging diagnostic procedures available, which are complementary to each other, the clinician needs to decide the best for the patient based on individual conditions. Radiologic imaging can show morphology, extent and possibility of malignancy, and assists in guided procedures. While nuclear medicine imaging brings in further clarity to the physiologic or functional status of the pathology, also providing therapeutic channels for treatment of thyroid conditions.

REFERENCES

1. Sholosh B, Borhani AA. Thyroid ultrasound part 1: technique and diffuse disease. Radiol Clin North Am. 2011; 49(3):391-416.
2. Castelins JA, van den Brekel MW, Mukherji SK, Lameris JS. Ultrasound of the neck. In: Som PM, Curtin HD (Eds). Head and Neck Imaging, 4th Edition. Boston, MA: Mosby; 2003:2181-2201.
3. Cox AE, LeBeau SO. Diagnosis and treatment of differentiated thyroid carcinoma. Radiol Clin North Am. 2011;49(3):453-62.
4. Henrichsen TL, Reading CC. Thyroid ultrasonography. Part 2: nodules. Radiol Clin North Am. 2011;49(3):417-24.
5. Blum M. Thyroid imaging. In: Groot LJ, Jameson JL (Eds). Endocrinology Adult and Pediatric: The Thyroid Gland, 6th Edition. Philadelphia: Saunders; 2013. pp. e152-70.
6. Leboulleux S, Girard E, Rose M, Travagli JP, Sabbah N, Caillou B, et al. Ultrasound criteria of malignancy for cervical lymph nodes in patients followed up for differentiated thyroid cancer. J Clin Endocrinol Metab. 2007;92(9):3590-4.
7. Cantisani V, Grazhdani H, Drakonaki E, D'Andrea V, Di Segni M, Kaleshi E, et al. Strain US elastography for the characterization of thyroid nodules: advantages and limitation. Int J Endocrinol. 2015;2015:908575.
8. Horvath E, Majlis S, Rossi R, Franco C, Niedmann JP, Castro A, et al. An ultrasonogram reporting system for thyroid nodules stratifying cancer risk for clinical management. J Clin Endocrinol Metab. 2009;94(5):1748-51.
9. Danese D, Sciacchitano S, Farsetti A, Andreoli M, Pontecorvi A. Diagnostic accuracy of conventional versus sonography-guided fine-needle aspiration biopsy of thyroid nodules. Thyroid. 1998;8(1):15-21.
10. Cibas ES, Ali SZ. The Bethesda system for reporting thyroid cytopathology. Am J Clin Pathol. 2009;132(5):658-65.
11. Cooper DS, Doherty GM, Haugen BR, Kloos RT, Lee SL, Mandel SJ, et al. Management guidelines for patients with thyroid nodules and differentiated thyroid cancer: The American Thyroid Association Guidelines Taskforce. Thyroid. 2006;16(2):109-42.
12. Frates MC, Benson CB, Charboneau JW, Cibas ES, Clark OH, Coleman BG, et al. Management of thyroid nodules detected at US: society of radiologists in ultrasound consensus conference statement 1. Radiology. 2005;237(3):794-800.
13. Thrall JH, Ziessman HA. Endocrine System. In: Nuclear Medicine: The Requisites. 2nd Edition. St. Louis: Mosby; 2001. pp. 363-88.
14. Taylor A, Schuster DM, Alazraki N. The Thyroid and Thyroid Cancer. In: A Clinician's Guide to Nuclear Medicine. Reston: Society of Nuclear Medicine; 2000. pp. 181-98, 325-41.
15. Haugen BR, Lin EC. Isotope imaging for metastatic thyroid cancer. Endocrinol Metab Clin North Am. 2001;30(2):469-92.
16. RD Lele. Nuclear medicine in thyroid disease. In: Principles and Practice of Nuclear Medicine and Correlation Medical Imaging, 1st Edition. Missouri: Jaypee Brothers Medical Publishers; 2009. pp. 207-24.
17. Datz FL. Endocrine system imaging. In: Handbook of Nuclear Medicine, 2nd Edition. St. Louis: Mosby; 1993. pp. 1-30.
18. Marcus C, Whitworth PW, Surasi DS, Pai SI, Subramaniam RM. PET/CT in the management of thyroid cancers. Am J Roentgenol. 2014;202(6):1316-29.
19. Alnafisi NS, Driedger AA, Coates G, Moote DJ, Raphael SJ. FDG PET of recurrent or metastatic 131I-negative papillary thyroid carcinoma. J Nucl Med. 2000;41(6):1010-5.

CHAPTER **10**

Surgery in Thyroid Disorders

PS Venkatesh Rao

INTRODUCTION

Theodor Kocher was the first surgeon to win the Nobel Prize in 1909 for his contributions to physiology, pathology, and surgery of the thyroid gland. He was able to reduce the mortality following thyroid surgery from approximately 50 to 1%. The focus of thyroid surgeons has always been on safe and adequate surgery with best cosmetic result. Inadequate thyroid surgery, complications, mortality, disabilities, and bad scars after thyroidectomy bring disrepute to surgery and reduce patient's acceptance of surgical management. Every effort should be made to explain postsurgical problems, need for thyroid and calcium supplement, and to make surgery safe, acceptable, and affordable. Endoscopic and robotic thyroid surgeries have not become popular due to their several limitations, constraints, and also cost.

MULTINODULAR GOITER

Indications for Surgery

Small asymptomatic nontoxic multinodular goiters may be observed with twice a year ultrasound scan. If any suspicious lesion is seen, a fine needle aspiration cytology (FNAC) should be done. The indications for total thyroidectomy for multinodular goiter are dyspnea, dysphagia, or dysphonia due to goiter, suspected malignancy, substernal (retrosternal/mediastinal) extension, displacement and or narrowing of trachea, significant growth in size, recurrence of a cyst after aspiration, neck discomfort, and cosmetic concern. Total thyroidectomy is preferred to radioactive iodine (RAI) ablation for toxic large multinodular goiters as the goiter persists and grows after RAI ablation.

Investigations

Investigations before surgery should include ultrasound scan, FNAC of any suspicious area on the ultrasound scan, chest and soft tissue neck X-ray, thyroid function tests, antithyroid antibodies, thyroglobulin, laryngoscopy examination, in addition to routinely done investigations prior to any major surgery. If the lower border of the goiter is not palpable, a contrast-enhanced computed tomography (CT) scan with three-dimensional (3D) rendering is desirable to assess the status of the mediastinal (substernal/retrosternal) extension of the goiter and plan the surgery.

Surgical Management

Total thyroidectomy includes identification and removal of all extensions of the thyroid, especially the retrosternal extension, the tubercles of Zuckerkandl on both sides and the pyramidal lobe. In patients with a short muscular neck, the goiter appears deceptively small as it grows inwards displacing and compressing vessels, trachea, and esophagus, especially when it grows through the thoracic outlet into the mediastinum. These goiters are prone to complications before and during surgery and difficult to remove compared to a huge goiter hanging out in a long-necked person with thin stretched muscles. If the larynx is displaced and trachea distorted, intubation for anesthesia and to relieve respiratory obstruction may not always be successful even with bronchoscopy assistance. Tracheostomy will then have to be done under local anesthesia. Total thyroidectomy will require thoracotomy if the goiter extends into the mediastinum below the upper level of the aortic arch. Long-standing tracheal compression by large multinodular goiters can lead to tracheomalacia due to weakening of tracheal cartilages, needing a temporary tracheostomy at surgery. Very rarely, even laryngomalacia may occur due to weakening of thyroid cartilage requiring placement of a stent. Hence, where indicated the possible need for thoracotomy, tracheostomy in addition to the possible complications of total thyroidectomy and need for lifelong thyroxine medication should be explained to the patient and written consent taken before surgery.

CASE 1

Multinodular goiter with pressure symptoms

A 50-year-old female in respiratory distress presented in the emergency room with a neck swelling since 20 years, dry cough and food getting stuck in the neck since 3 months and progressive dyspnea since 1 month. She had no hypo- or hyperthyroid symptoms. On examination, she had stridor, a large multinodular goiter, distended neck veins, active accessory muscles of respiration, and the right side much larger than the left with trachea grossly displaced to the left side and right carotid displaced posteriorly. Lower border of the goiter was not palpable. There were no palpable lymph nodes. She was clinically euthyroid. She had with her recent ultrasound scan, FNAC, chest and soft tissue neck X-ray reports. She had refused surgery earlier out of fear of loss of speech or death at surgery.

Basic blood tests including complete blood counts, coagulation tests, blood glucose, thyroid and renal function tests, hepatitis B surface antigen, human immunodeficiency virus, blood grouping, and cross match were done, high risk consent was taken for total thyroidectomy and tracheostomy and she was taken up for surgery immediately. After bronchoscopy-guided intubation failed, and as cervical plexus block was not feasible due to the goiter size, the surgeon infiltrated her with lignocaine on the lower neck on the left of the midline. Through a low neck skin crease incision, he divided the thyroid isthmus and performed a tracheostomy through which the patient was given general anesthesia. Total thyroidectomy was performed. All four parathyroids and their vascular supply, the external branch of the superior laryngeal nerve (EBSLN) and the recurrent laryngeal nerve (RLN) on both sides were preserved. Hemostasis and counts were checked and the wound sutured close and the tracheostomy tube left in situ. One unit of whole blood had to be transfused. Postoperative recovery was rapid and there was no voice change or hypocalcemia. The tracheostomy tube could be removed early (in 2 days) as there was no tracheomalacia.

SOLITARY THYROID NODULE

Indications for Surgery and Criteria for Suspecting Malignancy

Solitary thyroid nodule is usually asymptomatic even if malignant and is discovered on routine checkup. Others present as a progressively growing swelling in the neck. Most of these are benign and do not need surgery. Significant criteria for suspecting malignancy include age, family history of thyroid disease or cancer, previous head or neck irradiation, rapid rate of growth of the neck mass, dysphonia, dysphagia, and dyspnea. Symptoms of hyperthyroidism or hypothyroidism, history of use of iodine-containing drugs or supplements, and pain are also important for diagnosis and management. Examination should focus on location, consistency and size of the nodule, immobility, hoarseness of voice, presence of neck tenderness, cervical adenopathy, and presence of any distant metastases.

Factors Suggesting Increased Risk of Malignant Potential are:[1]
- History of head and neck irradiation
- Family history of medullary thyroid carcinoma, multiple endocrine neoplasia type 2, or papillary thyroid carcinoma
- Age less than 14 years or more than 70 years
- Male sex
- Growing nodule
- Firm or hard consistency
- Cervical adenopathy
- Fixed nodule
- Persistent dysphonia, dysphagia, or dyspnea.

Investigations

Ultrasound scan of the neck, FNAC, thyroid function tests, serum thyroglobulin, anti-thyroglobulin antibody, calcitonin, anti-thyroid peroxidase (TPO) antibody, chest X-ray (to detect unsuspected metastases) and laryngoscopic examination are part of the usual workup. A thyroid nodule with firm or hard consistency is associated with an increased risk of malignancy. Elastography has recently been applied in the diagnostic approach to nodular thyroid disease and has shown a high sensitivity and specificity in selected patients.[1] Thyroid scintigraphy is indicated in a single thyroid nodule with suppressed thyroid stimulating hormone (TSH) level. Fine needle aspiration cytology is not necessary if the nodule is hot.

Ultrasound features helpful in identifying potentially malignant thyroid nodules include microcalcifications, local invasion, lymph node metastases, a nodule that is taller than the width, and markedly reduced echogenicity.[2] Other features, such as the absence of a halo, ill-defined irregular margins, solid composition, and vascularity, are less specific but may be useful ancillary signs.[2] Apart from local extrathyroidal invasion, none of these features is individually pathognomonic of malignancy.[2] However, in combination, these features may lead to a diagnosis of malignancy and may direct attention to other suspicious nodules in need of further investigation.[2]

Fine needle aspiration cytology is the most accurate, cost-effective screening test for rapid diagnosis of thyroid swellings.[3] A recent study highlighted the greater diagnostic difficulties of thyroid cancer compared to other thyroid nodules on FNAC and suggested that clinicians must interpret the results of FNAC with caution and consider the routine use of ultrasound scanning to help guide FNAC.[4] Fine needle aspiration cytology has inherent limitations related not only to inadequate sampling but also, most importantly, to its inability to distinguish between benign and malignant follicular lesions in the absence of nuclear features of papillary carcinoma.[5] The indeterminate diagnosis of follicular neoplasm encompasses a number of heterogeneous thyroid lesions including cellular adenomatous nodule, follicular adenoma, and follicular carcinoma.[6] Another limitation of FNAC is the presence of false negative and positive results particularly with small tumors and when there is associated degenerative or inflammatory change in adjacent thyroid tissue.[5] Core needle biopsy and frozen section are not anymore helpful than FNAC in differentiating follicular adenoma from carcinoma.

Surgical Management

The choice between total thyroidectomy as a primary single procedure and hemithyroidectomy (followed by completion thyroidectomy, when biopsy is positive) has to be discussed with the patient. Most benign lesions, papillary and medullary carcinomas are usually diagnosed before surgery and offered appropriate surgery. For solitary nodules less than 1 cm without suspicious history or ultrasonography findings, follow-up observation with repeated clinical and ultrasound examination and TSH measurement in 6-18 months is advised[1] though many clinicians prefer to check with an ultrasound guided FNAC when feasible. For pressure symptoms and for a larger benign nodule, hemithyroidectomy (lobectomy plus isthmectomy) is performed with a review after biopsy is reported. For suspicious nodules, total thyroidectomy or hemithyroidectomy followed by completion thyroidectomy (if lesion is reported malignant on biopsy) is done. Total thyroidectomy with ipsilateral paratracheal lymphadenectomy is done if cancer is suspected to be spread to them. Lymphoma or metastatic lesion in the thyroid needs appropriate treatment for the primary condition and thyroidectomy if the lesion persists after that.

CASE 2

Solitary nodule with indeterminate cytology

A 24-year-old female presented with a progressive neck swelling since 6 months. She had no hypo- or hyperthyroid symptoms or any pressure symptoms. On examination, she had a 2-cm solitary firm nodule in the right thyroid lobe. Trachea and carotids were not displaced. There were no palpable lymph nodes. She was clinically euthyroid.

She underwent an ultrasound scan of the neck, FNAC, and laryngoscopic examination. Chest X-ray, tests for serum thyroglobulin, anti-thyroglobulin antibody, calcitonin, anti-TPO antibody, and thyroid function were done in addition to routine preoperative investigations. The scan confirmed presence of a solitary nodule with no enlarged lymph nodes. Fine needle aspiration cytology, was suggestive of a follicular lesion. Other investigations were reported as within normal range.

After detailed explanations to the patient and her parents about hemi- versus total thyroidectomy, a hemithyroidectomy was done. On histopathology examination, the lesion had the features of a follicular adenoma and hence, no further surgery was required. If the nodule had turned out to be a carcinoma, rest of the thyroid would have been excised at a second surgery (completion thyroidectomy).

THYROID CANCERS

Indications for Surgery

All well-differentiated thyroid carcinomas are primarily treated by surgery. Metastatic lesions usually need surgical excision. Poorly differentiated and anaplastic thyroid carcinomas may need surgery to decompress the trachea and provide tissue for biopsy. Prophylactic surgery is indicated in children with family history of medullary thyroid cancer found to have inherited the mutation in the RET proto-oncogene.

Investigations

Ultrasound-guided core needle biopsy is useful only to confirm the diagnosis of anaplastic carcinoma so as to offer radiotherapy instead of surgery. Contrast-enhanced CT scan with 3D rendering helps in assessment of the extent of tumor spread locally and to plan the surgery. Positron emission tomography scan is used to look for any distant metastases. Genetic studies are also done in medullary thyroid cancer.

Surgical Management

Surgery for well-differentiated thyroid carcinomas includes ipsilateral paratracheal node dissection in addition to total thyroidectomy. Metastasis to cervical nodes is managed by modified neck dissection. A total thyroidectomy with bilateral neck dissection is the standard treatment for medullary thyroid cancer. Involvement of neighboring structures like the trachea, esophagus, larynx, and blood vessels requires radical surgery and reconstruction where possible. Distant metastatic lesions are surgically excised where feasible. Isthmectomy is usually performed in anaplastic carcinoma to confirm the diagnosis and to relieve tracheal compression. Prophylactic total thyroidectomy is done for children with family history of medullary thyroid cancer found to have inherited the mutation in the RET proto-oncogene. This may be done in their first year of life for high-risk cases or up to the age of 10 years in lower-risk cases.

TOXIC GOITER

Indications for Surgery

Surgical therapy is preferred over RAI ablation for those toxic goiter patients who are young, pregnant, those with large nodules or with obstructive symptoms, those with dominant nonfunctioning or suspicious nodules, those in whom RAI therapy has failed, those with advanced ophthalmopathy and those who require a rapid resolution of the thyrotoxic state. Surgery is also offered to those who prefer surgery to RAI ablation[7] and in those parts of the world where RAI ablation facility is not available.

Investigations

Thyroid function tests, TSH receptor antibody (TSHrAb) and antithyroid antibodies are checked for diagnostic purpose. Nuclear scintigraphy with radioactive iodine-123 (^{123}I) or with technetium-99m (Tc-99m) helps determine the functional status of the thyroid. In Graves' disease, there is a homogeneous diffuse uptake; in thyroiditis, uptake is low; and in toxic nodular goiter, the scan usually reveals patchy uptake. Retrosternal extension of the thyroid gland containing toxic nodules also shows up on the scan. In an autonomously functioning (hot) solitary thyroid nodule, FNAC is not indicated. Such a nodule is ideally treated with RAI ablation.

Surgical Management

Restoring euthyroid state prior to surgery is desirable to help stabilize the hemodynamic status and avoid a thyroid storm. Euthyroidism can be rapidly accomplished with the potent inhibitors of the deiodination of thyroxine to triiodothyronine, iopanoic acid (500 mg twice a day), propylthiouracil, methimazole or carbimazole when necessary, and β-blockers.[8] Lugol's iodine (saturated solution of potassium iodide) is traditionally administered for a week before surgery to reduce vascularity of the thyroid. Preoperative Lugol's solution treatment was found to be a significant independent determinant of intraoperative blood loss.[9] Subtotal thyroidectomy results in rapid cure of hyperthyroidism in 90% of patients and allows for rapid relief of compressive symptoms[10] but there can be recurrence. Hence, total thyroidectomy is now the procedure of choice in both Graves' disease and toxic multinodular goiter to avoid any recurrence.[11] Risk of complications is higher because of vascularization and dense inflammation of the perithyroid tissues. Total thyroidectomy for persistent large goiter after I-131 ablation is very difficult and risky due to scarring; hence, toxic large goiters should be primarily operated upon.

OTHER SURGICAL PROBLEMS OF THYROID

Thyroglossal cyst is an embryological anomaly due to persistence of thyroid tissue along its path of descent. It presents as a swelling in the upper neck or a fistula. The entire developmental tract of the thyroid needs to be removed including the central portion of the hyoid cartilage by Sistrunk's operation to prevent recurrence.

Lingual thyroid is another embryological anomaly due to failure of thyroid to descend or persistence of thyroid tissue at its origin in the midline of the back of the tongue. It may be the only thyroid tissue in the absence of a normal thyroid. It may cause symptoms like dysphagia, dysphonia with stomatolalia (speech that is produced with clogged nostrils), upper airway obstruction, and hemorrhage, often with hypothyroidism. Endoscopic or surgical excision may be needed if thyroxine supplement fails to provide relief.

Thyroid abscess is rare and may be pyogenic or very rarely due to tuberculosis. It needs surgical drainage and appropriate antibiotics.

Trauma to neck and thyroid is another indication for surgery.

SURGICAL PROCEDURES AND APPROACH

Surgical procedures on the thyroid are:
- Total thyroidectomy for cancer, multinodular goiter, Graves' disease. Sternotomy may be required for large substernal (retrosternal) goiter if it extends into the mediastinum below the upper level of the aortic arch or is too large to extract from the neck. The rare intrathoracic goiter independent of the thyroid gland is another indication for sternotomy
- Total thyroidectomy with modified neck dissection for cancer with metastasis to cervical nodes. Resection-reconstruction of involved neighboring structures may be required
- Hemithyroidectomy (lobectomy plus isthmectomy) for unilateral benign lesions
- Isthmectomy to confirm the diagnosis and to relieve tracheal compression in solitary benign nodules of the isthmus and in Riedel's thyroiditis and anaplastic or inoperable carcinoma
- Sistrunk's operation for thyroglossal cyst
- Partial and subtotal thyroidectomy are not recommended anymore to avoid recurrence.[11]

Open Surgery

It is the traditional approach. Recent advances include use of:
- An incision high in the neck to hide the scar in the flexure skin crease and in the shadow of the jaw
- New energy devices like the ultrasonic 'Focus' are especially designed for ligatureless thyroid surgery (often referred to as sutureless thyroid surgery) and are associated with a shorter operative time, less blood loss, and less postoperative pain.[12] The low occurrence of hypocalcemia and RLN paresis confirms that Harmonic Focus can improve thyroidectomy efficiency without increasing the risk of complications.[13] Other ultrasonic and diathermy energy devices, e.g., LigaSure Small Jaw,[14] Thunderbeat,[15] BiClamp 150,[16] are available from competing companies but the original device is still preferred by this author
- Nerve monitoring equipment (Medtronic) during surgery to locate and test viability of EBSLN[17] and RLN or vagus nerve[18,19] has been promoted as a risk-minimizing tool
- Operating loupe to magnify fine structures like laryngeal nerves and parathyroid vasculature[20]
- Autotransplantation of the parathyroid,[21] if its vascular supply cannot be saved. The parathyroid is minced into tiny pieces in a suspension of buffered sodium lactate solution and the suspension drawn into syringe and injected into the sternomastoid muscle or a forearm flexor utilizing a syringe with a blunt tip needle
- Recurrent laryngeal nerve reconstructions when a segment infiltrated by cancer has to be excised or when the nerve is injured.[22]

Minimally Invasive Surgery

Indications

Minimally invasive surgery is suitable only for a small thyroid lobe (<20 mL) in the absence of adhesions due to previous neck surgery or cervical irradiation or thyroiditis in young patients without skin creases in the neck.

Procedures and Access

- Minimally invasive, video-assisted thyroidectomy (MIVAT) was first performed in Pisa in 1998 by Miccoli et al.[23] The technique is characterized by a unique central lower neck small open surgery incision with external retraction combined with use of special instruments and endoscope for visualization. There is a controversy about the validity and limited indications of this and other minimally invasive thyroidectomy techniques.[23] The results of MIVAT are similar to those of traditional thyroidectomy.[23]
- Video endoscopic thyroidectomy
  - Anterior chest access[24,25]
  - Axillary, nipple access (axillobilateral breast approach, bilateral axillary breast approach)[26,27]
  - Lateral neck access[28,29]
  - Retroauricular access[30,31]
  - Transoral access: Natural orifice surgery (totally transoral video-assisted thyroidectomy or endoscopic thyroidectomy using the oral vestibular approach or transoral video-assisted neck surgery)[32-34]

  These procedures differ from open surgery in the use of laparoscopy equipment to perform neck surgery through small incisions away from the visible front of the neck.

They differ from each other in the location of the incision and hence the direction from which the thyroid is approached. Described techniques are listed earlier and include incisions on the anterior aspect of upper chest or in the axillae and nipples, lateral aspect of the neck, behind the pinna, and the more recent incision in the anterior buccal sulcus. All these require creation of a subcutaneous tunnel from the site of the incision to the front of the neck and then through the deep fascia and muscles up to the thyroid gland. This leads to an extensive area of postoperative anesthesia or paresthesia
- Robot-assisted endoscopic surgery is done by a surgeon using a Da Vinci operating robot, usually through incision in the axilla, though the incision can be at any of the other locations listed earlier.[35] Robotic arms are far more flexible and maneuverable than the human arm, hence very suitable for surgery in a small space deep inside the body, e.g., radical prostatectomy. The 3D visualization is another major advantage in robotic surgery that has now become available for video endoscopic surgery with development of 3D laparoscopy equipment. Insufflation with gas is not required. The robot is expensive, and the disposable instruments needed make robotic surgery too expensive. Application of robotic technology for endoscopic thyroid surgeries would overcome the limitations of conventional endoscopic surgeries in the surgical management of thyroid cancer,[36] especially when lymph node dissection is required.

Advantages
- Small incision scars in less obvious locations in young patients without skin creases in the neck
- Magnified view helps the surgeon identify fine structures.

Limitations and Disadvantages
- Not suitable for large goiters, cancers, and those with adhesions due to previous neck surgery or cervical irradiation or thyroiditis
- Higher incidence of complications than open surgery
- More expensive
- More difficult for surgeon.

Use of Drain in Thyroid Surgery

Formerly, it was routine to have a drain placed in every patient undergoing thyroid surgery because of the fear of postoperative hematoma.[37] Now, they are selectively used for draining the thyroid bed in the presence of a large dead space, operation for a large substernal goiter, a large multinodular goiter, or for Graves' disease.[37] In these cases, tube drains attached to a suction bulb are used to reduce seroma formation. Seromas can get infected and can delay wound healing with poor cosmetic result.

COMPLICATIONS OF THYROIDECTOMY
- Significant postoperative bleeding can rarely cause stridor requiring immediate opening of the wound and evacuation of the hematoma
- A hoarse voice is usually due to edema in and around the larynx, sometimes due to traction injury to the RLN and occasionally due to permanent vocal cord paralysis following RLN injury. Laryngoscopy should be repeated in patients with dyspnea, hoarseness, or loss of voice quality. Bilateral RLN injury can lead to adduction of

both vocal cords and stridor and even asphyxia. The EBSLN injury paralyses the cricothyroid muscle and leads to changes in the pitch of the voice and an inability to make explosive sounds. A bilateral palsy presents as a tiring and hoarse voice
- Paresthesia, cramps, and tetany due to low blood calcium due to temporary or permanent hypoparathyroidism
- Rare injuries to trachea, esophagus, large vessels in the neck have also been reported
- Difficulty in swallowing due to inflammation in the neck around the esophagus
- Numbness of the skin on the neck following disruption of cutaneous sensory nerves when skin flaps are raised
- Other postoperative complications include tracheostomy, wound infection, thyrotoxic storm, myocardial infarction, atrial fibrillation, and stroke
- Recurrence of nodular goiter can occur from residual parts of thyroid or its extensions left at surgery or any thyroid rests or accessory thyroid tissue in the neck or mediastinum. Recurrence of toxicity occurs if a significant part of a toxic goiter is retained at surgery. Cancer can recur locally or as distant metastases
- The mortality rate is almost zero.

POSTOPERATIVE MANAGEMENT AND FOLLOW-UP

- Thyroid hormone replacement is started after the biopsy report rules out cancer. Thyroid stimulating hormone is used to monitor thyroxine dose. If cancer is present, RAI scan and ablation of residual thyroid tissue is done after a month and then thyroid hormone replacement is started. Follow-up by 6-monthly thyroglobulin assay is done and RAI scans are done if thyroglobulin levels keep rising. In patients with higher risk of recurrence, RAI scans are done every 6 months for 3 years and then yearly for 2 more years. Any recurrence of cancer is managed as per its location and nature
- Calcium and vitamin D supplement is necessary for hypocalcemia.

REOPERATIVE SURGERY

Indications

- Recurrence from residual thyroid tissue after partial or subtotal thyroidectomy for benign thyroid disease
- Recurrence from thyroid tissue missed at total thyroidectomy
- Completion total thyroidectomy when a partially removed thyroid gland is found to have differentiated thyroid cancer.

Problems and Prospects

Incidence of postoperative complications is higher after repeat thyroid surgery than in primary thyroid surgery because of devascularization of the parathyroid glands during the previous surgery, distorted RLN anatomy, strong postoperative adhesions,[38] and fusion of anatomical planes by dense scar tissue. Incidence increases in direct proportion to the the mean weight of the resected thyroid gland. Incidence also increases if during the previous surgery there was hyperthyroidism, and if bilateral thyroid exploration was done compared to unilateral exploration. In a French series,[38] the permanent morbidity rate after thyroid reoperation was 3.8% (2.2%), including 1.5% RLN palsy (0.5%) and 2.5% (1.8%) hypoparathyroidism compared to rates after primary thyroid surgery given in brackets here. A lateral neck approach is often used to avoid going through the previous scar. Total thyroidectomy for persistent large goiter after RAI ablation for toxicity or reduction of size, is more difficult than reoperation on the thyroid, with higher rate of complications because of extensive scarring that obscures anatomical planes, encloses parathyroids and RLNs, and comprises their vascularity.

CONCLUSION

Surgery is useful in the management of thyroid swellings including solitary nodules, multinodular goiter, thyroid cancers, and certain toxic goiters. To plan the surgery, investigations including thyroid function tests and other blood tests to detect any blood or coagulation disorder or organ malfunction, determining fitness for anesthesia and surgery, and imaging to delineate the surgical anatomy and alterations, should be performed. Fine needle aspiration cytology and occasionally biopsy to determine the pathology before deciding the extent of surgery and laryngoscopy to check vocal cords, larynx, and any likely problems with intubation form important aspects. Many other tests mentioned above are useful for diagnosis, deciding suitability for surgery, surgical planning, prognosis, and follow-up. Surgical procedures on the thyroid gland are total thyroidectomy for multinodular goiters, thyrotoxicosis, thyroid cancers; hemithyroidectomy for adenoma and solitary benign nodules in one lobe; isthmectomy for solitary benign nodules in the isthmus of thyroid and to relieve tracheal constriction in anaplastic or inoperable carcinoma. Radical procedures to remove involved nodes in the neck and neighboring structures are done in advanced thyroid cancers. Total thyroidectomy as a primary procedure is preferred over partial or subtotal thyroidectomy to avoid reoperation.

REFERENCES

1. Gharib H, Papini E, Paschke R, Duick DS, Valcavi R, Hegedüs L, et al. American Association of Clinical Endocrinologists, Associazione Medici Endocrinologi, and European Thyroid Association Medical Guidelines for Clinical Practice for the Diagnosis and Management of Thyroid Nodules. Endocr Pract. 2010;16 Suppl 1:1-43.
2. Hoang JK, Lee WK, Lee M, Johnson D, Farrell S. US Features of thyroid malignancy: pearls and pitfalls. Radiographics. 2007;27:847-60.
3. Caruso P, Muzzaferri EL. Fine needle aspiration biopsy in the management of thyroid nodules. Endocrinol. 1991;1:194-202.
4. Sandeep G Mistry, Navin Mani, Prad Murthy. Investigating the value of fine needle aspiration cytology in thyroid cancer, J Cytol. 2011 Oct-Dec; 28(4): 185–190.
5. Sinna EA, Ezzat N. Diagnostic accuracy of fine needle aspiration cytology in thyroid lesions. J Egypt Natl Canc Inst. 2012;24:63-70.
6. Saggiorato E, De Pompa R, Volante M, Cappia S, Arecco F, Dei Tos AP, et al. Characterization of thyroid 'follicular neoplasms' in fine-needle aspiration cytological specimens using a panel of immunohistochemical markers: a proposal for clinical application. Endocr Relat Cancer. 2005;12:305-17.
7. Grodski S, Stalberg P, Robinson BG, Delbridge LW. Surgery versus radioiodine therapy as definitive management for graves› disease: the role of patient preference. Thyroid. 2007;17:157-60.
8. Panzer C, Beazley R, Braverman L. Rapid preoperative preparation for severe hyperthyroid Graves› disease. J Clin Endocrinol Metab. 2004 May;89:2142-4.
9. Yilmaz Y, Kamer KE, Ureyen O, Sari E, Acar T, Karahalli O. The effect of preoperative Lugol›s iodine on intraoperative bleeding in patients with hyperthyroidism. Ann Med Surg (Lond). 2016;9:53-7.
10. Smith JJ, Chen X, Schneider DF, Nookala R, Broome JT, Sippel RS, et al. Toxic nodular goiter and cancer: a compelling case for thyroidectomy. Ann Surg Oncol. 2013;20:1336-40.
11. Rudolph N, Dominguez C, Beaulieu A, De Wailly P, Kraimps JL. The Morbidity of Reoperative Surgery for Recurrent Benign Nodular Goitre: Impact of Previous Unilateral Thyroid Lobectomy versus Subtotal Thyroidectomy. J Thyroid Res. 2014;2014:231857.
12. Miccoli P, Materazzi G, Miccoli M, Frustaci G, Fosso A, Berti P. Evaluation of a new ultrasonic device in thyroid surgery: comparative randomized study. Am J Surg. 2010;199:736-40.

13. Cheng H, Soleas I, Ferko NC, Clymer JW, Amaral JF. A systematic review and meta-analysis of Harmonic Focus in thyroidectomy compared to conventional techniques. Thyroid Res. 2015;8:15.
14. Hammad AY, Deniwar A, Al-Qurayshi Z, Mohamed HE, Rizwan A, Kandil E. A Prospective Study Comparing the Efficacy and Surgical Outcomes of Harmonic Focus Scalpel Versus LigaSure Small Jaw in Thyroid and Parathyroid Surgery. Surg Innov. 2016;23:486-9.
15. Van Slycke S, Gillardin JP, Van Den Heede K, Minguet J, Vermeersch H, Brusselaers N. Comparison of the harmonic focus and the thunderbeat for open thyroidectomy. Langenbecks Arch Surg. 2016;401(6):851-9.
16. Del Rio P, Lazzari G, Rossini M, Nisi P, Perrone G, Bonati E, et al. The use of energy devices for thyroid surgical procedures. Harmonic Focus versus Biclamp 150. Ann Ital Chir. 2015;86:553-9.
17. Barczyński M, Randolph GW, Cernea C. International Neural Monitoring Study Group in Thyroid and Parathyroid Surgery. International survey on the identification and neural monitoring of the EBSLN during thyroidectomy. Laryngoscope. 2016;126(1):285-91.
18. Dralle H. Intraoperative monitoring of the recurrent laryngeal nerve in thyroid surgery. World J Surg. 2008;32:1358-66.
19. Randolph GW, Dralle H; International Intraoperative Monitoring Study Group, Abdullah H, Barczynski M, Bellantone R, et al. Electrophysiologic recurrent laryngeal nerve monitoring during thyroid and parathyroid surgery: international standards guideline statement, Laryngoscope. 2011;121:S1-16.
20. Saber A, Rifaat M, Ellabban G, Gad MA. Total thyroidectomy by loupe magnification: a comparative study. Eur Surg. 2011;43(1):49-54.
21. Abd Elmaksoud M. Abd Elmaksoud, Iman G. Farahat, and Mahmoud M. Kamel. Parathyroid gland autotransplantation after total thyroidectomy in surgical management of hypopharyngeal and laryngeal carcinomas: A case series. Ann Med Surg (Lond). 2015;4(2):85-88.
22. Miyauchi A, Inoue H, Tomoda C, Fukushima M, Kihara M, Higashiyama T, et al. Improvement in phonation after reconstruction of the recurrent laryngeal nerve in patients with thyroid cancer invading the nerve. Surgery. 2009;146(6):1056-62.
23. Miccoli P, Berti P, Raffaelli M, Conte M, Materazzi G, Galleri D. Minimally invasive video-assisted thyroidectomy. Am J Surg. 2001;181(6):567-70.
24. Cho YU, Park IJ, Choi KH, Kim SJ, Choi SK, Hur YS, et al. Gasless endoscopic thyroidectomy via an anterior chest wall approach using a flap-lifting system. Yonsei Med J. 2007;48(3):480-7.
25. Kim YS, Joo KH, Park SC, Kim KH, Ahn CH, Kim JS. Endoscopic thyroid surgery via a breast approach: a single institution's experiences. BMC Surg. 2014;14:49.
26. Shimazu K1, Shiba E, Tamaki Y, Takiguchi S, Taniguchi E, Ohashi S, Noguchi S. Endoscopic thyroid surgery through the axillo-bilateral-breast approach. Surg Laparosc Endosc Percutan Tech. 2003;13:196-201.
27. Choe JH, Kim SW, Chung KW, Park KS, Han W, Noh DY, et al. Endoscopic thyroidectomy using a new bilateral axillo-breast approach. World J Surg. 2007;31(3):601-6.
28. Inabnet WB 3rd, Jacob BP, Gagner M. Minimally invasive endoscopic thyroidectomy by a cervical approach. Surg Endosc. 2003;17:1808-11.
29. Sebag F, Palazzo FF, Harding J, Sierra M, Ippolito G, Henry JF. Endoscopic lateral approach thyroid lobectomy: safe evolution from endoscopic parathyroidectomy. World J Surg. 2006;30(5):802-5.
30. Lee DY, Baek SK, Jung KY. Endoscopic thyroidectomy: retroauricular approach. Gland Surg. 2016;5(3):327-35.
31. Byeon HK, Holsinger FC, Tufano RP, Park JH, Sim NS, Kim WS, et al. Endoscopic retroauricular thyroidectomy: preliminary results. Surg Endosc. 2016;30:355-65.
32. Benhidjeb T, Wilhelm T, Harlaar J, Kleinrensink GJ, Schneider TA, Stark M. Natural orifice surgery on thyroid gland: totally transoral video-assisted thyroidectomy (TOVAT): report of first experimental results of a new surgical method. Surg Endosc. 2009;23(5):1119-20.
33. Wang C, Zhai H, Liu W, Li J, Yang J, Hu Y, et al. Thyroidectomy: a novel endoscopic oral vestibular approach. Surgery 2014;155(1):33-8.
34. Nakajo A, Arima H, Hirata M, Mizoguchi T, Kijima Y, Mori S, et al. Trans-Oral Video-Assisted Neck Surgery (TOVANS). A new transoral technique of endoscopic thyroidectomy with gasless premandible approach. Surg Endosc. 2013;27:1105-10.
35. Bhatia P, Mohamed HE, Kadi A, Kandil E, Walvekar RR. Remote access thyroid surgery. Gland Surg. 2015;4(5):376-87.
36. Kang SW, Jeong JJ, Yun JS, Sung TY, Lee SC, Lee YS, et al. Robot-assisted endoscopic surgery for thyroid cancer: experience with the first 100 patients, Surg Endosc. 2009;23(11):2399-406.
37. Shaha AR, Jaffe BM. Selective use of drains in thyroid surgery. J Surg Oncol. 1993;52(4):241-3.
38. Lefevre JH, Tresallet C, Leenhardt L, Jublanc C, Chigot JP, Menegaux F. Reoperative surgery for thyroid disease. Langenbecks Arch Surg. 2007;392(6):685-91.

CHAPTER 11

Thyroid Hormone Resistance Syndrome/ Resistance to Thyroid Hormone

Romesh Khardori, Jagdeesh Ullal, Smita Gupta

INTRODUCTION

The syndrome of reduced end-organ sensitivity to thyroid hormone (TH) was described in 1967.[1] Three clinically euthyroid or hypothyroid siblings with goiters, stippled epiphyses, and deaf mutism, but increased circulating protein-bound iodine formed the basis of this first report. Further investigations revealed that serum total and free TH levels were indeed high and that there were no binding protein abnormalities, and pituitary thyrotropin secretion [thyroid stimulating hormone (TSH)] was refractory to both endogenously secreted and exogenously administered TH.[2-4] This syndrome is usually suspected when elevated serum TH are found in conjunction with nonsuppressed TSH. In all subjects, the defect is most likely because complete insensitivity to TH is incompatible with life. The concept of hormone resistance dates back to more than 7 decades ago with the description of pseudohypoparathyroidism by Albright.[5] Even though Albright et al. were correct in their assumption in case of pseudohypoparathyroidism, they were wrong in proposing the eponym "Sebright bantam syndrome" since the female feathering (henny feathering) of Sebright bantam rooster is not due to androgen resistance but due to increased aromatase activity generating an excess of estrogen from testosterone.[6]

The first defect identified nearly 50 years ago yielded reduced sensitivity to TH and was given the name resistance to thyroid hormone (RTH or Refetoff syndrome). Its major cause is mutations in the thyroid hormone receptor β gene (*THRβ*). The spectrum of mutation in thyroid hormone receptor (TR) has now extended to *THRα* gene (*THRα*) [associated with a different phenotype owing to distinct THα receptor tissue distribution].

Thyroid hormone is essential for normal growth or development and metabolism. Much of TH actions are mediated by binding of triiodothyronine (T3), the major bioactive form of TH to nuclear TR. Two genes *THRα* and *THRβ* encode thyroid receptors, namely THRα and THRβ (also referred to as TRα and TRβ), generating different splice variants, such as TRα1, TRβ1, TRβ2 and TRβ3, that are highly efficient in T3 binding. These variants are expressed preferentially and disproportionately in different tissues (Table 1). Depending on dominant site of expression, mutations in the receptor will adversely affect tissue development and metabolism.

The variants TRα2 and TRα3 lack the ability to bind T3. The TRα and TRβ receptors have considerable homology. The deoxyribonucleic acid (DNA)-binding domain (DBD) of all TR isoforms is highly homologous. Thyroid hormone receptors were first

---

The author would like to acknowledge Ms Natalie Gray for typesetting, illustration and editorial assistance.

TABLE 1: Tissue distribution of thyroid hormone receptor isoforms

TRα1	TRβ1	TRβ2	TRβ3
Central nervous system	Liver	Hypothalamus	Liver
Heart	Kidneys	Pituitary	Kidneys
Bone	Thyroid	Thyroid	Lungs
Intestines	Skeletal muscle	Auditory system	–
Trophoblast	Trophoblast	Retina	–
Stromal cells, placenta	Stromal cells, placenta	–	–

isolated and described in 1986.[7] Thyroid hormone receptor belongs to the nuclear receptor super family [vitamin D receptor (VDR); estrogen receptor (ER); peroxisome proliferator-activated receptor (PPARs); retinoic acid receptor (RAR); and retinoid X receptor (RXR)]. The receptor has three main functional domains (Fig. 1): an amino terminal domain, a central DBD, and a carboxyl terminal ligand-binding domain (LBD). The LBD is critical for specificity of the receptor for its ligand and modulates its capacity to interact with other proteins.[8] Thyroid hormone receptors can constitutively bind to the thyroid hormone response elements (TREs) of T3 target genes, thus acting in ligand-independent mode and silencing downstream signaling. Activation function (AF)-1 domain of THR appears to be involved in determination of THR specificity for TREs. Activation function-2 region is important for T3 binding. Thyroid hormone receptors can homodimerize or form heterodimers with other TRs or nuclear receptor superfamily receptors such as RXRs, PPARs, and liver X receptors. Dimerization drives TR binding to specific TREs.

THYROID HORMONE RECEPTOR ISOFORMS AND GENE REGULATION

In spite of structural homology between TRα and TRβ proteins, patients with mutations in TRα have markedly different clinical presentation from those with mutations in *TRβ*. This suggests that there must be other factors (repressors, corepressors) that influence biological impact directly or indirectly. Unlike patients with TRβ mutations, patients with mutations in TRα do not have impairment in hypothalamus-pituitary-thyroid (HPT) axis.[9] Indeed, findings from studies in mouse model have identified TRβ as the receptor that modulates negative regulations of HPT axis.[10,11] Even though both TR proteins bind to the same TREs of T3-responsive genes, they also bind to unique sites to regulate expression of T3 target genes in an isoform specific manner.[12] What determines nature of binding when both isoforms TRα1 and TRβ1 are present in normal tissue is not clear.

Resistance to thyroid hormone (RTH) is better appreciated if one considers and captures the essence of function of TRs (Fig. 1). Thyroid hormone receptors are crucial docking sites for circulating thyroid hormone (T3). The binding of T3 to TR results in either increase or a decrease in the transcription of target genes. The binding of T3 occurs after the receptor has already interacted with the genomic TRE situated in TH target gene promoter regions. A receptor with ligand bound (liganded state) results in transcription of genes positively regulated by T3. In this state, corepressors bound to thyroid receptor are

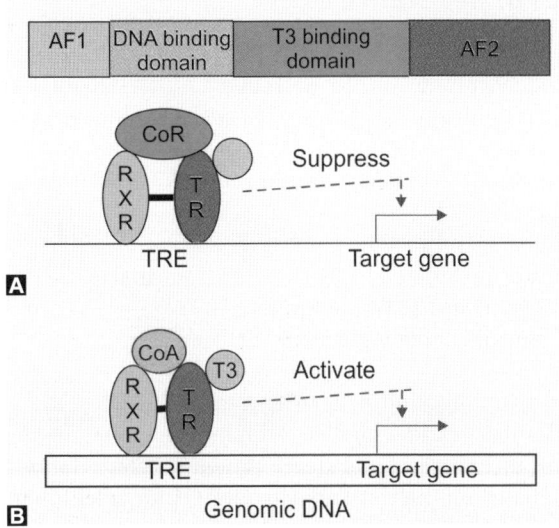

AF1, activation function 1; AF2: activation function 2; RXR, retinoid X-receptor; TR, thyroid hormone receptor; CoR, corepressor; CoA, coactivator; T3, triiodothyronine; TRE, thyroid hormone response element.

FIG. 1: Structure of thyroid hormone receptor. **A,** unliganded receptor state; **B,** liganded receptor state

displaced allowing an activated complex-mediated forward signaling and specific gene transcription. In the unliganded state (absence of T3), TR interacts with cofactors such as nuclear receptor corepressor 1 (N-CoR1) or nuclear receptor corepressor 2 (N-CoR2) and this complex acts as silencer of T3 responsive gene transcription. Any steps involved in hormonogenesis pathways can lead to a possible state of TH resistance such as:[13]

- Impaired function of TR
- Defective transport of TH into cell
- Defective conversion of thyroxine (T4) into T3
- Impaired translocation of T3 and TR to the nucleus
- Defective cofactor interaction with TR
- Possible defects in nongenomic pathways of TH decline.

Typically, RTH syndrome refers to patients with mutation in TRβ (RTHβ). Majority of patients with RTHb are heterozygous for mutation in TR resulting in production of mutant receptor that inhibits the function of wild type receptor "dominant negative effect". This inhibition of wild type receptor directs signaling through TRα receptors.

Patients with homozygous mutation in *TRβ* exhibit profound features of thyroid hormone resistance such as large goiter, hearing deficits, and severe dysregulation of HPT axis. By 2012, four cases of homozygous *THRβ* gene mutations were reported in literature.[14]

Previously, mutation of *TRα* was considered possibly lethal because of lack of any credible reports. However, in the past 2 years, four reports of cases with heterozygous mutations in *TRα* have come to attention. Mutations in both *TRα*1 and *TRα*2 have been reported.[15] These patients often have prominent growth retardations, poor motor coordination, abnormalities of gastrointestinal tract, weight gain, and speech impediment. We shall come to it later and describe features of more commonly encountered type first.

Clinical Features of Resistance to Thyroid Hormone Due to Defective *TRβ*

Resistance to thyroid hormone due to defective *TRβ* (RTHβ or RTβ) is inherited in autosomal dominant fashion and most cases are caused by mutations in *TRβ* gene (*THRβ*) located on chromosome 3.

Mutations are found in the carboxyl terminus on TRβ covering the LBD and adjacent hinge domain.

Patients with RTβ lack any specific clinical manifestations. It has been found in over 3,000 individuals from approximately 1,000 families. Cardinal features are:
- High free serum T4 and also T3 concentration
- Nonsuppressed (normal or higher) serum TSH
- Goiter
- Absence of usual symptoms and signs of thyrotoxicosis.

Common features that lead to medical attention may include learning disabilities, hyperactive behavior, tachycardia, and developmental delay. Goiter is seen in 66–95% of cases. Although about one-half of subjects in RTH have learning disability, mental retardation (intelligence quotient <60) is found in only 3% of cases.[16] Tachycardia is seen in 33–75% of cases. Recurrent ear and throat infections have been reported in 55% of cases. Growth and developmental disorders are reported in 18–47% of cases.[13] Impaired color vision may also be seen.

Diagnosis of RTH becomes challenging in the presence of concurrent thyroid disease that would independently alter THs, such as autoimmune hypothyroidism where subjects present with higher TSH levels. When suspecting thyroid hormone resistance, *TRβ* gene sequencing may be needed to confirm diagnosis.

As against mothers with hyperthyroidism, woman with RTH do not have increased frequency of premature labor, preeclampsia, still births, or perinatal loss. However, a 3-4-fold increase in the rate of miscarriages has been reported in affected women from a retrospective study of 167 members of an Arizona family with RTH.[17]

Clinical Features of Resistance to Thyroid Hormone Due to Defective *TRα*

In the past 4 years, 6 patients with 3 different mutations in the *TRα1* portion of the *THRα* gene located on chromosome 17 have been described and clinical features better explained including a recently reported variant with significant bone abnormalities.[9,15,18-23]

Features Include
- Delay in linear growth
- Delayed tooth eruption
- Severe constipation
- Bradycardia
- Decreased blood pressure
- Low insulin-like growth factor 1 (IGF-1) with insufficient growth hormone response to clonidine and L-dopa
- Elevated total and low density lipoprotein cholesterol
- Elevated sex hormone-binding globulin (SHBG) levels
- Circulating TSH levels are within normal range
- Slightly lower levels of free T4 (FT4)

- Slightly elevated levels of free T3 (FT3) or total T3
- Low reverse T3 (rT3) or elevated T3/rT3 ratio; it reflects increased deiodinase 1 or decreased deiodinase 3 activity.

Unlike patients with RTHβ, the HPT axis is minimally affected. Mild normocytic anemia with raised muscle creatine kinase levels are a consistent feature.

Differential diagnosis for high T3, low T4, and normal TSH includes:
- Dyshormonogenesis due to genetic or environmental causes such as iodine deficiency
- Resistance to TH
- Defects in *MCT8* gene—Allan-Herndon-Dudley syndrome.

Thyroglobulin levels are raised in dyshormonogenesis, whereas rT3 levels are normal. Goiter is a feature in dyshormonogenesis.

Functional analysis of *TRα1* mutants has shown that none of them are capable of T3 binding or stimulating expression of T3 responsive genes.

THERAPY

Treatment with levothyroxine (LT4) results in suppressed TSH and normalization of serum FT4 and rT3 while serum T3 remains elevated. Treatment with LT4 induced further rise in SHBG while serum creatine kinase levels decreased. In all patients, treatment has beneficial effects on constipation without any improvement in gut motility. Therapy raises serum IGF-1 and improves metabolic rate. There was no difference in body temperature. Cardiac response was blunted despite elevations in serum T3. Levothyroxine therapy or addition of growth hormone therapy did not have measurable impact on growth. In most cases, anemia persists following treatment, and relative to the changes in TH levels, changes in cardiac parameter, such as heart rate and indices of myocardial contraction, are disappointing.

DIAGNOSIS OF RESISTANCE TO THYROID HORMONE

Resistance to thyroid hormone should be considered in subjects with elevated TH levels in the setting of normal or elevated TSH. The presence of goiter and elevation of FT4 and FT3 with nonsuppressed TSH is diagnostic. All such patients should be tested for antibodies that may interfere with hormone measurements. Measurement of reverse T3 and thyroglobulin help in assessing degree of TSH elevation. Often, TSH may be "normal" and goiter out of proportion to TSH elevation suggesting its enhanced bioactivity.[24]

Differential Diagnosis
- Assay artifact: interfering antibodies
- Thyroid stimulating hormone secreting pituitary tumor (TSHoma).

For assay interference, different techniques are available to rule it out. A discussion with laboratory staff may be in order to sort it out.

Thyroid stimulating hormone secreting pituitary tumors must be excluded. Diagnosis of resistance to TH can be substantiated by the following:
- Absence of elevation of serum concentration of α pituitary glycoprotein subunit
- Stimulations of TSH following administration of thyrotropin releasing hormone (TRH): TRH stimulation test
- Absence of discernable pituitary tumor on imaging

- Suppressibility of TSH with supraphysiologic doses of T_3: liothyronine (LT3) suppression test
- Presence of thyroid test abnormalities compatible with RTH in other family members.

Thyrotropin Releasing Hormone Stimulation Test

This test measures response of serum TSH to administration of synthetic TRH. After a dose of 4 µg/kg of TRH is administered by rapid intravenous injection, TSH response peaks between 15 and 40 minutes (increment is on average five times the basal level). No increment in TSH is seen in patients with TSH-secreting adenomas. Flushing and urge to urinate may be experienced following the administration of TRH.

Levotriiodothyronine Suppression Test

This test requires close supervision. Details of protocol have been published by Weiss and Refetoff in their review in 1993.[16] The test involves administration of three incremental doses of LT3 each for 3 days. A TRH test is performed at baseline and at the time of the administration of the last LT3 dose for each three doses. Magnitude of thyroid gland suppression can be gauged by measurement of thyroglobulin and T4, while peripheral tissue response is assessed by measurement of cholesterol, creatine kinase, SHBG, ferritin, and osteocalcin.

Thyroid Color Flow Doppler Sonography:

Intrathyroidal blood flow as assessed by color flow Doppler sonography (CFDS) and quantitated by measuring peak systolic velocity (PSV) is markedly increased in thyrotoxic states caused by Graves' disease, toxic uninodular, or multinodular goiter, but not hyperthyroidism induced by ingestion of exogenous TH or destructive thyroiditis. The intrathyroidal vascularity depends on TSH receptor activation by TSH or TSH receptor antibody. Increased CFDS is seen in both TSHoma and RTH. Following T3 suppression, CFDS pattern and PSV normalizes in patients with RTH but not in those with TSH secreting pituitary adenoma.[25]

OTHER CAUSES OF THYROID HORMOINE RESISTANCE

Cell Membrane Thyroid Hormone Transport Defects

Thyroid hormone does not passively diffuse across the cell membrane. Several classes of molecules that serve as membrane transporters have been identified. Amongst these, the X-linked monocarboxylate transporter 8 (MCT8) remains the most specific TH transporter.[26,27] Mutations in the *MCT8* (*SLC C16A2*) gene generates a phenotype of complex and severe neurodevelopmental defect and elevated serum T3, low rT3, low or normal T4 with normal or elevated TSH.[28,29] The LT3 suppression test shows reduced pituitary sensitivity to LT3. The ratio of T3 or rT3 is characteristically high in MCT8 deficiency. Aspiration pneumonia is the most common cause of death in affected males.

Thyroid Hormone Metabolism Defect

Intracellular TH metabolism is regulated by three selenoprotein iodothyronine deiodinases. Their expression varies according to cell type. Enzymatic activity of deiodinases depends on the presence of rare amino acid selenocysteine located in the center of molecule. Although alterations of TH in man are typically acquired such as "low T3 syndrome" of nonthyroidal illness,[30] first inherited thyroid hormone metabolism defect was reported in 2005.[31] It is caused by recessive mutations in *SBP2* gene affecting selenoprotein synthesis that include selenoenzymes deiodinases. Affected individuals have deployed growth and abnormal thyroid tests: high total and FT4, low T3 and high rT3, and slightly elevated serum TSH. Delayed bone age is characteristic of this disorder. It is also associated with absence of goiter.

At the 10th International Workshop on Resistance to Thyroid Hormone and Thyroid Hormone Action that took place in 2012 in Quebec City of Canada, a new nomenclature for inherited forms of impaired sensitivity to TH was proposed. It identified following categories:[32]
- Thyroid hormone cell membrane transport defects
- Thyroid hormone metabolism defects
- Thyroid hormone action defects.

For extensive discussion of the topic, the reader is directed to a selected review given under "Advanced Reading Section" other than the references cited within the text.

TREATMENT OF RESISTANCE TO THYROID HORMONE

It is important to make correct diagnosis before embarking on treatment. An asymptomatic patient with milder elevation of TH may need cautious observation and follow-up only. If evidence of TH deprivation exists in face of elevated TH, medical treatment should be considered, often in the form of LT3 replacement. Often, biochemical profile in different forms of TH resistance states reveals a relative state of hyperthyroxinemia. It is important to consider other clinical disorders where a similar profile may be encountered such as:
- ↑Thyroxin binding globulin—TBG (↑ T4, T3, rT3, normal TSH and FT4, FT3)
- ↑ Transthyretin (↑ T4, normal T3, ↑ rT3, normal TSH, FT4, FT3)
- Familial dysalbuminemic hyperthyroxinemia (↑ T4, ↑ rT3, n TSH, NF4 by dialysis)
- Acute non-thyroidal illness (↑ T4, ↓↓ T3, ↑ rT3, n TSH).

A well-compensated clinically euthyroid state does not require any treatment. Concern about long-standing unrestrained thyrotrope stimulation may be a theoretical concern for possibility of developing pituitary adenoma. So far, there is only one report of pituitary adenoma in a patient with resistance to TH syndrome.[33] When TH therapy is contemplated, it should be kept in mind that dosage of thyroid hormone (LT4) required to attain necessary TH may be quite high.

In patients with tachycardia, atenolol can be effectively used. It is preferred over propranolol because it does not interfere with conversion of T4 to T3, an undesirable effect in those with classical RTH syndrome. Regarding suppression of goiter, LT4, or high dose LT3 on alternate days can be quite successful.

CONCLUSION

Thyroid hormone resistance syndrome(s) occur with less frequency in communities all across the globe. Its biochemical and clinical course may be challenging, and a careful history including family history may offer clues. Often free circulating TH levels are elevated with normal, high normal, or elevated TSH. Patients may have phenotypic features that suggest tissue hormone deprivation. Treatment with LT4 or LT3 should be considered on case by case basis. Where in doubt, a referral to laboratory offering genetic testing should be considered.

CASE 1

A 56-year-old Caucasian female presented to endocrine clinic with history of long-standing goiter and persistently elevated levels of FT4 and FT3, and unsuppressed TSH without any symptoms of hyper- or hypothyroidism. Her laboratory data revealed the following:
- TSH: 9.7 mIU/mL (normal range 0.3–5.5)
- Free T4: 2.6 ng/dL (normal range 0.8–2.0)
- Free T3: 6.9 pg/mL (normal range 2.3–4.3)
- Thyroid antibodies including thyroperoxidase and TSH receptor antibody were negative
- No sellar mass seen on magnetic resonance imaging
- Normal serum concentration α-subunit of pituitary glycoprotein.

Patient had smooth thyroid enlargement with no bruit overheard. Pemberton sign was negative and all ocular movements were intact. She had resting heart rate of 100 beats/min. She claimed to have moderate hearing impairment. She stated that she knew of other family members with abnormal thyroid.

She was presumed to have resistance to TH. This was further confirmed by normal TSH response to TRH stimulation test, absence of elevated SHBG and suppression of TSH with supraphysiologic doses of LT3.

Genomic DNA was isolated from peripheral blood. Sample was sent to referral center and a heterozygous missense mutation was reported in exon 10, with c.1293G>A transition. This mutation localizes to cluster one at codon 346 of the LBD of *THRβ* gene.

REFERENCES

1. Refetoff S, DeWind LT, DeGroot LJ. Familial syndrome combining deaf-mutism, stippled epiphyses, goiter and abnormally high PBI: possible target organ refractoriness to thyroid hormone. J Clin Endocrinol Metab. 1967;27:279-94.
2. Refetoff S, DeGroot LJ, Benard B, et al. Studies of sibship with apparent hereditary resistance to the intracellular action of thyroid hormone. Metabolism. 1972;21:723-56.
3. Benarl J, Refetoff S, DeGroot LJ. Abnormalities of triiodothyronine binding to lymphocytes and fibroblast nuclei from a patient with peripheral resistance to thyroid hormone action. J Clin Endocrinol. 1978;47:1266-72.
4. Refetoff S, DeGroot LJ, Barsano CP. Defective thyroid hormone feedback regulation in the syndrome of peripheral resistance to thyroid hormone. J Clin Endocrinol Metab. 1980;51:41-5.
5. Albright F, Burnett CH Smith PH, Parson W. Pseudohypoparathyroidism- an example of 'Seabright Bantam syndrome'. Endocrinology. 1942;30:922-32.
6. George FW, Wilson JD. Pathogenesis of henny feathering trait in the Sebright bantam chicken. J Clin Invest. 1980;66:57-65.
7. Sap J, Munoz A, Damm K, Goldberg Y, Ghysdael J, Leutz A, et al. The c-erb-A protein is a high affinity receptor for thyroid hormone. Nature. 1986;324:635-40.
8. Figueira AC, Saidemberg DM, Souza PC, Martínez L, Scanlan TS, Baxter JD, et al. Analysis of agonist and antagonist effect of thyroid hormone receptor conformation by hydrogen/deuterium exchange. Mol Endocrinol. 2011;25:15-31.
9. Bochukova E, Schoenmakers N, Agostini M, Schoenmakers E, Rajanayagam O, Keogh JM, et al. A mutation in the thyroid hormone receptor alpha gene. N Engl J Med. 2012;366:243-9.
10. Gauthier K, Chassande O, Plateroti M, Roux JP, Legrand C, Pain B, et al. Differential functions for the thyroid hormone receptor TRalpha and TRbeta in the control of thyroid hormone production and postnatal development. EMBO J. 1999;18:623-31.
11. Abel ED, Ahima RS, Beers ME, Elmquist JK, Wondisford FE. Critical role for thyroid hormone receptor beta2 in the regulation of para-ventricular thyrotropin releasing hormone neurons. J Clin Invest. 2001;107:1017-23.
12. Chatonnet F, Guyot R, Benoit G, Flamant F. Genome-wide analysis of thyroid hormone receptors shared and specific functions in neuronal cells. Proc Natl Acad Sci USA. 2013;110:E766-75.
13. Weiss RE, Refetoff S. Syndrome of Resistance to Thyroid Hormone. In: Wondisford FE, Radovick S (Eds). Clinical Management of Thyroid Disease. Philadelphia: Saunders/Elsevier; 2009. pp. 299-315.
14. Ferrara AM, Onigata K, Ercan O, Woodhead H, Weiss RE, Refetoff S. Homozygous thyroid hormone receptor b mutations in resistance to thyroid hormone: three new cases and review of the literature. J Clin Endocrinol Metab. 2012;97:1328-36.

15. Moran C, Agostini M, Visser WE, Schoenmakers E, Schoenmakers N, Offiah AC, et al. Resistance to thyroid hormone caused by mutation in thyroid hormone receptor (TR)α1 and TRα2: clinical, biochemical and genetic analyses of three related patients. Lancet Diabetes Endocrinol. 2014;2:619-26.
16. Refetoff S, Weiss RE, Usala SJ. The syndrome of resistance to thyroid hormone. Endocr Rev. 1993;14:348-99.
17. Anselome J, Cao D, Karrison T, Weiss RE, Refetoff S. Fetal loss associated with excess thyroid hormone exposure. JAMA. 2004;292:691-5.
18. Van Mullem AA, Visser TJ, Peeters RP. Clinical consequences of mutations in thyroid hormone receptor-α1. Eur Thyroid J. 2014;3:17-24.
19. Van Mullem A, van Heerebeck R, Chrysis D, Visser E, Medici M, Andrikoula M, et al. Clinical phenotype and mutant TRalpha1. N Engl J Med. 2012;366:1451-3.
20. Van Mullem A, Chrysis D, Ethimaidou A, Chroni E, Tsatsoulis A, de Rijke YB, et al. Clinical phenotype of new type of thyroid hormone resistance caused by mutation of TRα1 receptor: Consequences of LT4 treatment. J Clin Endocrinol Metab. 2013;98:3029-38.
21. Moran C, Schoenmakers N, Agostini M, Schoenmakers E, Offiah A, Kydd A, et al. An adult female with resistance to thyroid hormone mediated by defective thyroid hormone receptor alpha. J Clin Endocroinol Metab. 2013;98:4254-61.
22. Espiard S, Savagner F, Flamant F, Vlaeminck-Guillem V, Guyot R, Munier M, et al. A novel mutation in THRA gene associated with an atypical phenotype of resistance to thyroid hormone. J Clin Endocrinol Metab 2015;100:2841-8.
23. Moran C, Chatterjee K. Resistance to thyroid hormone due to defective thyroid receptor alpha. Best Pract Res Clin Endocrinol Metab. 2015;29(4):647-57.
24. Persani L, Asteria C, Tonacchera M, Vitti P, Krishna V, Chatterjee K, et al. Evidence for the secretion of thyrotropin with enhanced bioactivity in syndrome of thyroid hormone resistance. J Clin Endocrinol Metab. 1994;78:1034-9.
25. Bogazzi F, Manetti L, Tomisti L, Rossi G, Cosci C, Sardella C, et al. Thyroid color flow doppler sonography: An adjunctive tool for differentiating patients with inappropriate thyrotropin (TSH) secretion due to TSH secreting pituitary adenoma or resistance to thyroid hormone. Thyroid. 2006;16:989-95.
26. Hennemann G, Docter R, Friesema EC, de Jong M, Krenning EP, Visser TJ. Plasma membrane transport of thyroid hormone and its role in thyroid hormone metabolism and bioavailability. Endocr Rev. 2001;22:451-76.
27. Friesema EC, Ganguly S, Abdalla A, Manning Fox JE, Halestrap AP, Visser TJ. Identification of monocarboxylate transporter 8 as a specific thyroid hormone transporter. J Biol Chem. 2003;278:40128-35.
28. Dumitrescu AM, Liao XH, Best TB, Brockmann K, Refetoff S. A novel syndrome combining thyroid and neurological abnormalities is associated with mutations in monocarboxylate transporter gene. Am J Hum Genet. 2004;74:168-75.
29. Friesema EC, Grueters A, Biebermann H, Krude H, von Moers A, Reeser M, et al. Association between mutations in thyroid hormone transporter and severe X-linked psychomotor retardation. Lancet. 2004;364:1435-7.
30. Koenig RJ. Regulation of type1 iodothyronine deiodinase in health and disease. Thyroid. 2005;15:835-40.
31. Dumitrescu AM, Liao XH, Abdullah MS, Lado-Abeal J, Majed FA, Moeller LC, et al. Mutations in SECISBP2 result in abnormal thyroid hormone metabolism. Nat Genet 2005;37:1247-52.
32. Refetoff S, Bassett JH, Beck-Peccoz P, Bernal J, Brent G, Chatterjee K, et al. Classification and proposed nomenclature for inherited defects of thyroid hormone action, transport, and metabolism. J Clin Endocrinol Metab. 2014;99:768-70.
33. Safer JD, Cohan SD, Fraser LM, Wondisford FE. A pituitary tumor in a patient with thyroid hormone resistance: a diagnostic dilemma. Thyroid. 2001;11:281-91.

CHAPTER 12

Interpreting Thyroid Hormone Results

Kaushik Pandit

INTRODUCTION

Thyroid disorders in its florid form are easily recognized. However, barring that rarity, most disorders of thyroid function requires a measurement of the thyroid gland secreted hormones, thyroxine (T4) and triiodothyronine (T3), and measurement of the pituitary hormone controlling the secretion of the thyroid hormones (TH), thyroid stimulating hormone (TSH). In any given individual, the level of the hormones T3 and T4 remain relatively constant over time, and thereby reflecting the set-point of the hypothalamo-pituitary-thyroid (HPT) axis in that individual.[1] A reasonable deviation from this condition, therefore, calls for a pathological state as an explanation. It is all the more important to appreciate that the population reference ranges for T4 and T3 are quite wide (especially for T4) and may preclude a correct interpretation of minor disease state based only on the serum T4 and T3 levels. Therefore, the level of the hormone which is homeostatically linked to the T4 and T3 levels, namely TSH remains the principal test to assess thyroid dysfunction, and therefore, TSH is invariably included in a thyroid function test (TFT).

PHYSIOLOGICAL BASIS OF THYROID HORMONES IN THYROID ILLNESS

The production of TH—T4 and T3 are homeostatically tightly regulated by the influence of pituitary secreted TSH and that in turn controlled by the hypothalamus secreted hormone thyrotropin releasing hormone (TRH). The thyroid gland secretes 85–90% T4 and 10–15% T3 in a euthyroid state. Both T4 and T3 are strongly bound (>99.5%) to circulating proteins, e.g., thyroid binding globulin (TBG), albumin, and transthyretin. The cellular entry of TH especially in some organs like brain and also the cellular efflux of TH from thyroid gland is dependent on specific membrane proteins [e.g., monocarboxylate transporter 8 (MCT8)].

Triiodothyronine is the principal bioactive hormone. Conversion of T4 to T3 at peripheral intracellular site, is controlled by another set of enzymes called deiodinases (DIOs), which therefore regulates the action of the TH at the cellular level. Of the various DIOs, DIO1 (hepatic type) controls the peripheral conversion of T4 to T3, DIO2 converts T4 to T3 in the hypothalamus and pituitary, thereby playing the central role in negative feedback regulation of the HPT axis; in contrast DIO3 converts T4 to reverse T3 (rT3), thereby limiting the action of the TH.[2]

The pituitary secretion of TSH is under strict negative feedback loop with the circulating T3 and T4 levels. In a given population, the reference range for the T4 and T3 is pretty wide, whereas in a normal individual, the variation of the T4 and T3 is very narrow. In a diseased thyroid state, the perturbation in the T4 and T3 making the person hyper, or hypothyroid may not be appreciably ascertained merely from the level of T4 and T3 when compared in relation to the population reference range. In contrast, the TSH gets elevated or suppressed to a greater magnitude by this seemingly little change in the T4 and T3. Therefore, TSH has been traditionally been regarded as the frontline screening test for detection of hypo, or hyperthyroidism.[1]

The THs exert their actions through their effect on the gene transcription. For this to happen, they need to ingress inside the cells through transporter proteins present on the cell surface. These proteins are members of several transporter families that include the organic anion-transporting polypeptide OATP1C1, the MCT8 and MCT10, the L-type amino acid transporters LAT1 and LAT2 and the bile acid transporter SLC10A1. These membrane transporters are also responsible for the efflux of the TH from the thyroid follicular cells. These transporters also influence the balance between secretion of T4 and T3.[3] The importance of TH transport is underscored by the phenotype of patients with Allan-Herndon-Dudley syndrome, which is associated with mutations in the X-linked MCT8 transporter. Male patients manifest a marked neurologic phenotype, including poor muscle tone, impaired speech, and severe mental retardation.[4]

There are two different types of nuclear thyroid hormone receptors (THR), which mediate most of the actions of the TH at the cellular level. There are two different THR genes (*THRα, THRβ*), which exist on chromosomes 17 and 3, respectively. The *THRα* gene, located on chromosome 17, has one product, THRα1 that is able to bind T3 and another product, α2, which is incapable of binding T3. However, the *THRβ* gene, located on chromosome 3, expresses two T3-binding isoforms, *TRβ1* and *TRβ2* that mainly differ in their tissue distribution. The TRα1 is the predominant isoform in the central nervous system, myocardium, colon, and skeletal muscle; *TRβ1* is highly expressed in the liver and kidney; *TRβ2* plays a major role in negative feedback regulation at the level of the hypothalamus and pituitary.[5,6]

HOW TO INTERPRET THE RESULTS?

Interpretation of a TFT is dependent on the background knowledge of the interplay between TH and TSH, in the physiological state and its deviation in the various pathological states. The seven different patterns of TFT that are possible and the plausible explanations of each pattern and the pathological states associated with should be considered for interpretation of a TFT. Further testing to unravel the pathology should be based on this baseline TFT interpretation (Fig. 1).

It is important to appreciate that despite the fact, TSH remains the frontline test for detection of various thyroid disorders, at times a single estimated TSH fails to depict the ongoing thyroid disease status (Box 1).

Fallacies in the Thyroid Hormone Results

Some clinical conditions require a detailed analysis of the pathophysiology to interpret the TFT and avoid the pitfalls in the interpretation of TFTs in such situations.

Disorders of Thyroid

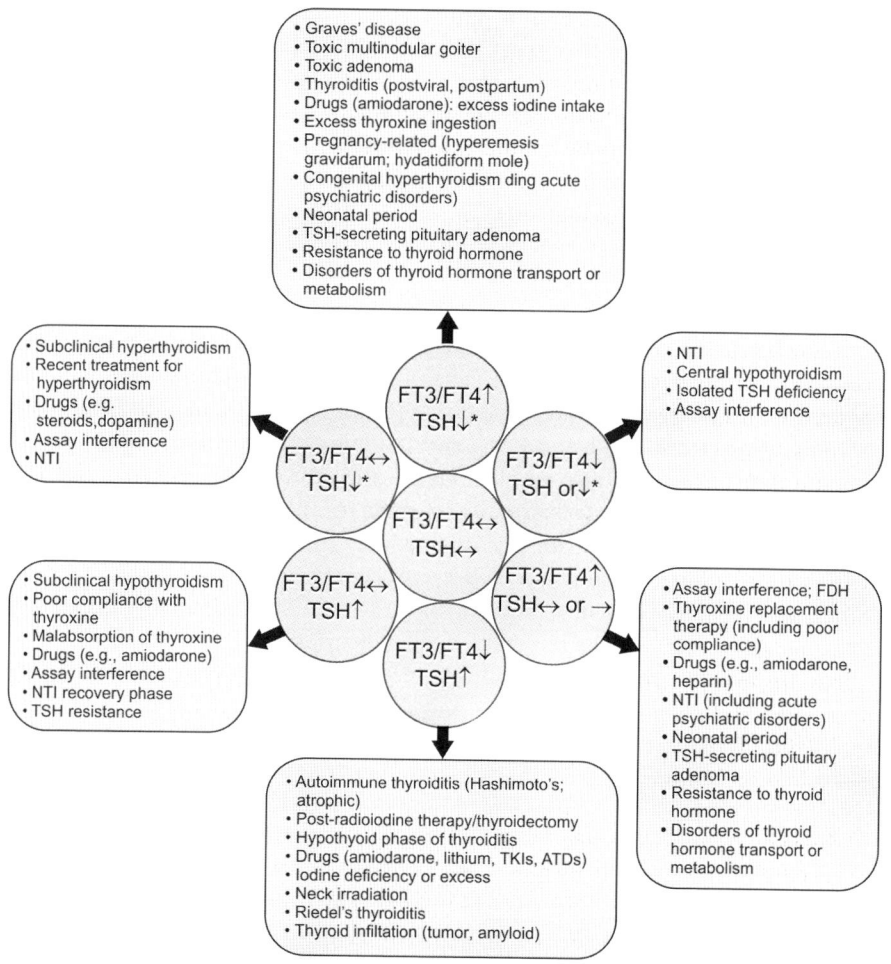

ATDs, antithyroid drugs; FDH, familial dysalbuminemic hyperthyroxinemia; FT3, free triiodothyronine; FT4, free thyroxine; NTI, nonthyroidal illness; TKIs, tyrosine kinase inhibitors; TSH, thyroid stimulating hormone.

FIG. 1: Different patterns of thyroid function tests and their causes

Source: Adapted from Koulouri O, Gurnell M. How to interpret thyroid function tests. Clin Med (Lond). 2013;13(3):282-6. © 2013 Royal College of Physicians.

Box 1: Conditions where a single measurement of thyroid stimulating hormone may not unravel the complete picture of thyroid dysfunction[8]
- Recent treatment for thyrotoxicosis (thyroid stimulating hormone may remain suppressed even when thyroid hormone concentrations have normalized)
- Nonthyroidal illness
- Thyroid stimulating hormone assay interference
- Central hypothyroidism (e.g., hypothalamic or pituitary disorders)
- Thyroid stimulating hormone-secreting pituitary adenoma (thyrotropinoma or TSHoma)
- Resistance to thyroid hormone
- Disorders of thyroid hormone transport or metabolism

RESISTANCE TO THYROID HORMONES

The classical form of resistance to thyroid hormone (RTH) is due to mutations in the THRB locus, which is inherited in an autosomal dominant fashion. It is characterized by elevated TSH and T3 levels. Interestingly, the T3 tissue response was altered to different degrees in RTH patients, from severe thyrotoxicosis to hypothyroidism. The clinical signs and symptoms suggest that there is inhibition of endogenous functional THRs by the mutant receptor through a "dominant-negative effect". This explains the lack of negative feedback in the HPT axis, which causes elevation in TSH and TH circulating levels.[9] The majority of RTH mutations cause resistance to TH in most tissues, a characteristic of the generalized form of RTH (GRTH), even though TH levels are elevated. However, few patients have been described with RTH mutations that were associated with central resistance to T3 (CRTH), and those individuals seem to have preserved peripheral sensitivity to T3.[10]

In contrast, *THRα* mutation leads to nonclassical RTH. They usually present with delay of linear growth and tooth eruption, low serum insulin-like growth factor-1 (IGF-1) levels, reduced muscle tone, impaired fine-motor coordination, dry skin, slow reflexes, and severe constipation. The heart rate and blood pressure were also low and which do not respond to T4 treatment.[11,12]

NONTHYROIDAL ILLNESS

Nonthyroidal illness (NTI), which is also known as sick euthyroid syndrome, remains the commonest pitfall in the interpretation of any TFT. Any serious acute or chronic illness leads to a state of adaptive secondary hypothyroidism, wherein there is low T3 level. In prolonged or severe illness, there is additional drop in T4 level, leading to a low T3 and low T4 situation. The inhibition of type 1 DIO activity in the liver leads to situation of low T3 level and inhibition of metabolism of rT3 leading to a high level of rT3.[13]

A marked decrease in T3 and T4 may not bode well for the patient, in fact, it has been postulated to increase mortality, especially if the T4 level goes below 4 g/L.[14,15]

The serum TSH in contrast, is either normal or low, signifying thereby that there is diminution of intrapituitary T4 to T3 conversion. Some analysts believe the low TSH is the driver for the low T3 syndrome. Thyroid stimulating hormone level, however, increases during the recovery phase of NTIs.[16,17]

The changes in the level of the TH (especially for T3) and TSH may start appearing as early as 24 hours after the onset of the underlying primary disorder. Nonthyroidal illness, which is heterogeneous with a variety of abnormal TFT patterns is also dynamic and changes its pattern with time.[18,19]

In the initial days, it is the T3, which is decreased and with the prolongation of the illness, the T4 level also goes down. This decrease of serum TH levels is seen in starvation, sepsis, surgery, myocardial infarction, cardiopulmonary bypass, bone marrow transplantation, and in fact probably any severe illness can be an example of it.[20,21]

Pari passu, there is also a change in the level of the TSH. The TSH level becomes "inappropriately" normal or low. The T4 to T3 conversion is reduced because of the inhibited action of DIOs. The serum T4 level goes down in prolonged illness primarily because of the reduction in TBG. However, a very low level of T4 to the tune of 2 µg/dL is a reliable poor prognostic factor.

PSYCHIATRIC ILLNESSES

Psychiatric conditions may be caused by thyroid disorders, and therefore, TFTs are routinely ordered in psychiatric illnesses. Psychiatric disorders on the other hand leads to changes in TH and interpreting a TFT requires a background knowledge of the changes in the TFT caused by psychiatric illness. Acute psychiatric decompensation leads to transient increase in TH, especially T4 or Free T4 (FT4) index. This at times is associated with increased T3 as well, in contrast to the NTI. Hypothyroxinemia has also been noted in acute psychiatric disorders, albeit much less frequently than the hyperthyroxinemia.[22]

In contrast to depression and psychotic disorders, panic disorders are not associated with any change in the TH level or change in TFT. Therefore, an elevated TH with panic disorder would suggest the presence of thyrotoxicosis.[23]

Lithium is a commonly used agent in psychiatric disorders and it is known to alter the TFT. The quantum of effect is also significant, with a hazard ratio of 2.31 for development of hypothyroidism,[24] and in a retrospective study, 36% of patients of bipolar disorders who were put on lithium developed abnormal TSH and/or FT4 index,[25] the effects have been noted to be more prominent and prevalent in females.[26]

PREGNANCY

Pregnancy causes a physiological change in the TH levels in the blood. The increase in the level of TBG, caused by excess hepatic synthesis of this protein, which in turn is caused by the excess amount of estrogens in normal pregnancy as well as decreased degradation because of excess sialylation of this protein during pregnancy.[27,28]

The elevated level of TBG during pregnancy leads to increased amount of bound TH, [though the Free T3 (FT3) and FT4 levels remain relatively normal] ultimately leading to increased level of total T3 and total T4 in the blood. The increase in total T4 level undergoes a change to the tune of 50% compared to the nonpregnant state.[29,30]

Longitudinal studies conducted during pregnancy reveal significant fluctuations in free TH levels throughout pregnancy, although these concentrations generally remain within normal reference limits. The FT4 and FT3 levels may be slightly increased in the first trimester at between 6 and 12 weeks and may fall progressively throughout gestation, often to levels below the nonpregnant assay specific reference ranges. This pattern is uniformly constant regardless of the FT4 assay method used. Thus, the reductions in free TH levels in late pregnancy is an inexplicable but a real phenomenon that cannot be accounted for by the pregnancy-induced changes in serum albumin, nonesterified fatty acids, or TBG.[31]

There is a concomitant change in the TSH level as well. The placenta secretes a large amount of human chorionic gonadotropin (hCG) into the circulation, which because of its molecular mimicry with TSH, acts on the TSH receptor of the thyroid follicular cells. This leads to increased generation and output of the TH during pregnancy and consequently leading to a suppressed TSH level. In its most extreme form (hyperemesis gravidarum), affected women may become overtly thyrotoxic with a fully suppressed TSH.[32] At times, it becomes difficult to differentiate between it and the common thyroid disease namely, Graves' disease, and in such a situation, one may need to measure the presence of TSH-receptor antibody (TRAβ) level to bring clarity into the situation. The hCG level peaks in between the 9 and 14 weeks of gestation and this clearly correlates with the reduced TSH levels measured during the first trimester of pregnancy.[33]

Serum TSH level dip to a very low level during the first trimester of pregnancy, between 0.03 and 2.5 mIU/L. In the second and third trimester, greater variance is seen, although the lower limit of "normal" remains below what would be expected for nonpregnant individuals. Therefore, mildly suppressed TSH in pregnancy should be considered as safe and consistent with physiology. There is a suggestion of using a "trimester specific" reference range of TSH level in pregnancy. This, however, is susceptible to a significant extent of ethnicity specific variation.[34,35]

ASSAY INTERFERENCE

Thyroid Stimulating Hormone Measurement

The commonly used TSH measurement techniques use the standard immunometric double antibody sandwich technique, in which one antibody attaches with the TSH molecule and the solid phase (capture antibody) and the other one attaches with the TSH and the signal (detection antibody). There will be considerable interference in case of presence of human anti-animal antibodies (HAA) in the patient's serum. Therefore, a HAA, which retards the binding of TSH to either detection or capture antibody will cause "negative interference" leading to falsely low TSH reading in the sample. In contrast, presence of HAA which can cross-link with the detection and capture antibody (in absence of TSH molecule) will lead to "positive interference" and leads to falsely high TSH reading.

The presence of assay interference in TSH measurement is suspected if the results differ with two different antibody pairs, measurement varies with polyethylene glycol (PEG) precipitation of interfering antibody or nonlinear TSH measurement with sample dilution.[36,37]

Free Thyroxine or Triiodothyronine Measurement

Measurement of minute amounts of FT4 and FT3 compared to the large amounts of total T4 and T3 throws two important challenges. Firstly, the amount of free hormone is very small (<0.05%) compared to the total hormone present in the sample, and the size of T4 and T3 are too small to use the double antibody sandwich assay technique. Therefore, "competition assays" are used instead, where labeled T4 (the tracer) competes with serum T4 for a fixed number of anti-T4 antibody binding sites. Free hormone assays are designed in such a way that the equilibrium between T4 and its binding proteins is conserved during measurement, so that the amount of tracer displaced reflects the "free" rather than "total" hormone concentration.[36]

The assay interference occurs in situations where there is artifactual elevation of FT4 or FT3 because of displacement of T4 or T3 from their binding sites in carrier proteins by agents like heparin. Positive interference by presence of HAA directly binds to tracers or negative interference by presence of blocking antibody to tracers. There may be presence of variant TH binding proteins (e.g., albumin in familial dysalbuminemic hyperthyroxinemia) with altered affinity for T4. In situations of suspected assay interference, a two-step (back titration) assay method should be employed to avoid the pitfall. If the problem persists, hormone measurement following equilibrium dialysis (ED) remains the gold standard for eliminating FT4 assay interference.[38-41]

DRUG EFFECTS

Many drugs cause alterations in the tests of the thyroid function in a euthyroid individual. These need to be kept in mind while interpreting the TFTs in patients receiving such pharmaceutical agents. The effect of lithium and heparin has already been described earlier. In addition, amiodarone cause significant changes in the TFT. Amiodarone contains a large amount of iodine in its structure and can inhibit T4 to T3 conversion by inhibiting the enzyme DIO1, and may cause elevation of FT4 (the FT3, therefore, remains normal). It may cause transient elevation of TSH as well, which however recedes with time. Amiodarone, is also known to cause two types of thyrotoxicosis, the type 1 variety caused by large iodine load leading to thyroid autonomy and type 2 caused by destructive thyrotoxicosis. In a minority of patients, however, it may also cause hypothyroidism.[8]

Propylthiouracil, glucocorticoids, propranolol, and iodinated contrast media or iodine-containing supplements also does diminish the peripheral T4 to T3 conversion via a similar mechanism to amiodarone, leading to elevated FT4 with normal TSH, and FT3 levels are usually normal.[42]

Immune modulators, e.g., highly active antiretroviral therapy in human immunodeficiency virus, interferon-α in chronic hepatitis C may lead to raised FT4 and suppressed TSH and conversely tyrosine kinase inhibitors, e.g., sunitinib, sorafenib may lead to a situation of hypothyroidism with diminished FT4 and raised TSH.[8]

CASE STUDY

CASE 1

A 23-year-old woman presented with palpitation and anxiety for the last 1 year. There was no history of weight loss, excessive sweating, or increased hunger. On examination, she had grade 2 diffuse goiter and tachycardia. The TFT revealed FT3 10.3 pmol/L (reference range: 3.5–7.8 pmol/L), FT4 42.7 pmol/L (reference range: 9.0–25.0 pmol/L) and TSH 1.94 mIU/L (reference range: 0.4–4.0 mIU/L). She was advised to undergo thyroid ablation with 10 mci radioiodine. A repeat TFT was done 4 weeks later, which showed the FT3 9.9 pmol/L, FT4 44.6 pmol/L, and TSH 2.21 mIU/L, respectively. Magnetic resonance imaging scan of the pituitary was done, which showed no definite adenoma in the pituitary. Four of the siblings of the patient are called in (all of whom are healthy and asymptomatic) and their TFTs are performed. Three of the four showed similar patterns of raised FT3 and T4 and normal level of TSH.

A person presenting with tachycardia, anxiety, palpitation, and presence of diffuse goiter raises a possibility of thyrotoxicosis, especially Graves' disease. The elevated FT3 and FT4 supports the diagnosis, but a normal TSH goes strongly against it. However, the treating team ignored the logic and had advised radioiodine ablation for a misdiagnosed Graves' disease, which expectedly failed to alleviate the problem. A possibility of TSHoma was entertained based on the biochemical parameters and a MRI scan was done. Though, a raised FT3 and FT4 and normal TSH level does support the diagnosis, the situation is a rare one. Rather, a commoner situation to entertain would be the entity TH resistance with a similar biochemical profile. At times, though it becomes difficult to separate the two clinical entities, and one needs to go for some special tests. TSHomas are known to cosecrete significant amount of pituitary glycoprotein α subunit along with TSH. In fact, a raised molar ratio of α subunit or TSH of greater than 1.0 is strongly suggestive of the presence of micro TSHoma in the pituitary. Other peripheral markers are at times helpful, e.g., elevated sex hormone binding globulin (SHBG) is seen in TSHoma, which may help to discriminate in this situation. The important discrimination may come from information of similar biochemical TH profile in siblings in cases of RTH, as this is an autosomal dominant condition.

CASE 2

A 62-year-old man with diabetes and hypertension was admitted in hospital with central chest pain and respiratory distress. He was diagnosed to have acute myocardial infarction and congestive heart failure. Appropriate cardiac intervention managed the acute cardiac ischemic event but the congestive heart failure did not improve much. A battery of routine tests at the time of admission was done which included (as part of the hospital protocol) a TFT. The TFT read T3 62 ng/dL (reference range: 80–180 ng/dL), T4 11.3 µg/dL (reference range: 4.6–12.0 µg/dL), and TSH 3.26 mIU/L (Reference range: 0.4–4.0 mIU/L). The patient's heart failure status deteriorated and the treating cardiologist became wary of the deranged TFT and its implication on the outcome of the heart failure and sought an endocrine consultation. The endocrinologist wanted another TFT be done to rule out laboratory aberration being the cause. A repeat TFT 4 days later showed T3 17 ng/dL, T4 2.6 µg/dL, and TSH 1.49 mIU/L. The treating cardiologist was made aware of the situation and no active thyroid intervention was ruled out. The patient's condition deteriorated further in the next 2 days and he expired.

The initial TFT suggested a state of low T3 and normal T4 and TSH suggestive of a situation of NTI. This was because of diminished peripheral deiodination of T4 to T3 by inhibition of DIO1 in the liver. This is usually seen in the initial phase of the illness. The repeat test 4 days later showed further diminution of T3 and reduced T4 with normal TSH. The reduced T3 suggests further suppression of DIO1. The reduction of T4, however, is because of diminished TBG and usually in proportion to the degree and duration of the illness. The altered biochemical profile signifies a diminished serum hormone level and the patient is biochemically hypothyroid, which is a beneficial physiologic response (on a teleological sense) and should not be altered by treatment. However, studies have noted that a low T4, especially if less than 4 µg/dL signifies an increased risk of mortality.

CONCLUSION

Interpretations of TFT require background knowledge of the HPT axis physiology, the factors governing the TH actions at the cellular level, and the different patterns of TFTs that may be encountered in clinical practice.

Correct interpretation of TFT is fundamental to establish the correct diagnosis when clinical features and TFT results appear discordant or incongruous.

ADDENDUM

Recently, attention has been drawn to analytical error in assays involving streptavidin-biotin interaction resulting in erroneous results that appear robust when taken out of any consideration of contrary clinical findings. This is more likely to appear in some patients who consume biotin as a supplement. Elevated thyroid antibody titers (TPO, TgA), thyrotropin receptor antibody (TRab), free T4, and free T3 have been reported. Such patients may be misdiagnosed as Graves' disease patients and treated unnecessarily with risk of possible adverse outcomes. Therefore, when symptom complex and laboratory data do not match, patients should be asked whether they are taking biotin supplement.[43]

REFERENCES

1. Andersen S, Pedersen KM, Bruun NH, Laurberg P. Narrow individual variations in serum T4 and T3 in normal subjects: a clue to the understanding of subclinical thyroid disease. J Clin Endocrinol Metab. 2002;87(3):1068-72.
2. Bianco AC, Kim BW. Deiodinases: implications of the local control of thyroid hormone action. J Clin Invest. 2006;116(10):2571-9.
3. Visser WE, Friesema EC, Visser TJ. Minireview: thyroid hormone transporters: the knowns and the unknowns. Mol Endocrinol. 2011;25(1):1-14.
4. Schwartz CE, Stevenson RE. The MCT8 thyroid hormone transporter and Allan-Herndon-Dudley syndrome. Best Pract Res Clin Endocrinol Metab. 2007;21(2):307-21.
5. Mitsuhashi T, Tennyson GE, Nikodem VM. Alternative splicing generates messages encoding rat c-erbA proteins that do not bind thyroid hormone. Proc Natl Acad Sci U S A. 1988;85(16):5804-8.
6. Williams GR. Cloning and characterization of two novel thyroid hormone receptor beta isoforms. Mol Cell Biol. 2000;20(22): 8329-42.
7. Koulouri O, Gurnell M. How to interpret thyroid function tests. Clin Med (Lond). 2013;13(3):282-6.
8. Koulouri O, Moran C, Halsall D, Chatterjee K, Gurnell M. Pitfalls in the measurement and interpretation of thyroid function tests. Best Pract Res Clin Endocrinol Metab. 2013;27(6):745-62.
9. Refetoff S, Weiss RE, Usala SJ. The syndromes of resistance to thyroid hormone. Endocr Rev. 1993;14(3):348-99.
10. Brucker-Davis F, Skarulis MC, Grace MB, Benichou J, Hauser P, Wiggs E, et al. Genetic and clinical features of 42 kindreds with resistance to thyroid hormone. The National Institutes of Health Prospective Study. Ann Intern Med. 1995;123(8):572-83.
11. Moran C, Schoenmakers N, Agostini M, Schoenmakers E, Offiah A, Kydd A, et al. An adult female with resistance to thyroid hormone mediated by defective thyroid hormone receptor . J Clin Endocrinol Metab. 2013;98(11):4254-61.
12. van Mullem A, van Heerebeek R, Chrysis D, Visser E, Medici M, Andrikoula M, et al. Clinical phenotype and mutant TRalpha-1. N Engl J Med. 2012;366(15):1451-3.
13. Kaptein EM. Clinical relevance of thyroid hormone alterations in nonthyroidal illness. Thyroid Int. 1997;4:22-25.
14. Maldonado LS, Murata GH, Hershman JM, Braunstein GD. Do thyroid function tests independently predict survival in the critically ill? Thyroid. 1992;2(2):119-23.
15. De Marinis L, Mancini A, Masala R, Torlontano M, Sandric S, Barbarino A. Evaluation of pituitary-thyroid axis response to acute myocardial infarction. J Endocrinol Invest. 1985;8(6):507-11.
16. Faber J, Kirkegaard C, Rasmussen B, Westh H, Busch-Sørensen M, Jensen IW. Pituitary-thyroid axis in critical illness. J Clin Endocrinol Metab. 1987;65(2):315-20.
17. Kaptein EM, Grieb DA, Spencer CA, Wheeler WS, Nicoloff JT. Thyroxine metabolism in the low thyroxine state of critical nonthyroidal illnesses. J Clin Endocrinol Metab. 1981;53(4):764-71.
18. Docter R, Krenning EP, de Jong M, Hennemann G. The sick euthyroid syndrome: changes in thyroid hormone serum parameters and hormone metabolism. Clin Endocrinol (Oxf). 1993;39(5):499-518.
19. Beckett GJ. Thyroid function and thyroid function tests in nonthyroidal illness. CPD Bulletin. Clin Biochem. 2006;7:107-16.
20. McIver B, Gorman CA. Euthyroid sick syndrome: An overview. Thyroid. 1997;7(1):125-32.
21. Hennemann G, Docter R, Krenning EP. Causes and effects of the low T3 syndrome during caloric deprivation and non-thyroidal illness: an overview. Acta Med Austriaca. 1988;15 Suppl 1:42-5.
22. Arem R, Cusi K. Thyroid function testing in psychiatric illness: Usefulness and limitations. Trends Endocrinol Metab. 1997;8(7):282-7.
23. Stein MB, Uhde TW. Thyroid indices in panic disorder. Am J Psychiatry. 1988;145(6):745-7.
24. Shine B, McKnight RF, Leaver L, Geddes JR. Long-term effects of lithium on renal, thyroid, and parathyroid function: a retrospective analysis of laboratory data. Lancet. 2015;386(9992):461-8.
25. Fagiolini A, Kupfer DJ, Scott J, Swartz HA, Cook D, Novick DM, et al. Hypothyroidism in patients with bipolar I disorder treated primarily with lithium. Epidemiol Psichiatr Soc. 2006;15(2):123-7.
26. Tsui KY. The impact of Lithium on thyroid function in Chinese psychiatric population. Thyroid Res. 2015;8:14.
27. Glinoer D, Gershengorn MC, Dubois A, Robbins J. Stimulation of thyroxine-binding globulin synthesis by isolated rhesus monkey hepatocytes after in vivo beta-estradiol administration. Endocrinology. 1977;100(3):807-13.
28. Ain KB, Mori Y, Refetoff S. Reduced clearance of thyroxine-binding globulin (TBG) with increased sialylation: a mechanism for estrogen-induced elevation of serum TBG concentration. J Clin Endocrinol Metab. 1987;65(4):689-96.
29. Whitworth AS, Midgley JE, Wilkins TA. A comparison of free T4 and the ratio of total T4 to T4-binding globulin in serum through pregnancy. Clin Endocrinol (Oxf). 1982;17(3):307-13.

30. Osathanondh R, Tulchinsky D, Chopra IJ. Total and free thyroxine and triiodothyronine in normal and complicated pregnancy. J Clin Endocrinol Metab. 1976;42(1):98-104.
31. Sapin R, d'Herbomez M. Free thyroxine measured by equilibrium dialysis and nine immunoassays in sera with various serum thyroxine-binding capacities. Clin Chem. 2003;49(9):1531-5.
32. Glinoer D, de Nayer P, Bourdoux P, Lemone M, Robyn C, van Steirteghem A, et al. Regulation of maternal thyroid during pregnancy. J Clin Endocrinol Metab. 1990;71(2):276-87.
33. Ballabio M, Poshychinda M, Ekins RP. Pregnancy-induced changes in thyroid function: role of human chorionic gonadotropin as a putative regulator of maternal thyroid. J Clin Endocrinol Metab. 1991;73(4):824-31.
34. Soldin OP, Soldin D, Sastoque M. Gestation-specific thyroxine and thyroid stimulating hormone levels in the United States and worldwide. Ther Drug Monit. 2007;29(5):553-9.
35. Korevaar TI, Medici M, de Rijke YB, Visser W, de Muinck Keizer-Schrama SM, Jaddoe VW, et al. Ethnic differences in maternal thyroid parameters during pregnancy: The Generation R Study. J Clin Endocrinol Metab. 2013;98(9):3678-86.
36. Després N, Grant AM. Antibody interference in thyroid assays: a potential for clinical misinformation. Clin Chem. 1998;44(3):440-54.
37. Verhoye E, Van den Bruel A, Delanghe JR, Debruyne E, Langlois MR. Spuriously high thyrotropin values due to anti-thyrotropin antibodies in adult patients. Clin Chem Lab Med. 2009;47(5):604-6.
38. Bartalena, L, Robbins J. Variations in thyroid hormone transport proteins and their clinical implications. Thyroid. 1992;2(3):237-45.
39. Cartwright D, O'Shea P, Rajanayagam O, Agostini M, Barker P, Moran C, et al. Familial dysalbuminemic hyperthyroxinemia: a persistent diagnostic challenge. Clin Chem. 2009;55(5):1044-6.
40. Stevenson HP, Archbold GP, Johnston P, Young IS, Sheridan B. Misleading serum free thyroxine results during low molecular weight heparin treatment. Clin Chem. 1998;44(5):1002-7.
41. Holm SS, Hansen SH, Faber J, Staun-Olsen P. Reference methods for the measurement of free thyroid hormones in blood: evaluation of potential reference methods for free thyroxine. Clin Biochem. 2004;37(2):85-93.
42. Stockigt JR, Lim CF. Medications that distort in vitro tests of thyroid function, with particular reference to estimates of serum free thyroxine. Best Pract Res Clin Endocrinol Metab. 2009;23(6):753-67.
43. Piketty ML, Polak M, Flechtner I, Gonzales-Briceño L, Souberbielle JC. False biochemical diagnosis of hyperthyroidism in streptavidin-biotin-based immunoassays: the problem of biotin intake and related interference. Clin Chem Lab Med. 2017;55(6):780-88.

CHAPTER 13

Thyroid-associated Orbitopathy

Rajesh Rajput

INTRODUCTION

Thyroid-associated orbitopathy (TAO), also known as Graves' ophthalmopathy, is an autoimmune disease seen in patients with dysfunction of thyroid gland in which the orbital and periocular soft tissues are primarily affected with secondary effects on the eye.[1] Although TAO is usually seen in background of Graves' disease, around 10% of the patients had no evidence of Graves' disease and most of such patients have autoimmune hypothyroidism or thyroid antibodies. The onset of TAO usually occurs within the year before or after the diagnosis of thyrotoxicosis in two third of the cases but in some it precede the diagnosis of thyrotoxicosis by several years, accounting for some cases of euthyroid ophthalmopathy.[2] The diagnosis of euthyroid ophthalmopathy can be confirmed by estimation of (thyrotropin) TSH receptor antibodies which are usually present in high titer in such cases.[3] Most cases of Graves' disease have little or no clinical evidence of ophthalmopathy, however, enlarged extraocular muscles seen typically in this disease is usually seen in almost all the cases with ultrasound or CT of the orbit. It is more common in females; however, the gender difference in incidence rate decreases as severity of TAO increases. The female to male ratio was 9.3:1 in patients with mild ophthalmopathy, 3.2:1 in those with moderate ophthalmopathy, and 1.4:1 with severe ophthalmopathy. The prevalence of TAO in patients with hyperthyroidism was significantly higher in Europeans (42%) compared to Asians (7.7%).[4] Various risk factors that increases the risk and severity of TAO includes genetic predisposition to develop TAO, cigarette smoking, advanced age, stress, TSH receptor antibody levels, and type of treatment for hyperthyroidism.[5-8] Out of all these risk factors, cigarette smoking is identified as the strongest modifiable risk factor for development of TAO. Other related autoimmune diseases like diabetes mellitus, myasthenia gravis are seen more commonly in these patients and when present increases the severity of TAO including the chances to develop dysthyroid optic neuropathy (DON).

CASE 1

A 48-year-old woman presented with complaint of palpitations, tremulousness, and weight loss from the last 3 month. Her mother and aunt had hypothyroidism. Clinical and biochemical examination was suggestive of hyperthyroidism. She was put on antithyroid medication. Recently, she noticed increasing redness and prominence of both the eyes. Eye examination revealed restriction of abduction in both eyes and supraduction in the left eye. She was diplopic in upgaze and in left gaze and clinical activity score was five. A diagnosis of hyperthyroidism with thyroid eye disease was made. Computed tomography (CT) scan demonstrated enlargement of muscles with diminution of fat around the optic nerve. She was put on antithyroid medication and given the clinical progression and increasing inflammatory features an intravenous methylprednisolone was instituted, and patients responded to it with marked decrease in clinical activity score.

CASE 2

A 55-year-old man presented with complaint increasing prominence of eyes, grittiness from last 2 month. He was a known case of hyperthyroidism from past many years and was taking treatment for it. His thyroid function test was within normal limits. Eye examination revealed clinical activity score of 4 with proptosis of 24 mm in both the eyes. In view of evidence of inflammation as suggested by clinical activity score, a course of intravenous methylprednisolone was stared. The patient responded to methylprednisolone but was much worried about proptosis and diplopia now. After several months with no evidence of disease progression, reconstructive surgery was undertaken to decompress the orbit. Fat decompression with medial and lateral wall removal was performed in a bilateral fashion. The patient proptosis improved but required additional surgery to improve the diplopia which was present prior to the decompression surgery.

PATHOGENESIS

Thyroid-associated orbitopathy is an autoimmune disease and with common the association of TAO with hyperthyroidism, it is likely that thyroid and orbital tissues share a common antigen.[9] The various candidate antigen includes thyroglobulin, the TSH receptor, insulin-like growth factor-1 receptor, or extraocular muscle antigens but none has been identified with certainty in all the cases.[10] Genetic factors also plays an important role in the pathogenesis of Graves' disease with certain human leukocyte antigens (HLAs) haplotypes like HLA-B8, DR3, and DQA1*0501 seen more commonly in such patients compared to control population. The presence of these haplotypes increases the susceptibility to develop the disease while presence of HLA-DR β1*07 may offer protection. In a study done in 81 Brazilian TAO patients and 161 normal controls, HLA-DRB1*16 allele was present in higher frequency in patients major extraocular muscle involvement whereas patients with minor extraocular muscle involvement were found to have a higher frequency of the HLA-DRB1*03 allele.[11]

Antigen antibody interaction within the orbit causes lymphocytic infiltration of the orbital tissue and release of various cytokines, e.g., tumor necrosis factor, interleukin 1. Orbital fibroblast are extremely sensitive to cytokines and are believed to be the primary target and effector cells in TAO. Once activated, these orbital fibroblast secretes hyaluronic acid, a glycosaminoglycan (GAG), which by hyperosmotic shift, cause tissue edema in the extraocular muscles. The orbit is a pear-shaped box with an anterior opening accommodating the eye globe with its muscles with stalk of the pear represented by optic nerve. In TAO, early in the disease process an active phase of inflammation is present which result in increase in orbital volume resulting from the swelling of extraocular muscles and fat. The increased orbital volume causes forward protrusion of the eye resulting in proptosis and at the narrow posterior apex of the orbit causes compression of the optic nerve. The resulting edema and inflammation if not treated in time will cause tissue damage and fibrosis, with restriction in extraocular motility and lagophthalmos. Even if not identified timely and treated, the inflammation and edema subsides within 1–2 years of the onset and is followed by a more quiescent, fibrotic phase predominated by scarring of the orbital tissues.[11,12]

Apart from genetic predisposition and autoimmunity, smoking is identified as an important modifiable risk factor that increases the incidence and severity of TAO. Graves' disease patients who smoke have a five times higher risk of developing TAO than those who do not. *In vitro* studies have shown that orbital fibroblasts when exposed to cigarette extract have a dose-dependent significant increase in GAG production and adipogenesis. There is also enough evidence to suggest that cessation of smoking will reduces the risk of worsening of the orbitopathy and increases the chance of having a favorable response to treatment.[8]

CLINICAL MANIFESTATIONS

Since 80–85% of the patients with TAO has associated hyperthyroidism, 10% hypothyroidism and 5–10% have euthyroid ophthalmopathy, majority of these patients have goiter and clinical signs and symptoms suggestive of hyperthyroidism.[13,14] The eye symptoms and signs are usually bilateral but unilateral signs are found in up to 10% of the cases. The earliest manifestation of ophthalmopathy are sensation of grittiness, eye discomfort, photophobia, and lacrimation secondary to the wide palpebral aperture combined with poor blinking, leading to increased tear evaporation, and poor maintenance of tear film on the eye. The ocular manifestations of TAO include eyelid retraction, proptosis, chemosis, periorbital edema, and altered ocular motility. The eyelid retraction causing a staring appearance is the most common eye sign seen in majority of patients is not specific for Graves; ophthalmopathy. Lid retraction is caused by sympathetic over activity and stimulation and contraction of Muller's and levator muscle. Normally, the location of the upper lid is 1–1.5 mm below the superior limbus and, therefore, if the white of the cornea is seen above the corneoscleral limbus, eyelid retraction of at least 1.5 mm is present. The lower lid is usually at the level of inferior limbus and its retraction is less common and is not seen without concomitant retraction of the upper eyelid. Although lid retraction is nonspecific and can be seen in any form of thyrotoxicosis, flare over lateral side of the retracted upper eyelid almost pathognomic for TAO. Other common finding includes periorbital edema, scleral injection, chemosis, lid lag (i.e., failure of the upper eyelid to follow the eyeball movement on vertical downward movement), and incomplete eyelid closure (lagophthalmos). A characteristic conjunctival finding in TAO is focal injection over insertion of lateral or medial rectus muscle. The engorged vessels do not extend to corneoscleral limbus. About one-third of the patients develops proptosis which is best judged clinically by visualization of sclera between lower border of the iris and lower eyelid. Another way by which physician can ascertain presence of it is by standing behind the seated patient and looking downward from above to ascertain the extent to which eyes protrudes beyond plane of the forehead. Proptosis should be ideally measured and recorded by Hertel's exopthalmometer and if severe will result in corneal exposure and damage. The Hertel exopthalmometer measures the distance between lateral angle of the bony orbit and an imaginary perpendicular tangent to the most anterior part of cornea. The upper limit of normal is 18–20 mm for Whites, 20–22 mm for Blacks, and 16–18 mm for Asians. A difference in reading of more than 2 mm between the two eyes is suggestive of proptosis. Proptosis measurement is affected by systemic nonthyroidal illness, with recession seen wasting disorders and forward bulge in obesity, chronic obstructive airway disease and Cushing's disease. Proptosis of up to 25 mm has also been described as familial trait. Proptosis also needs to be differentiated from pseudoproptosis in which pseudoretraction of the eyelid occurs in response to ptosis in the normal appearing contralateral eye. In 5–10% of patients, the muscle swelling is so severe that it results in diplopia especially on looking up and laterally. The most commonly affected muscle is Inferior rectus followed by medial, superior, levator, and lateral rectus. The most serious manifestation of TAO is compression of optic nerve at leading to DON is seen in around 5% of cases. Dysthyroid optic neuropathy causes decrease in vision, color vision, contrast sensitivity, relative afferent papillary defect (Marcus Gunn pupil), papilledema, peripheral field defects, and, if untreated, may result in permanent loss of vision. Various objective measurements used for each eye includes documentation of maximum lid fissure width, assessment of exposure keratitis with rose Bengal or fluorescein, quantification of extraocular muscle function with use of Hess chart or Maddox rod test, measurement of intraocular pressure, and measurement of visual acuity, fields, and color vision. Farnsworth-Munsll panel detects subtle acquired color vision defects better than the pseudoisochromatic color plate system. It is also important to remember that 7–8% of males has some degree of congenital red-green color blindness. Various eponymous signs are associated with TAO are described in table 1.[13-15]

TABLE 1: Various eponymous signs associated with thyroid-associated orbitopathy

Eye sign in thyroid-associated orbitopathy	Description
Dalrymple's sign	Unnatural degree of separation between margins of two eyelid, i.e., widened palpebral fissure
Von Graefe's sign	Lid lag of the upper eyelid on downward gaze
Collier's sign	Lower lid retraction
Gifford's sign	Difficulty in eversion of upper lid
Boston's sign	Jerky movements of upper lid on lower gaze
Enroth's sign	Edema especially of the upper eyelid
Kocher's sign	Eye globe lag on supraduction
Mobius sign	Imperfect power of convergence
Stellwag's sign	Diminished frequency of blinking and imperfect closure of the lids during the act
Joffroy's sign	Absent creases in the forehead on superior gaze
Vigouroux sign (eyelid fullness)	Eyelid fullness
Ballet sign	Restriction of one or more extraocular muscles
Jendrassik's sign	Abduction and rotation of eyeball is limited also
Knies' sign	Uneven pupillary dilatation in dim light
Snellen-Rieseman's sign	When placing the stethoscope's capsule over closed eyelids a systolic murmur could be heard
Suker's sign	Inability to maintain fixation on extreme lateral gaze
Topolanski's sign	Around insertion areas of the four rectus muscles of the eyeball a vascular band network is noticed and this network joints the four insertion points
Wilder's sign	Jerking of the eye on movement from abduction to adduction

Disorders of Thyroid

Since TAO is a self-limiting disease with an active phase which is amenable to anti-inflammatory and immunosuppressive treatment followed by a variable length of time to a chronic phase where only surgical treatment is indicated, it is useful to classify the patient into active and or chronic phase. Also, when disease is active, one should try to establish the severity of this active phase so as to plan an appropriate therapy. Many classifications and scoring systems have been used to assess the extent and severity of eye involvement in TAO. The NO SPEC is a mnemonic used to describe one such scheme of eye changes used in many studies (Table 2).[16] In 1981, Van Dyke refined the class 2 NO SPECS soft tissue findings with the mnemonic RELIEF (Box 1).[17] However NO SPEC has some limitations which includes that it did

TABLE 2: NO SPEC classification

Class	Grade	Description
Class 0		No signs or symptoms
Class 1		Only signs (limited to upper lid retraction and stare, with or without lid lag)
Class 2		Soft tissue involvement (edema of conjunctivae and lids, conjunctival injection, etc.)
	0	Absent
	A	Minimal
	B	Moderate
	C	Marked
Class 3		Proptosis
	0	<23 mm
	A	24–25 mm
	B	25–27 mm
	C	≥28 mm
Class 4		Extraocular muscle involvement (usually with diplopia)
	0	Absent
	A	Limitation of movement in extremes of gaze
	B	Evident restriction of movement
	C	Fixed eyeball
Class 5		Corneal involvement (primarily due to lagophthalmos)
	0	Absent
	A	Stippling of cornea
	B	Ulceration
	C	Clouding
Class 6		Sight loss (due to optic nerve involvement)
	0	Absent
	A	20/20–20/60
	B	20/27–20/200
	C	<20/200

Box 1: RELIEF classification of soft tissue signs and symptoms	
• Resistance to retropulsion	• Injection over the horizontal rectus muscle insertions
• Edema of conjunctiva and caruncle	• Edema of the eyelids
• Lacrimal gland enlargement	• Fullness of the eyelids

not describe the eye changes fully, patients may fall into more than 1 particular class, patients do not necessarily progresses from one class to another and lastly patients with vision loss due to optic nerve involvement may not have proptosis or other signs of severe disease. Another simple classification is describing TAO patients into two categories—type I and type II. Type I is characterized by minimal inflammation and restrictive myopathy while type II is characterized by significant orbital inflammation and restrictive myopathy, however, again these two forms are not mutually exclusive and did not describe about severity of disease.[18] To overcome challenges and shortcomings associated with various classifications and to identify the patients with active disease at the earliest who can best be treated with drugs, Mourits et al.[19] developed a widely used clinical activity score (CAS) based on 10 items (Table 3). The score of more than or equal to 4 has been helpful for predicting inflammatory changes and the outcome of immunosuppressive treatment in patients with TAO. A modified version of this CAS using seven items is recommended by European Group on Graves' Orbitopathy (EUGOGO),[20] in which one point each is given for presence of spontaneous retro bulbar pain, pain on up or down eye movement, eyelid erythema, conjunctival injection, chemosis, swelling of caruncle, and eyelid edema or fullness; a score of more than or equal to 3/7 signified active disease and justify the use of anti-inflammatory treatment. The severity TAO is graded into three stages as recommended by EUGOGO (Table 4) and patients with active diseases (CAS of ≥3/7) and moderate-to-severe TAO should be treated with anti-inflammatory/immunosuppressive therapy.

Based on suggestions given by international working groups, Dolman and Rootman[21] devised a classification system known by the acronym VISA. The four disease endpoints included in this classification system includes Vision, Inflammation, Strabismus, and Appearance/exposure (VISA). The changes in these four parameters can be used in outdoor setting to assess the improvement and to guide and assess therapy. Each section records subjective and measurable objective inputs that aid in planning ancillary testing and treatment. Vision is tested to rule out optic neuropathy. Subjectively, this is described early on as episodes of greying out with and without color desaturation. On examination, abnormalities in visual acuity, color vision assessment, relative afferent papillary defect, or peripheral visual field assessment may be detected. Inflammation is assessed by modified CAS which includes pain, redness, swelling, and impaired visual function. The CAS consists of two conjunctival signs, two eyelid signs, and two orbital signs and the maximum score is 8. A score of 4 or more is suggestive of active eye disease

TABLE 3: Clinical activity score of thyroid-associated ophthalmopathy

Pain	1.	Painful, oppressive feeling on or behind the globe during the last 2 weeks
	2.	Pain on attempted up, side or down gaze during the last 4 weeks
Redness	3.	Redness of the eye lids
	4.	Diffuse redness of the conjunctiva covering at least one quadrant
Swelling	5.	Swelling of the eyelids
	6.	Chemosis
	7.	Swollen caruncle
	8.	Increase of proptosis ≥2 mm during a period of 1–3 months
Impaired function	9.	Decrease of eye movements in any direction ≥5 during a period of 1–3 months
	10.	Decrease of visual acuity of ≥1 line on the Snellen chart during a period of 1–3 months

TABLE 4: Severity grading of thyroid-associated ophthalmopathy

Severity of thyroid-associated orbitopathy	Description

Mild	- Features of Graves' ophthalmopathy have only a minor impact on daily life insufficient to justify immunosuppressive or surgical treatment
	- These patients usually have only one or more of the following:
	  ○ Minor lid retraction (<2 mm)
	  ○ Mild soft tissue involvement
	  ○ Exophthalmos <3 mm above normal for race and gender
	  ○ Transient or no diplopia
	  ○ Corneal exposure responsive to lubricants

Moderate to severe	- Absence of sight-threatening Graves' ophthalmopathy but sufficiently severe to have impact on daily life justifying the risks of immunosuppression (if active) or surgical intervention (if inactive)
	- Usually have any one or more of the following:
	  ○ Lid retraction ≥2 mm
	  ○ moderate or severe soft tissue involvement
	  ○ proptosis ≥3 mm above normal for race and gender
	  ○ Inconstant or constant diplopia

Sight-threatening	- Dysthyroid optic neuropathy and/or corneal breakdown - Require immediate intervention

and thus is more likely to respond to anti-inflammatory/immunosuppressive treatment. The disadvantage of CAS is it is still very subjective in nature with a large inter-observer variation. The advantage of CAS is it is inexpensive and can be done instantly in a clinic. The symptoms for strabismus include a progression from no diplopia, diplopia in horizontal or vertical gaze, intermittent diplopia in primary gaze, and constant diplopia in primary gaze. Strabismus can be measured objectively by prism cover testing in different gaze directions and graded from 0° to >45° in four directions, using the Hirschberg principle. Objective measures of appearance change include eyelid retraction, proptosis, and documentation of redundant skin and fat prolapse. Measures of exposure include corneal staining or ulceration. Photographs can document the appearance changes.

NATURAL HISTORY OF THYROID-ASSOCIATED ORBITOPATHY

The natural history of TAO is characterized by a period of progression over 3–6 months followed by a plateau phase over next 12–18 months and then gradual improvement particularly in soft tissue changes.[13] Majority of patients with mild disease do not require any specific treatment except local measures for symptomatic relief and have a self-limiting course. However 5–10% of the patients have more aggressive course requiring urgent intervention in active phase especially if corneal ulceration or optic nerve involvement is present. Soft tissue changes such as chemosis and swelling of the lid improves in majority of patients over a short period of follow-up, while lid retraction takes time to subside. Strabismus regresses spontaneously in only 30–40% of cases without specific therapy and persist due to fibrosis of the extraocular muscles. Proptosis persist in up to 90% of the patients to some degree.[22]

TREATMENT OF THYROID-ASSOCIATED ORBITOPATHY
Proper management of TAO includes general measures and specific management of TAO.

General Management
The risk factors associated with development of severe TAO includes nonmodifiable risk factors like older age and male gender and modifiable risk factors like smoking and suboptimal control of thyroid function. Evidence suggests that smoking cessation is associated with an improved TAO outcome therefore all patients with TAO should be advised to stop smoking.[23]

Since both hyperthyroidism and hypothyroidism aggravates TAO, euthyroidism should be achieved and maintained in all the patients.[24] Choice of treatment to achieve euthyroidism in hyperthyroid patient include antithyroid drugs, radioiodine ablation, and surgery. Antithyroid drugs and surgical thyroidectomy have no influence on the course of TAO, radioiodine ablation, however, is associated with increased risk of exacerbations of TAO. Thyroid ablation with radioiodine is associated with release of putative thyroid antigen into the circulation resulting in exacerbation of autoimmune process and ophthalmopathy.[22,25] However, as radioiodine ablation eventually eradicates the thyrocytes and associated the TSH receptor immune response, radioiodine might have long term beneficial effect on TAO. The risk of exacerbation of TAO with use of radioablation can be minimized by short course of steroid therapy and avoiding post-treatment hypothyroidism.[25] Currently, there is no consensus on the best suitable steroid regimen with respect to the issues that when it should be initiated, how long it should continue after radiation therapy and the initial and cumulative dose. European Group on Graves' Orbitopathy[20] suggests that prednisolone in dose of 0.3–0.5 mg/kg/day orally should be started 1–3 days after radioactive iodine and then dosage is to be tapered gradually until withdrawal at about 3 months. The others recommends starting prednisolone in a dose of 0.5 mg/kg/day to be started one month before radioiodine treatment and then gradually to be tapered and stopped over next 3 months.

Specific Treatment of Thyroid-associated Orbitopathy
Supportive Measures
For symptomatic relief from corneal drying, patients can be advised to use methylcellulose containing lubricant eye drops during day time and lubricant ointment and taping of the eyelid at night. For troublesome lid retraction topical adrenergic blocking agent such as 5% guanethidine sulfate eye drops can be used for some time. However, these are not used widely and rarely used now a days due to side effects like worsening of ocular redness and pain. Botulinum toxin have also been used for treatment of upper lid retraction. Patients with symptomatic diplopia should be given prisms if appropriate. Worsening of diplopia and soft tissue changes at night result from dependent edema, which can be benefitted from elevation of head end of the patient. While driving one should use sunglasses or tinted glasses to avoid photophobia and damage to the cornea.[25]

Disorders of Thyroid

Medical Management of Thyroid-associated Orbitopathy

The choice of treatment depends on whether the patient has active inflammatory or quiescent fibrotic phase of the disease. The patients with mild disease needs observation, symptomatic treatment, and maintenance of euthyroid status since majority of them will recover on its own.

Patients with active disease (CAS of ≥3/7) and moderate-to-severe TAO requires treatment with anti-inflammatory and immunosuppression drugs to prevent development of exposure keratopathy, debilitating strabismus, and sight-threatening optic neuropathy.

Various drugs used for treatment of TAO includes glucocorticoids, immunosuppressive drugs (cyclosporine, azathioprine, cyclophosphamide, methotrexate, etc.), somatostatin analog, intravenous immunoglobulin, anti-ß cell therapy (rituximab), pentoxifylline, and orbital radiotherapy.[26,27]

Both oral and intravenous steroid have been used to treat active, moderate to severe TAO and DON. The principal advantage with steroid therapy is that it is fast acting and cost effective. The exact mechanism of immunosuppressive and anti-inflammatory effect of glucocorticoids include inhibition of T and B lymphocyte infiltration and activation, decrease in the effect of inflammatory cytokines and the production of GAG's by the fibroblasts of the orbit.[27] Till now, no universally accepted guidelines for the treatment of TAO with systemic steroid therapy have been set up, and various centers across the globe uses their own schedule. The most commonly used schedule for oral glucocorticoid includes using prednisolone at a dose of 1–2 mg/kg body weight for 6–8 weeks or until soft tissues has subsided followed by a gradual decrease in dose by no more than 5–10 mg every two weeks until a maintenance dose of 5–7.5 mg/day has been reached. In good number of cases, reduction in dosage/withdrawal result in exacerbation, which requires increase in dosage and slowing of tapering rate. Improvement in soft tissue inflammation begins within first few days and typical course range from 3 to 12 months.[28] For the last few years, systemic steroid therapy with the use of intravenous methylprednisone pulses has become widely used. A large systematic review and meta-analysis concluded that intravenous pulse corticosteroids were significantly better at reducing the CAS and were associated with fewer adverse events than oral steroids although there was no difference between the groups in terms of proptosis, diplopia, lid aperture, and visual acuity. Nagayama et al.[29] described the first treatment protocol where 1 g of methylprednisone intravenous is given for 3 days, with the repeat of treatment for the next 3–7 weeks and total cumulative dose of 9–21 g. Since then, many modifications of this method have been recently described in literature. Kahaly et al.[30] revealed the 12-week therapy, with only one pulse weekly, as effective as giving three pulses per week. The rationale behind this was that effect of even single massive dose of steroid is observed for at least 6 weeks and causes the disappearance of dendritic cells responsible for antigen presentation and initiating the immunological response by inhibiting their production and differentiation in the marrow and apoptosis of the precursors of those cells. Furthermore, there is a risk of fulminant hepatic failure if the cumulative dose of methylprednisolone exceeds 8 g.[31] Based on these observations, EUGOGO[20] recommends that the cumulative dose of methylprednisolone should not exceed 8 g and the regimen for administration of methylprednisone is 15 mg/kg (maximum 1.0 g) once a week for 4 weeks, then 7.5 mg/kg once a week for the next 8 weeks. This is followed by additional oral therapy with prednisone at a dose of 10–40 mg/daily for 2 months after finishing intravenous treatment. Concomitant antiresorptive agents with bisphosphonate should be also considered for patients treated with oral or intravenous steroid for more than 3 weeks. The various side effects associated with such a long-term steroid therapy include cushingoid syndrome, hyperglycemia, hypertension, steroid-induced psychosis, susceptibility to infections, and electrolyte imbalance. Furthermore, there is a substantial relapse rate once steroids are discontinued, and up to 30–35% of patients have no response whatsoever. The predictors of clinical response to steroid therapy include high clinical activity score, high signal intensity on T1-weighted magnetic resonance imaging, increased orbital uptake of radiolabelled somatostatin analogs, and duration of disease. Depot subconjunctival or retro bulbar corticosteroid injections had been used by few as a mean of attaining high local concentration of drug and minimizing the systemic side effects but patient discomfort, risk associated with it and lack of benefit beyond conventional regimen limit practical utility of this approach.

In patients not responding to glucocorticoid therapy or relapsing following stoppage or tapering of glucocorticoid, steroid sparing agents, i.e., immunosuppressant's drugs like cyclosporine, azathioprine, cyclophosphamide, and methotrexate have been used with moderate success. Cyclosporine inhibits helper T-cell proliferation and cytokine production prevent cytotoxic T-cell activation and suppresses immunoglobulin production by B lymphocytes. Recurrence was seen only in 5% of the patient given both steroid and cyclosporine as compared to almost in 50% of patients in prednisolone group only. In another study, prednisolone was found to be superior to cyclosporine as a single agent but nearly 60% of the patients who did not respond to either drug alone showed response with combination therapy.[32] Other drugs like low dose treatment with methotrexate, azathioprine, and cyclophosphamide have been tried with some success, however, all these drugs have yet to prove their efficacy.[33] Presently, immunosuppressive therapy is to be used only in conjunction with steroid therapy in patients not responding to steroid therapy or who are relapsing while on maintenance dosage of steroid or as steroid sparing agent to minimize side effects associated with long-term steroid therapy.

Other Medical Therapies

Additional therapies like somatostatin analog, intravenous immunoglobulin, anti-ß cell therapy (rituximab), and pentoxifylline have been tried with no clear benefit over conventional steroid therapy and the number of the patients studies with these were too small to draw a definite conclusion.[28,34,35]

Rituximab is a human/murine chimeric monoclonal antibody that targets CD20, a transmembrane protein expressed on the surface of pre-B and mature B lymphocytes.[36] Beta cells are highly efficient antigen-presenting cells and preliminary work has shown that blocking the CD20 receptor on B-lymphocytes with rituximab affects the clinical course of TAO, by reducing inflammation and the degree of proptosis. Salvi et al.,[37] in a double-blind, randomized trial, compared rituximab with intravenous methylprednisolone in patients with active moderate to severe Graves' orbitopathy (GO) and concluded that rituximab is associated with better therapeutic outcome as compared to with iv methylprednisolone, even after a lower rituximab dose. The better eye motility outcome, visual functioning of the quality of life assessment, and the reduced number of surgical procedures in patients after rituximab seem to suggest a disease-modifying effect of the drug. Stan et al.,[38] in a prospective, randomized, double-masked, placebo-controlled trial, studies the effect of two rituximab infusions (1,000 mg each) given 2 weeks apart in 25 patients with active moderate to severe GO. The authors concluded that rituximab offered no additional benefit over placebo in patients with active and moderate to severe GO. So, currently there is insufficient evidence to support the use of rituximab in patients with TAO and there is a need for a large randomized control trials, investigating rituximab versus placebo or corticosteroids in patients with active TAO to make adequate judgment on the efficacy and safety of this novel therapy for this condition.

Orbital Radiotherapy

The rationale for use of radiation therapy for TAO is that lymphocytes which are primarily involved in pathogenesis are extremely radiosensitive. The usual dose for treatment of the retro-orbital area is 2,000 rads (20 Gy) given in equally divided 10 doses over two weeks by lateral ports angled 5 degrees posteriorly to prevent radiation to anterior chamber and retina.[39] The beneficial effect start appearing within 1–4 weeks and can continue for as long as one year after the completion. However, the value of orbital radiation remains controversial and in a meta-analysis of three trials, orbital radiation was no better than sham radiation for improvement in clinical activity score, though it was better for diplopia. Trials of combined radiation and glucocorticoid therapy have suggested that the combination may be more effective than either alone.[40] Potential side effects include temporary hair loss of the temples, transient worsening of soft tissue changes and uncommonly cataract, mild retinopathy, and transient blindness due to injury to the optic nerve.[41]

Surgical Management of Thyroid-associated Orbitopathy

Approximately 5% of patients with TAO may require surgical intervention. Unless compressive optic neuropathy or severe corneal exposure is present, surgery is generally delayed during the active inflammatory phase of TAO and is usually performed during the quiescent cicatricial phase of the disease. The two major indications for orbital decompression surgery in active disease includes failure of glucocorticoid therapy, rituximab, or orbital irradiation to halt progression of the ophthalmopathy and when there is immediate threat to vision either by ulceration or infection of the cornea or by changes in the retina or optic nerve.[25,28] The orbit may be decompressed by removing the lateral wall, the roof, or the medial wall and the floor and excellent results are seen with substantial reduction in proptosis and edema. However, diplopia usually does not improve and may worsen, so that eye muscle surgery is almost always needed later.

During chronic quiescent phase of the disease surgery is indicated for marked proptosis, strabismus, and lid deformity. It is beyond the scope of this article to discuss the different methods of eye muscle surgery in treating TAO but if the patient has marked proptosis, strabismus, and lid deformity, then the sequence of surgery is very important. First surgery to be performed is orbital decompression followed by strabismus surgery followed by lid-lengthening surgery and lastly blepharoplasty.

CONCLUSION

Thyroid-associated orbitopathy is a self-limiting autoimmune disease associated with dysthyroidism but mainly hyperthyroidism. Proper management of TAO requires multidisciplinary team approach with therapeutic options like local supportive measures, corticosteroids, external beam radiation, and steroid-sparing immunosuppressive agents for reducing the inflammation during active disease, and surgery for correcting the residual abnormalities secondary to fibrosis in the inactive state of the disease. Despite availability of various drugs and surgical options, much needs to be explored about is exact pathogenesis and optimal treatment.

REFERENCES

1. Ing E, Abuhaleeqa K. Graves' ophthalmopathy (thyroid-associated orbitopathy). Clin Surg Ophthalmol. 2007;25:386-92.
2. Prabhakar BS, Bahn RS, Smith TJ. Current perspective on the pathogenesis of Graves' disease and ophthalmopathy. Endocr Rev. 2003;24:802-35.
3. Wiersinga WM, Bartalena L. Epidemiology and prevention of Graves' ophthalmopathy. Thyroid. 2002;12:855-60.
4. Burch HB, Wartofsky L. Graves' ophthalmopathy: Current concepts regarding pathogenesis and management. Endocr Rev. 1993;14:747-93.
5. Bartley GB, Fatourechi V, Kadrmas EF, Jacobsen SJ, Ilstrup DM, Garrity JA, et al. The incidence of Graves' ophthalmopathy in Olmsted County, Minnesota. Am J Ophthalmol. 1995;120:511.
6. Wiersinga WM, Prummel MF. Pathogenesis of Graves' ophthalmopathy--Current understanding. J Clin Endocrinol Metab. 2001;86:501-3.
7. Frecker M, Stenszky V, Balazs C, Kozma L, Kraszits E, Farid NR. Genetic factors in Graves' ophthalmopathy. Clin Endocrinol (Oxf). 1986;25:479.
8. Perros P, Crombie AL, Matthews JN, Kendall-Taylor P. Age and gender influence the severity of thyroid-associated ophthalmopathy: a study of 101 patients attending a combined thyroid-eye clinic. Clin Endocrinol (Oxf). 1993;38:367.
9. Prummel MF, Wiersinga WM. Smoking and risk of Graves' disease. JAMA. 1993;269:479.
10. Salvi M, Zhang ZG, Haegert D, Woo M, Liberman A, Cadarso L, et al. Patients with endocrine ophthalmopathy not associated with overt thyroid disease have multiple thyroid immunological abnormalities. J Clin Endocrinol Metab. 1990;70:89.
11. Bahn RS. Understanding the immunology of Graves' ophthalmopathy. Is it an autoimmune disease? Endocrinol Metab Clin North Am. 2000;29:287.
12. Akaishi PM, Cruz AA, Silva FL, Rodrigues Mde L, Maciel LM, Donadi EA. The role of major histocompatibility complex alleles in the susceptibility of Brazilian patients to develop the myogenic type of Graves' orbitopathy. Thyroid. 2008;18:443-7.
13. Perros P, Kendall-Taylor P. Natural history of thyroid eye disease. Thyroid. 1998;8:423-5.
14. Gleeson H, Kelly W, Toft A, Dickinson J, Kendall-Taylor P, Fleck B, et al. Severe thyroid eye disease associated with primary hypothyroidism and thyroid-associated dermopathy. Thyroid. 1999;9:1115-8.
15. Bartley GB, Fatourechi V, Kadrmas EF, Jacobsen SJ, Ilstrup DM, Garrity JA, et al. Clinical features of Graves' ophthalmopathy in an incidence cohort. Am J Ophthalmol. 1996;121:284-90.
16. Werner SC. Classification of the eye changes of Graves' disease. Am J Ophthalmol. 1969;68:646-8.
17. Van Dyk HJ. Orbital Graves' disease. A modification of the "NO SPECS" classification. Ophthalmology. 1981;88:479-83.
18. Ing E, Abuhaleeqa K. Graves' Ophthalmopathy (thyroid-associated orbitopathy). Clinical and Surgical Ophthalmology. 2007;25:386-92.
19. Mourits MP, Koornneef L, Wiersinga WM, Prummel MF, Berghout A, van der Gaag R. Clinical criteria for the assessment of disease activity in Graves' ophthalmopathy: A novel approach. Br J Ophthalmol. 1989;73:639-44.
20. Dolman PJ, Rootman J. VISA Classification for Graves' orbitopathy. Ophthal Plast Reconstr Surg. 2006;22:319-24.
21. Bartalena L, Baldeschi L, Dickinson AJ, Eckstein A, Kendall-Taylor P, Marcocci C, et al. Consensus statement of the European group on Graves' orbitopathy (EUGOGO) on management of Graves' orbitopathy. Thyroid. 2008;18:333-46.
22. Eckstein A, Quadbeck B, Mueller G, Rettenmeier AW, Hoermann R, Mann K, et al. Impact of smoking on the response to treatment of thyroid associated ophthalmopathy. Br J Ophthalmol. 2003;87:773-6.
23. Prummel MF, Wiersinga WM, Mourits MP, Koornneef L, Berghout A, van der Gaag R. Effect of abnormal thyroid function on the severity of Graves' ophthalmopathy. Arch Intern Med. 1990;150:1098-101.
24. Azzam I, Tordjman K. Clinical update: treatment of hyperthyroidism in Graves' ophthalmopathy. Pediatr Endocrinol Rev. 2010;7 Suppl 2:193-7.
25. Bartalena L, Marcocci C, Bogazzi F, Panicucci M, Lepri A, Pinchera A. Use of corticosteroids to prevent progression of Graves' ophthalmopathy after radioiodine therapy for hyperthyroidism. N Engl J Med. 989;321:1349-52.
26. Bartalena L, Pinchera A, Marcocci C. Management of Graves' ophthalmopathy: reality and perspectives. Endocr Rev. 2000;21:168-99.
27. Bartalena L, Marocci C, Bogazzi F, Bruno-Bossio G, Pinchera A. Glucocorticoid therapy of Graves' ophthalmopathy. Exp Clin Endocrinol. 1991;97:320-7.
28. Stiebel-Kalish H, Robenshtok E, Hasanreisoglu M, Ezrachi D, Shimon I, Leibovici L. Treatment modalities for Graves' ophthalmopathy: systematic review and metaanalysis. J Clin Endocrinol Metab. 2009;94:2708-16.
29. Nagayama Y, Izumi M, Kiriyama T, Yokoyama N, Morita S, Kakezono F, et al. Treatment of Graves' ophthalmopathy with high-dose intravenous methylprednisolone pulse therapy. Acta Endocrinol. (Copenh). 1987;116(4):513-8.

30. Kahaly GJ, Pitz S, Hommel G, Dittmar M. Randomized, single blind trial of intravenous versus oral steroid monotherapy in Graves' orbitopathy. J Clin Endocrinol Metab. 2005;90:5234-40.
31. Marinò M, Morabito E, Brunetto MR, Bartalena L, Pinchera A, Marocci C. Acute and severe liver damage associated with intravenous glucocorticoid pulse therapy in patients with Graves' ophthalmopathy. Thyroid. 2004;14:403-6.
32. Prummel MF, Mourits MP, Berghout A, Krenning EP, van der Gaag R, Koornneef L, et al. Prednisone and cyclosporine in the treatment of severe Graves' ophthalmopathy. N Engl J Med. 1989;321:1353-9.
33. Smith JR, Rosenbaum JT. A role for methotrexate in the management of non-infectious orbital inflammatory disease. Br J Ophthalmol. 2001;85:1220-4.
34. Bartalena L. What to do for moderate-to-severe and active Graves' orbitopathy if glucocorticoids fail? Clin Endocrinol (Oxford). 2010;73:149-52.
35. Krassas KE, Dumas A, Pontikides N, Kaltsas T. Somatostatin receptor scintigraphy and octreotide treatment in patients with thyroid eye disease. Clin Endocrinol (Oxf). 1995;42:571-80.
36. El Fassi D, Nielsen CH, Hasselbalch HC, Hegedüs L. The rationale for B lymphocyte depletion in Graves' disease. Monoclonal anti-CD20 antibody therapy as a novel treatment option. Eur J Endocrinol. 2006;154:623.
37. Salvi M, Vannucchi G, Currò N, Campi I, Covelli D, Dazzi D, et al. Efficacy of B-cell targeted therapy with rituximab in patients with moderate to severe Graves' orbitipathy: A radomized controlled study. J Clin Endocrinol Metab. 2015;100(2):422-31.
38. Stan MN, Garrity JA, Carranza Leon BG, Prabin T, Bradley EA, Bahn RS. Randomized trial of rituximab in patients with Graves' orbitopathy. J Clin Endocrinol Metab. 2015;100(2):432-41.
39. Bartalena L, Marcocci C, Pinchera A. Orbital radiotherapy for Graves' ophthalmopathy. J Clin Endocrinol Metab. 2004;89:13-4.
40. Ng CM, Yuen HK, Choi KL, Chan MK, Yuen KT, Ng YW, et al. Combined orbital irradiation and systemic steroids compared with systemic steroids alone in the management of moderate-to-severe Graves' ophthalmopathy: a preliminary study. Hong Kong Med J. 2005;11:322-30.
41. Marcocci C, Bartalena L, Rocchi R, Marino M, Menconi F, Morabito E, et al. Long term safety of orbital radiotherapy for Grave's ophthalmopathy. J Clin Endocrinol Metab. 2003;88:3561-6.

CHAPTER 14

Juvenile Hypothyroidism

Puthezhath SN Menon, Madhava Vijayakumar

INTRODUCTION

In children, deficiency of thyroid hormone is much more commonly observed than hyperfunction of the thyroid. Hypothyroidism may manifest at birth or many years later. In older children, most cases are asymptomatic and abnormal thyroid function tests detected during evaluation are often the only indication for starting treatment. Many require prolonged or even lifelong treatment.[1]

HISTORICAL PERSPECTIVES

Hypothyroidism is an ancient disease. Endemic goiter and cretinism were prevalent in many parts of the world for more than 3000 years as depicted by ancient sculptors of goitrous dwarfs and in ancient Egyptian paintings. In comparison, sporadic goiter is a relatively new disorder, with various descriptions in the 18th and 19th century medical textbooks. Cretinism and goiter were noted in Alpine regions in 16th century, but was first described in detail in England in 1871.[2] Treatment with thyroid extract began in early 20th century in Europe first by injections and later by oral extracts, before more refined preparations became available.[3,4] Chronic autoimmune thyroiditis (Hashimoto's thyroiditis) was described for the first time in 1912.[5] Edward Kendall isolated thyroxine (T4) in crystalline form in 1912 leading to later elucidation of its structure.[6] The observation that circulating triiodothyronine (T3) is derived mainly from peripheral monodeiodination of T4 was noted in 1970.[7] The genes for the β-subunit of thyroid stimulating hormone (TSH) and TSH receptor were cloned in 1988 and 1989, respectively, paving the way for elucidation of genetic abnormalities leading to hypothyroidism.[8] The knowledge thus generated culminated in the introduction of neonatal screening and early treatment of congenital hypothyroidism.[9]

EPIDEMIOLOGY

Hypothyroidism is seen in around 0.3% of school-going children. The average age at presentation to a physician before the introduction of newborn screening was around 4 years as shown in a study from North India.[10] Subtle signs and symptoms of congenital hypothyroidism are often missed by parents; and children are detected as hypothyroid at a later age in underdeveloped countries where newborn screening is not universally available. Proportionate short stature is the common initial reason for referral. Dysgenesis and ectopia account for most children with late onset congenital hypothyroidism in both iodine-deficient and iodine-sufficient areas.[11,12] Euthyroid goiter is a common presentation at this age. Subclinical hypothyroidism is seen in about 2% of older children and adolescents. There is a striking female predilection with a female to male ratio of 2:1.[13] Chronic lymphocytic goiter is the commonest type of juvenile hypothyroidism.

ETIOLOGY

Box 1 lists the common causes of juvenile hypothyroidism. Juvenile hypothyroidism may result from various congenital or acquired defects in T4 production. Even with excellent neonatal screening facilities, some cases of congenital hypothyroidism due to ectopic or dysgenetic thyroid gland, and some cases of inborn errors of T4 metabolism (dyshormonogenesis) often escape detection during neonatal period and become symptomatic at a later age.[11] Hypothyroidism can also result from surgical removal of thyroid tissue, irradiation of thyroid gland, iodine deficiency and ingestion of goitrogenic substances. Certain infiltrative diseases (e.g., histiocytosis) can also lead to hypothyroidism at a later age. In critically ill children, hypothyroidism may occur as a progression of non-thyroidal illness state.[14]

Box 1: Causes of juvenile hypothyroidism

- Congenital hypothyroidism, late onset
  - Ectopic thyroid
  - Dysgenesis (hypoplasia)
  - Dyshormonogenesis
- Acquired primary hypothyroidism
  - Autoimmune thyroiditis
  - Autoimmune polyglandular syndromes
  - Hypothyroidism associated with type 1 diabetes mellitus
  - Hypothyroidism associated with chromosomal syndromes: Down syndrome, Klinefelter syndrome, Turner syndrome, Williams syndrome
- Endemic goiter: Iodine deficiency
- Drug-induced hypothyroidism: Amiodarone, aminoglutethimide, anticonvulsants (phenobarbitone, phenytoin, valproate), antithyroid drugs (methimazole, propylthiouracil), iodine-containing cough syrups, lithium, thalidomide
- Environmental goitrogens: Cassava, sweet potato, broccoli, cabbage, cauliflower
- Removal of thyroid: Irradiation, thyroid surgery, radioiodine
- Systemic infiltrative diseases: Cystinosis, histiocytosis
- Nonthyroidal illness syndrome (euthyroid sick syndrome)
- Hypothalamic and pituitary disorders (central hypothyroidism)
  - Multiple pituitary hormone deficiencies: Transcription factor defects involving *PIT1*, *PROP1*, *LHX3*, or *HESX1* genes
  - Isolated thyrotropin-releasing hormone deficiency
  - Tumors: Craniopharyngioma, meningioma
  - Infections: Meningoencephalitis, tuberculosis, toxoplasmosis
  - Cranial irradiation
  - Head trauma
  - Malignancies: Leukemia
  - Inflammatory disorders: Sarcoidosis
  - Iron deposition: Hemolytic anemia (thalassemia), hemochromatosis

Hypothyroidism resulting from either pituitary (secondary hypothyroidism) or hypothalamic (tertiary hypothyroidism) hormone deficiencies is collectively termed as central hypothyroidism. In this group of diseases, there are often other pituitary or hypothalamic hormone deficiencies as well.[15]

AUTOIMMUNE THYROIDITIS

Autoimmune thyroiditis (AIT) is the most common cause of hypothyroidism in older children and adolescents.[16,17] It is also the most common cause of acquired hypothyroidism at any age. Autoimmune thyroiditis is characterized by lymphocytic infiltration of thyroid gland and also by the presence of antibodies against thyroperoxidase (TPO) and thyroglobulin (TG). Even though it is reported in children younger than 3 years, its incidence increases exponentially after 6 years and reaches its peak in adolescence.[18]

Etiology

Autoimmune thyroiditis is influenced by genetic factors as indicated by high incidence in twins, siblings (20-fold increase) and children of affected parents (30-fold increase). This shows the importance of screening for antithyroid antibodies in family members of patients with AIT for early detection of thyroid dysfunction. Genetic etiology is described in around 75% of cases with environmental factors acting as triggering agents. Both antibody-mediated and cell-mediated injuries damage the thyroid. Autoimmune thyroiditis commonly affects adolescents with girls being affected four times more common.

Immunopathogenesis

Autoimmune thyroiditis is one of the most common organ-specific autoimmune diseases. Defects in the cell-mediated immune mechanism are of paramount importance in causing cell damage and death. Activated T-helper (CD4+) cells react with thyroid antigens leading to both T-helper 1 (Th1) and T-helper 17 (Th-17) responses resulting in release of various cytokines which help in leukocyte migration as well as increased secretion of complement factors and other mediators. The thyroid cells are damaged as a consequence of apoptosis combined with T-cell mediated cytotoxicity. In addition to cell-mediated immune mechanisms, AIT is characterized by the secretion of antibodies to various antigens of thyroid origin of which most important are TPO, TG, and TSH receptor. Measurement of the antibodies to TPO and TG are used in the diagnosis of AIT and is closely related to disease activity. Anti-TSH receptor antibodies of the blocking type may contribute to hypothyroidism in a minority of adults with the atrophic AIT, but this has not been proven in children. However, their measurement in adolescent girls serves as a marker of development of transient congenital hypothyroidism in the offspring. Antibodies against sodium-iodide symporter (NIS), pendrin, T4 and T3 are also produced.[19]

The characteristic histological features include diffuse lymphocytic infiltration, atrophic follicles, and fibrosis. The gland of atrophic thyroiditis is small, with lymphocytic infiltration and fibrous replacement of the parenchyma.

Genetic analysis has identified several genes responsible for occurrence, progression and severity of AIT including human leukocyte antigens (HLA-DR), CD40, CTLA-4 (cytotoxic T-lymphocyte antigen-4), PTPN-22 (protein tyrosine phosphatase non-receptor-22), TG, and TSH receptor.[16,20]

Environmental factors triggering the autoimmune process include iodine excess, smoking, stress, low selenium, irradiation, pollution, and infections. Some drugs such as interferon-α, interleukin-2, lithium, and amiodarone as well as drugs used in the treatment of human immunodeficiency virus (HIV) infection trigger an immune response. Various infectious agents implicated in this disorder include *Helicobacter pylori, Borrelia burgdorferi, Yesinia enterocolitica*, retroviruses, coxsackievirus and hepatitis C virus (HCV). Many environmental industrial pollutants have thyroid disrupting properties. These include hydrocarbons, fluorinated chemicals, phthalates, and bisphenol-A. Radiation exposure is also a triggering agent for inducing thyroid autoantibodies. Evidence suggests that environmental factors trigger an immune process in genetically susceptible children.[21]

Course and Evolution

Box 2 describes the various modes of clinical presentations of autoimmune hypothyroidism in young children. At diagnosis, some children and adolescents with AIT may be asymptomatic. Autoimmune thyroiditis in children usually presents in two different clinical types. Majority turns up with thyroid enlargement (Hashimoto's thyroiditis); very few present with nongoitrous hypothyroidism, also called as atrophic thyroiditis or primary myxedema.[16,22] Often they are diagnosed during the work-up of growth disorders or unrelated problems or screening of high-risk groups, i.e., screening of family members. Goitrous variety is more common in young children.[23] Both are characterized by circulating autoantibodies. Patients may be euthyroid or may have subclinical or overt hypothyroidism.[24]

In some cases, they may present initially in a thyrotoxic phase. This is due to the discharge of already formed thyroid hormones from the thyroid gland; damaged by lymphocytic infiltration.[25] Rarely, it may coexist with Graves' disease, producing a hyperthyroid picture (Hashitoxicosis). Graves' disease and Hashimoto's thyroiditis share a number of common etiological factors.[18] There are few reports on monozygotic twins in whom one had Graves' disease and the other had hypothyroidism secondary to Hashimoto's thyroiditis.[26] Familial cooccurrence of Graves' disease and Hashimoto's thyroiditis is reported from India.[27] In general, younger the age of presentation, more severe is the thyroid dysfunction.

The natural history of AIT in children and adolescents is not fully known. Very few studies are there on the spontaneous evolution of the disease.[28,29] Children who initially present as euthyroid gradually deteriorate into a hypothyroid state by 3–5 years (50%) or remain as euthyroid. Presence of goiter and very high levels of anti-TPO or anti-TG antibodies are factors which may predispose to progression into a hypothyroid state. Thyroid stimulating hormone level at baseline is not a useful marker to predict disease evolution.[17,30] A similar trend is seen in children who present initially with subclinical hypothyroidism. Half of the children with subclinical hypothyroidism develop overt hypothyroidism and the remaining half will eventually become euthyroid. Elevated

Box 2: Clinical presentations of autoimmune hypothyroidism	
• Euthyroidism and goiter	• Hyperthyroidism and goiter
• Subclinical hypothyroidism and goiter	• Atrophic thyroiditis
• Hypothyroidism and goiter	

TSH at presentation is the best predictor of development of future hypothyroidism. In children presenting with initial hyperthyroidism, resolution to euthyroid state is seen on follow up (within 8 months to 1 year).[31,32]

Usually, the deterioration from euthyroid state to a hypothyroid state is an irreversible process due to progressive thyroid cell damage. However, some children may spontaneously revert to euthyroid state after several years. This effect is due to a fall in the thyroid-stimulation blocking antibodies with time.

Autoimmune Encephalitis (Hashimoto's Encephalopathy)

Hashimoto's encephalopathy is a rare complication of AIT. This is believed to be due to immunologic cross-reactivity with the brain tissue. This entity is characterized by remitting and relapsing encephalopathy, with very high levels of anti-TPO antibodies. The disease is characterized by seizures, myoclonus, tremor, decreasing level of consciousness, psychiatric manifestations (e.g., hallucinations), stroke-like symptoms, and ataxia. Around 50% of affected children have hypothyroidism, while the rest are euthyroid. Cerebrospinal fluid studies show elevated proteins with occasional pleocytosis. Electroencephalogram usually shows generalized slowing. Magnetic resonance imaging brain may be normal or show diffuse white matter abnormalities and meningeal enhancement. Most children respond well to the treatment with steroids.[33]

Associated Diseases

Autoimmune thyroiditis may be associated with other autoimmune diseases such as type 1 diabetes mellitus, Addison disease, pernicious anemia, vitiligo, alopecia, and celiac disease. Children with congenital rubella have increased prevalence of autoimmune thyroid disease. Thyroiditis may be a part of autoimmune polyglandular syndromes (APS). Hypothyroidism is associated with chromosomal anomalies such as Down syndrome, Turner syndrome, Klinefelter syndrome, and Noonan syndrome, some of which are discussed below.

Down Syndrome

Down syndrome is characterized by increased incidence of both congenital and acquired hypothyroidism.[34] It is often diagnosed late because Down syndrome by itself produces short stature and mental subnormality. Several mechanisms are postulated to explain the increased incidence of congenital hypothyroidism in this disorder. These include immaturity of hypothalamic-pituitary-thyroid (HPT) axis, inappropriate TSH secretion, TSH insensitivity, and reduced TSH bioavailability, all resulting in raised TSH and low T4 levels. Many children have mild hypothyroidism or isolated hyperthyrotropinemia (subclinical hypothyroidism). Down syndrome is also associated with high incidence of autoimmune hypothyroidism with one-third of the cases showing positive anti-TPO antibodies during adolescence with about 10% developing overt hypothyroidism. Many of these children have subclinical hypothyroidism. The autoimmune regulator gene (*AIRE-1*) located on chromosome 21 is believed to be the cause for high incidence of AIT in Down syndrome.[35]

Turner Syndrome

Around one-third of patients with Turner syndrome develop hypothyroidism and nearly half of the cases of hypothyroidism are diagnosed by less than 18 years of age. In most cases, the hypothyroidism is autoimmune in origin. It is attributed to an upregulation of proinflammatory cytokines.[36] At least 40% of children with Turner syndrome develop antithyroid antibodies and a few (10%) show features of overt hypothyroidism. The hypothyroidism appears to be less severe. A karyotype to rule out Turner syndrome should be performed if a short girl with hypothyroidism has any of the following features—hearing impairment, cardiac defects, or ovarian failure.

Type 1 Diabetes Mellitus

Autoimmune thyroiditis is the most common autoimmune disease associated with type 1 diabetes mellitus in children and adolescents. About 20% of adolescents affected with type 1 diabetes have antithyroid antibodies.[37] Girls are more frequently affected. Only a small proportion of these children develop clinical hypothyroidism. The interval between the diagnosis of diabetes and development of hypothyroidism is usually 5 years. At least one-fourth of the children and adolescents with type 1 diabetes demonstrate antithyroid antibodies during the course of illness. Autoimmune thyroiditis accompanying type 1 diabetes is associated with worse glycemic control and lipid profile as well as a lower insulin requirement.[38] When type 1 diabetes and thyroid disease coexist, the possibility of associated adrenal deficiency should be thought of. The warning clinical features are decreasing insulin requirements, increased pigmentation of skin and buccal mucosa, weakness, low blood pressure, and an unusual liking for salt. They may also present with features of acute adrenal insufficiency.

Other Diseases

Autoimmune thyroiditis is often associated with other autoimmune diseases such as celiac disease, Addison disease, alopecia or pernicious anemia. Many of the cases of hypothyroidism are subclinical with mildly elevated TSH, normal T4 or free thyroxine (FT4) levels and often positive anti-TPO antibodies.

Box 3 lists the recommendations for thyroid screening in various clinical conditions in children and adolescents.

Box 3: Recommendations for screening for thyroid disorders in various clinical conditions	

• Down syndrome
  ○ At birth
  ○ 6 months
  ○ 1 year
  ○ Every year thereafter
• Turner syndrome
  ○ 4 years or at the time of diagnosis (if diagnosed at >4 years)
  ○ Every year thereafter
	• Type 1 diabetes mellitus
	  ○ 4 years or at the time of diagnosis (if diagnosed at >4 years)
	  ○ Every year thereafter

AUTOIMMUNE POLYGLANDULAR SYNDROMES

Type 1 APS is characterized by autoimmune polyendocrinopathy, candidiasis, and ectodermal dysplasia (APECED). Autoimmune thyroiditis is seen in 10% of APS-1. This is usually seen in childhood and is caused by a mutation in the *AIRE* gene. Autoimmune polyglandular syndromes 2 consists of two entities. Carpenter syndrome is characterized by AIT and type 1 diabetes mellitus. Schmidt syndrome is a combination of AIT and Addison disease. Autoimmune thyroiditis is seen in 75% of cases of APS-2 and is usually seen in older children. Another syndrome termed as immunodysregulation polyendocrinopathy enteropathy X-linked syndrome includes AIT, diabetes mellitus, and colitis.[39]

CONGENITAL HYPOTHYROIDISM: LATE PRESENTATION

Due to the existence of universal neonatal screening program in many countries, a lion's share of congenital hypothyroidism is detected and treated in the newborn period itself. However, some newborn infants with ectopic and hypoplastic thyroid glands or inborn errors of thyroid hormone synthesis may be missed and diagnosed late in childhood or adolescence. Unilateral agenesis or hypoplasia also escapes detection in early childhood. In countries like India, where routine neonatal screening is not practiced in most states, many cases of thyroid dysgenesis go unrecognized in infancy.[10] There is a striking female preponderance with a male to female ratio of 1:2. Majority of cases are sporadic, but genetic causes have been detected in at least 2% of cases. The major mutations include those involving *TTF-1/NKX2.1, TTF2,* and *PAX8* genes.

IODINE DEFICIENCY (ENDEMIC GOITER AND CRETINISM)

All over the world, around 2 billion individuals suffer from iodine deficiency. Of these, 285 million are school-going children, indicating that about one-third of all school-going children are iodine deficient. About 25% of them reside in Southeast Asian countries. Worldwide, 40 million neonates, of whom 14 million are in India, are at risk of intellectual and developmental compromise due to iodine deficiency.

Of the total body content of 10–15 mg of iodine, nearly 75% is located in the thyroid gland of which 90% is organically bound to TG. Iodide is actively absorbed by the thyroid gland. It is oxidized to iodine and reacts with amino acid tyrosine in the TG moiety to form monoiodotyrosine (MIT) and diiodotyrosine (DIT). Monoiodotyrosine and DIT combine to form T4 and T3. Table 1 provides the currently recommended daily intake of iodine in various age groups of children.[40]

Severe iodine deficiency in pregnancy increases the chance of stillbirths, abortions, and congenital anomalies in newborn babies of which endemic cretinism is the most severe form. Three types of iodine deficiency-induced cretinism are described in children in iodine-deficient endemic areas.[40] These include hypothyroid cretinism, neurologic cretinism, and a combination of both. Milder degree of brain damage resulting in reduced cognitive capacity may affect a significant number of the population. Many children present with simple goiter which initially is diffuse and homogenous in texture but gradually become nodular. Table 2 describes the spectrum of iodine deficiency disorders associated with iodine intake with respect to mean urinary iodine concentrations.[41]

TABLE 1: Recommended daily intake of iodine in various age groups

Age group	Recommended daily intake (µg)
Up to 5 years	90
6–12 years	120
Above 12 years	150
Pregnant and lactating women	250

TABLE 2: Spectrum of iodine deficiency diseases associated with relation to iodine intake

Mean urinary iodine concentration (µg/L)	Deficiency status	Disease spectrum
<25	Severe iodine deficiency	• Cretinism • Goiter • Hypothyroidism
25–50	Moderate iodine deficiency	• Low intelligence quotient • Goiter • Hypothyroidism • Short stature
50–100	Mild iodine deficiency	• Goiter • Hypothyroidism

Iodine Excess

An excess intake of iodine can also result in thyroid dysfunction in children in two ways. It may precipitate AIT in susceptible individuals. It can also produce direct blockade of the gland (Wolff-Chaikoff effect). It is postulated that increased iodination of TG increases its immunoreactivity. Iodine also generates reactive oxygen metabolites.[21]

Other Nutrient Deficiencies

Selenium is a cofactor for the enzyme deiodinase and its deficiency is associated with impaired peripheral conversion of T4 to T3.[42] Iron deficiency reduces heme-dependent TPO activity and decreases the efficacy of iodine.[43] Vitamin A deficiency increases TSH stimulation and goiter through decreased vitamin A-mediated suppression of the pituitary TSH–βgene. Zinc deficiency may cause elevation of TSH especially in Down syndrome, which normalizes following zinc administration.

GOITROGENS

Goitrogens mainly act by competing with iodine for uptake by the thyroid gland. Many of them contain cyanogenic glycosides that are metabolized to thiocyanates. Examples include cassava, linseed, sorghum, and sweet potato. Others contain glucosinolates, examples being cruciferous vegetables such as cabbage, cauliflower, broccoli, turnips, and rapeseed. Soy contains flavonoids which impair TPO activity. Perchlorate, an industrial pollutant, acts as competitive inhibitor of sodium iodide symporter and disulfides reduce iodine uptake by the thyroid gland. Smoking during breastfeeding results in low iodine levels in breast milk.[44]

DRUGS CAUSING HYPOTHYROIDISM

Administration of various drugs to children may lead to hypothyroidism. The commonest among them are expectorants and nutritional supplements containing iodide. Anticonvulsants such as phenobarbitone, phenytoin, and sodium valproate often cause mild or subclinical hypothyroidism. Other drugs include lithium, tyrosine kinase inhibitors, drugs used in HIV infection such as zidovudine and stavudine, interferon-α, and thalidomide. Table 3 lists the common drugs which affect thyroid function and the mechanism involved in thyroid dysfunction.

TABLE 3: Drugs causing hypothyroidism and the mechanism of action

Drugs	Mechanisms of thyroid dysfunction
Glucocorticoids	TSH suppression, inhibition of peripheral conversion of T4
Propranolol	Inhibition of peripheral conversion of T4
Iodinated contrast agents	Inhibition of hormone synthesis and secretion
Povidone iodine	Inhibition of hormone synthesis and secretion
Amiodarone	Inhibition of peripheral conversion of T4 by inhibiting enzyme deiodinase
Phenobarbitone	Increased T4 clearance
Dopamine	TSH suppression
Opiates	TSH suppression
Benzodiazepines	Inhibition of peripheral conversion of T4
Sulfonamides	Inhibition of hormone synthesis
Furosemide	Interaction with serum binding proteins

T4, thyroxine; TSH, thyroid-stimulating hormone.

THYROID ABNORMALITIES IN CRITICALLY ILL CHILDREN

In healthy children, thyroid hormones released from the thyroid gland are T4 (90%) and T3 (10%). In circulation, only 0.03% of T4 and 0.3% of T3 are present in free forms, the remaining is bound to carrier proteins, mainly thyroid-binding globulin (TBG), thyroid-binding prealbumin and albumin. In the target cells, T4 is mainly converted to T3, which is the active form of the hormone and small amount is converted into inactive form namely reverse T3 (rT3).

During acute illness or during surgery, the level of T3 shows a decreasing trend and rT3 level shows an opposite change. This is followed by a fall in T4 levels. The rate of fall in T4 is directly proportional to the severity of illness and is often taken as a prognostic marker of the disease outcome and mortality. Thyroid stimulating hormone levels show a transient rise during the initial hours of acute illness, but as the illness becomes prolonged, TSH level gradually falls. Once the disease settles down, plasma levels of these hormones improve.

Peripheral conversion of T4 to T3 is brought about by the enzyme iodothyronine deiodinase. Abnormal action of iodothyronine deiodinase enzymes is regarded as the main reason for this change. There are three types of deiodinases, viz., D1, D2, and D3. Of these, D2 mostly converts T4 to T3 and is mainly seen in brain, pituitary gland and skeletal muscles. D3 is an inactivating enzyme which converts T4 to rT3. This enzyme is usually seen in brain and skin but is the commonest deiodinase enzyme in the fetal tissue and placenta where it protects the fetus from the damaging effects of excess T3. D1 catalyzes both these reactions. An increased activity of D3 is found in critical illness.[45] Plasma level of selenium, a mineral which is essential for peripheral deiodination, is found to be low in critical illness which adds to the abnormal function of deiodinase.

As the duration of illness gets prolonged, central suppression of HPT axis sets in resulting in low T3 and TSH. Moreover, many of the drugs used in the treatment of the illness may also alter the thyroid hormone levels. Important among these are corticosteroids, propranolol, amiodarone, barbiturates, iodinated contrast agents, dopamine, benzodiazepines, and frusemide.

These changes in thyroid hormones during illness are also called as "sick euthyroid syndrome", "nonthyroidal illness syndrome", or "low T3 syndrome". Usually these changes are transient and the hormonal levels gradually normalize as the patient recovers.[46]

CENTRAL HYPOTHYROIDISM

Central hypothyroidism is due to deficient stimulation by TSH of a normal thyroid gland. It may occur due to disorders of pituitary gland (secondary hypothyroidism) or hypothalamus (tertiary hypothyroidism).[47] Prevalence is about 1:100,000 individuals. Sex distribution is 1:1. Majority of the cases are associated with multiple pituitary hormone deficiencies associated with mutations in genes (*TRHR, POU1F1, PROP1, HESX1, SOX3, LHX3, LHX4,* and *TSHB*), craniopharyngioma, and previous irradiation for brain tumors or as a result of hematological malignancies. The hypothalamic-pituitary-growth hormone axis is highly vulnerable to radiation damage. Thyroid stimulating hormone deficiency starts to occur when radiation doses exceed 30 Gy.

Growth hormone replacement therapy in the initial phase is also recognized as a possible cause of unmasking central hypothyroidism in susceptible children.[48]

Central hypothyroidism is often missed if TSH is used as the only screening test for thyroid dysfunction. Serum TSH levels may vary from normal to subnormal.

CLINICAL PRESENTATION

The course of juvenile hypothyroidism is usually insidious. Many children present with asymptomatic goiter detected during a physical examination (e.g., Hashimoto's thyroiditis and dyshormonogenesis). Occasionally, there is a sensation of fullness in the anterior neck or mild tenderness (Fig. 1). As the disease progresses, subclinical followed by clinical hypothyroidism appears. Symptoms of hypothyroidism may be subtle, even with marked biochemical derangement. Non-goitrous variety of hypothyroidism includes primary myxedema, thyroid dysgenesis and central types of hypothyroidism.

A carefully plotted growth chart is a valuable early tool in the diagnosis of hypothyroidism. A dip in the height velocity and a mild increase in weight may be the first indication for checking thyroid hormone levels.

Unlike in congenital hypothyroidism, severe mental retardation is not a feature of acquired hypothyroidism. Some may present with subjective symptoms such as weakness, lethargy, tiredness, excessive sleepiness, cold intolerance, constipation, or

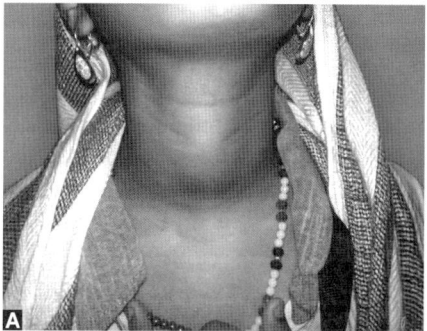
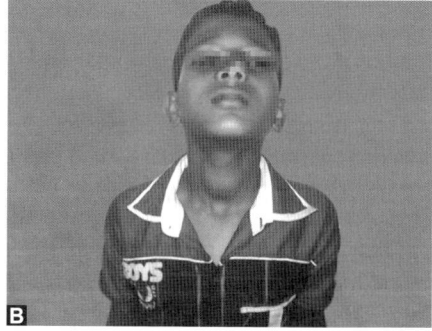

FIG. 1: A, A 10-year-old girl with autoimmune thyroiditis: note the diffuse goiter in the neck; **B,** An 11-year-old boy with autoimmune thyroiditis

dry skin. Many have mild obesity but morbid obesity is extremely uncommon. If the disease process is longstanding and of severe variety, affected children have a classical hypothyroid facies characterized by small nasal bridge and immature body proportions. Dental and skeletal maturation are delayed.

Quite a few of children with longstanding untreated primary hypothyroidism develop delayed puberty, but a few present with precocious pubertal development (Van Wyk and Grumbach syndrome).[49] They have accelerated breast development without corresponding sexual hair development. Galactorrhea (due to hyperprolactinemia) is seen in some children. Some adolescent girls experience irregular menstrual bleeding. Rarely a few manifest with abdominal distension and ovarian mass.

Unexplained anemia is a clinical feature in children and improvement occurs only after specific replacement therapy. Anemia is often the first sign of hypothyroidism and it may be microcytic, macrocytic and normocytic.[50]

Symptoms suggestive of raised intracranial tension, e.g., headache, vomiting, and visual defects, are seen in those with intracranial space occupying lesions such as craniopharyngioma.

Important findings in physical examination include bradycardia, decreased pulse pressure, short stature, delayed dentition, overweight, puffiness of face, dull facial expression, coarse hair, underdeveloped nostrils, and dry skin.

Palpation of thyroid gland is an important aspect of clinical examination. Box 4 highlights the various steps to be followed in the palpation of thyroid gland in children.

Children with Hashimoto's thyroiditis usually have thyroid enlargement with characteristic features. The gland is diffusely enlarged, non-tender, and feels firm and rubbery. Surface is classically described as pebbly (bosselated). Occasionally, asymmetric enlargement is seen. A palpable Delphian node may be noted above the isthmus. The gland is asymmetric and lobular, but nodular in one-third of cases.

Clinically palpable single thyroid nodule (>1 cm on ultrasonography) is more likely to be malignant in children. This is more likely in children who have received previous radiation therapy. Multinodular goiter is relatively rare. Table 4 describes the differentiating clinical features between AIT and malignancy (thyroid carcinoma) in children.

Delayed relaxation time of deep tendon reflexes may be seen in severe types of the disease. Muscular hypertrophy is seen in Kocher-Debre-Semelaigne syndrome along with myxedema and short stature. Maldevelopment of femoral epiphyses produces a waddling gait in long-standing congenital hypothyroidism. Table 5 lists the differentiating clinical features from late onset congenital hypothyroidism and acquired hypothyroidism.

Box 4: Steps in palpation of thyroid gland

- Patient should look up and swallow
- The movement of thyroid is visualized, the margins are marked, and size and symmetry are assessed
- As a rule of thumb, size of the gland (in grams) equals the patient's age in years multiplied by 0.5
- Thyroid is palpated best with the examiner standing behind the child and palpating the neck with fingertips
- Size, consistency (soft or firm), texture (smooth or irregular), symmetry, tenderness, and the details of any nodule are assessed
- Always palpate the regional nodes and the Delphian node situated in the isthmus
- If the thyroid gland is not palpable, search for an ectopic position, including the base of the tongue and the line of descend of thyroid gland

Central Hypothyroidism

Children with pituitary or hypothalamic disorders usually have features of other endocrine deficiencies.[47] Children with panhypopituitarism present with short stature, failure to thrive, midline defects, micropenis, delayed puberty, amenorrhea and polyuria, and have delayed skeletal maturation. Clinical features due to hypothyroidism are similar to those with primary hypothyroidism but of milder nature. In some children, growth failure may be the only manifestation. Table 6 lists the clinical features which help to differentiate central from primary hypothyroidism.

Iodine Deficiency Disorders

Adolescents in iodine deficient areas often present with thyroid enlargement. This is a marker of iodine deficiency. A total goiter rate [TGR (grade 1 and 2)] of 5% or more in 6-12 years-old school children is a public health problem. Severity of endemicity

TABLE 4: Differentiating clinical features between autoimmune thyroiditis and malignancy (thyroid carcinoma)

Clinical features	Autoimmune thyroiditis	Thyroid carcinoma
Thyroid gland	• Diffuse enlargement • Firm consistency with smooth surface • Uniform enlargement	• Solitary • Firm/hard nodule
Mobility	• Freely mobile	• Fixed to adjacent tissues
Hoarseness of voice (compression of recurrent laryngeal nerve)	• Never	• Occurs, but rare in children
Regional lymph nodes	• Not enlarged	• Enlarged

TABLE 5: Differentiating clinical features from late onset congenital hypothyroidism and acquired hypothyroidism

Clinical features	Congenital (late presentation)	Acquired (autoimmune)
Thyroid enlargement	Absent (95%)	Present (80%)
Scholastic backwardness or mental retardation	Present	Absent
Short stature	Severe	Mild
Delayed bone age	Marked	Mild
Coarse facial features	Present	Absent or mild

TABLE 6: Clinical features differentiating central from primary hypothyroidism

Clinical features	Primary hypothyroidism	Central hypothyroidism
Goiter	May be present	Absent
Features of other pituitary hormone deficiencies: Micropenis, hypoglycemia, polyuria, midline defects	Absent	May be present
Symptoms of hypothyroidism: Constipation, coarse facies, dry skin, bradycardia, cold intolerance	Present	Absent or mild involvement

TABLE 7: World Health Organization staging of goiter

Grade	Thyroid gland status
1	No palpable or visible goiter
2	Palpable goiter: A goiter that is palpable but not visible when the neck is in the normal position
3	Visible goiter: A goiter that is clearly visible when the neck is in the normal position and is consistent with an enlarged thyroid on palpation
A thyroid gland is considered as goitrous when each lateral lobe has a volume greater than the terminal phalanx of the thumbs of the subject being examined.	

is classified based on the percentage of TGR. Total goiter rate of 5–20% indicates mild endemicity, whereas 20–30% suggests moderate endemicity and more than 30% shows severe endemicity. Table 7 provides the World Health Organization's recommended staging of goiter.

Endemic cretinism is the most severe form of iodine deficiency disorder. Overlapping of clinical features is common in neurologic and myxedematous syndromes. Neurological syndrome is characterized by subnormal intelligence, deaf mutism, delayed motor development, abnormal gait, and pyramidal signs. Myxedematous syndrome is associated with myxedema, and delayed somatic and sexual development.[51]

INVESTIGATIONS

Table 8 provides the serum concentrations of T3, free T3, T4, FT4, and TSH in various age groups.[15]

Thyroid Hormones

In primary hypothyroidism, serum TSH is elevated and is the most sensitive or gold standard screening test. Recent immunometric assays using chemiluminescent reagents are very sensitive. In children with primary hypothyroidism, TSH is elevated and the

TABLE 8: Serum concentrations of T3, free T3, T4, free T4, and TSH in various age groups

Age group	T3 (ng/dL)	Free T3 (pg/mL)	T4 (µg/dL)	Free T4 (ng/dL)	TSH (µU/mL)
Cord blood	14–86	–	6.6–15	1.2–2.2	1–20
1–7 days	36–316	1.3–6.1	11–22	2.2–5.3	1–39
1–4 weeks	105–345	2.2–8.0	8.2–17	0.9–2.3	0.5–6.5
1–12 months	105–245	2.5–7.0	5.9–16	0.8–2.1	0.5–6.5
1–5 years	105–269	2.8–5.2	7.3–15	0.8–2.0	0.5–8
6–10 years	94–241	2.8–5.2	6.4–13	0.8–2.0	0.5–8
11–15 years	83–213	2.9–5.6	5.5–12	0.8–2.0	0.6–8
16–20 years	80–210	2.4–5.0	4.2–12	0.8–2.0	0.5–6

T3, triiodothyronine; T4, thyroxine; TSH, thyroid-stimulating hormone.

Source: Modified from Rivkees SA. Thyroid diseases in children and adolescents. In: Sperling MA (Ed). Pediatric Endocrinology, 4th edition. Philadelphia: Elsevier Saunders; 2014. pp. 446-7.

values range from mild elevation to higher than 1,000 μU/mL. In general, the degree of elevation correlates with severity of hypothyroidism. Children with serum levels in the range of 5–15 μU/mL have the milder form of the disease. In central hypothyroidism, TSH values are suppressed or low normal. Low serum levels of FT4 or T4 levels are seen in overt hypothyroidism, while in subclinical hypothyroidism, these levels are normal. Thyrotropin-releasing hormone (TRH) stimulation test helps to differentiate between hypothalamic and pituitary types. If T4 and T3 are elevated in the presence of elevated TSH, it indicates thyroid hormone resistance. In conditions such as nephrotic syndrome, since TBG is lost in urine, T4 levels will be low, but FT4 levels remain normal.[52] While interpreting the value of TSH, always refer to age-related cut off values. The time of blood sampling is also important because there is a nocturnal surge in TSH levels.[53]

Thyroid stimulating hormone levels are occasionally slightly increased in exogenous obesity, leading to overdiagnosis and treatment with levothyroxine (L-thyroxine). Serum T3 also shows mild elevation due to increased T4 to T3 conversion. Morbid obesity is not a usual feature of hypothyroidism and exogenous obesity causes increase in linear growth whereas hypothyroidism produces growth suppression.[54]

Thyrotropin-releasing hormone stimulation test: This is used to distinguish between secondary (pituitary) and tertiary (hypothalamic) hypothyroidism. The details are given in box 5.

Thyroid Autoantibodies

Serum levels of anti-TPO or anti-TG antibodies are elevated in AIT. Anti-TPO antibodies are the most sensitive screen for AIT, with very little benefit gained by the additional measurement of anti-TG antibodies.[55] About 90% of affected children have positive anti-TPO antibodies, but only 50% have raised anti-TG levels. When both tests are used, about 95% of affected children will demonstrate antibody positivity. Older the age, greater the chances of antibody positivity, hence the importance of repeated measurements in suspected cases. The levels decrease with long-term treatment with L-thyroxine.

Box 5: Thyrotropin-releasing hormone stimulation test

- Indication:
  - To distinguish between secondary and tertiary hypothyroidism
- Procedure:
  - A bolus dose of thyrotropin-releasing hormone (5–7 μg/kg; maximum of 200 μg) is given as intravenous bolus
  - TSH and T4 (or free T4) levels are measured at 0, 20, 40 and 60 minutes after injection
- Interpretation:
  - Pituitary dysfunction (secondary hypothyroidism): Flat (blunt) response. TSH fails to rise after TRH stimulation
  - Hypothalamic dysfunction (tertiary hypothyroidism): Delayed response. Basal TSH is slightly elevated. TSH levels are raised in all other samples but levels at 20 minutes are lower than the levels at 60 min
  - Primary hypothyroidism: Early response. TSH response is high from 20-min samples onwards (5–10 times higher than the basal value)
- Precautions:
  - Results may not be accurate in sick children (non-thyroidal illness) or severely malnourished children

TSH, thyroid-stimulating hormone; T4, thyroxine.

24-hour Urinary Iodine

In areas where iodine deficiency is prevalent, 24-hour urinary iodine measurement is a good marker of iodine intake. Twenty four hour urinary iodine more than 100 µg/L is a marker of iodine sufficiency. Iodine levels less than 25, 25–50, and 50–100 µg/L are considered as severe, moderate or mild deficiency, respectively, in a given population. Thyroid stimulating hormone levels in neonates are also used as a marker of iodine deficiency in susceptible populations. If more than 3% of neonates have elevated TSH concentration more than 5 µU/mL, then that population is iodine deficient.

Lipid Profile

Hypothyroidism results in an increase in serum cholesterol, which is largely accounted for by an increase of low-density lipoprotein cholesterol.[56]

Imaging

Radiology of the left hand is conventionally performed to assess the bone age. Bone age is very much delayed in late-onset congenital hypothyroidism. Epiphyseal dysgenesis is a classical feature of hypothyroidism in childhood and is best seen in the head of femur and humerus. In longstanding cases of congenital hypothyroidism, skull shows poorly developed base with delayed closure of fontanels resulting in a large head, widely set orbits, and a short, flat nasal bone. In addition, longstanding cases of hypothyroidism produce pituitary hypertrophy, which causes enlargement of sella turcica.[57]

Ultrasonography of Thyroid

Ultrasonography is the most useful imaging modality. It provides anatomical information of the gland whereas scintigraphy provides functional information. It is a useful investigation to diagnose dysgenesis or ectopic gland (scintigraphy is more sensitive). Inborn errors of thyroid metabolism (dyshormonogenesis) are characterized by enlarged thyroid and the lobes have a convex appearance laterally. Thyroid imaging is not essential for diagnosing AIT, but it helps to rule out thyroid nodules. Thyroid scan may be normal in the early phases of AIT. As the disease progresses, ultrasound shows characteristic diffuse, heterogeneous and coarse echotexture with multiple discrete hypoechoic nodules that may reach a diameter of 6 mm, suggestive of infiltration and fibrosis. These reduced echo levels advance as the disease progresses.[57]

Thyroid nodules are rare in children. Incidental ultrasound finding of a cyst with less than 1 cm in size probably represents degenerated follicles containing serous or colloid fluid and not a nodule. A nodule (>1 cm) with predominantly cystic appearance is usually benign. Solid nodule, calcification, and hypoechogenicity are features of malignant variety. As discussed earlier, clinically detected nodules are more likely to be malignant in children.[58]

Radioisotope Studies

Radioisotope study is rarely indicated in the evaluation of hypothyroidism in children. The main indication for a radioisotope study in children is to locate an ectopic gland or confirm agenesis (Fig. 2). It is also useful in thyroid dysgenesis and diagnosis of inborn errors of thyroid metabolism. In dyshormonogenesis, scintigraphy shows an enlarged gland in the normal position with increased isotope uptake. Normally, the isotope is

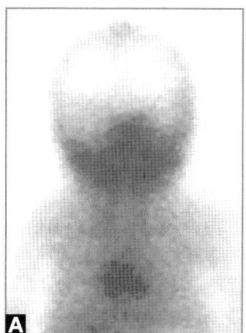 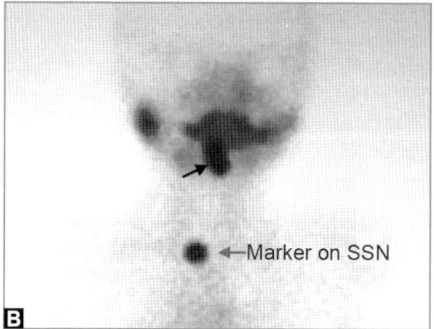

FIG. 2: A, Technetium scan showing agenesis of thyroid gland (note absence of concentration of the isotope in the neck); **B,** technetium scan showing ectopic thyroid (sublingual; note the arrows for location of suprasternal node and sublingual locations) *(For color version, see Plate 7)*

homogeneously distributed throughout both lobes of the gland. Isotope study shows marked reduction in content throughout the affected gland in AIT. The distribution of isotope is irregular and patchy. Irregular areas of relatively diminished and occasionally increased uptake are characteristic of large multinodular goiters. Thyroid nodules are described as "hot", "warm", and "cold" according to their isotope-concentrating ability relative to the surrounding normal parenchyma. Hot nodules are usually benign and cold, or hypofunctioning nodules are malignant.

Biopsy

Biopsy of the thyroid is rarely indicated in Hashimoto's thyroiditis. Prominent nodules of size more than 1 cm should undergo histologic studies.

Flowchart 1 describes the sequential algorithmic steps usually performed in a case of juvenile hypothyroidism.

MANAGEMENT

The management guidelines for congenital hypothyroidism were summarized recently.[59] L-thyroxine is the treatment of choice. It is given as a single daily dose. It should be taken on empty stomach at least 30 minutes before food intake for maximum absorption.

Rapid achievement of euthyroidism is not attempted in older children. If full dose is administered at the time of diagnosis, children generally experience undesired side effects such as irritability, restlessness, decreased attention span, insomnia, and headache. Hence, it is advised to start with a small dose (25 µg/day) for the first 2–4 weeks. The dose is gradually increased every 2–4 weeks until the maximum desired dose is attained. Thyroid stimulating hormone should be kept at lower range (0.5–2 µU/mL) and T4 at an upper range of age-related cut off. A general guideline for assessing the optimum dose of L-thyroxine is given in table 9. The rate of absorption and metabolism vary among children. Hence, optimum dosage should be determined in each child with titration of the dose with serial measurement of TSH, T4, and/or FT4. Children with central hypothyroidism require lesser dose compared to children with primary hypothyroidism.

Children should not take iron or calcium containing medications along with T4. Soy-based formula and high fiber diets also reduce the absorption of T4. Drugs such as phenobarbitone, carbamazepine, phenytoin, estrogen preparations, and rifampicin increase hepatic metabolism of T4, thus increasing its requirement.

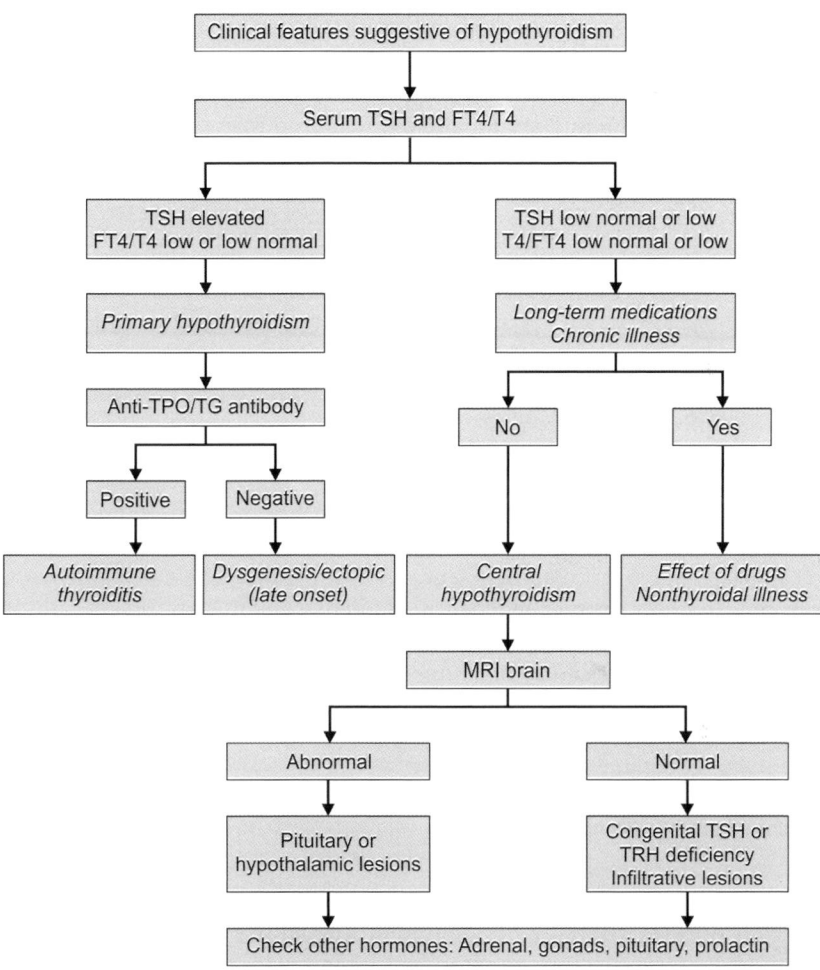

TRH, thyrotropin releasing hormone; T3, triiodothyronine; T4, thyroxine; FT4, free thyroxine; TSH, thyroid stimulating hormone; MRI, magnetic resonance imaging; TPO, thyroperoxidase; TG, thyroglobulin.

FLOWCHART 1: Approach to a case of juvenile hypothyroidism—based on laboratory evaluation

TABLE 9: Requirement of levothyroxine in different age groups

Age group	Daily dosage (µg/kg)
<6 months	6–10
6–12 months	5–8
1–5 years	4–6
5–12 years	3–5
12–18 years	2–3

Follow Up

The patient should be monitored at regular intervals with thyroid hormone levels (TSH and T4 or FT4) for titration of the dosage and for monitoring clinical improvement or development of adverse reactions. Initially, they should be monitored once in 2–4 months and later at every 6 months. Thyroid hormone levels should be repeated whenever the child becomes symptomatic in between the scheduled intervals. They should also be done 4–6 weeks after any dose change.

Majority of children with hypothyroidism require lifelong treatment. However, one-fourth of the patients with autoimmune hypothyroidism may revert to euthyroid state. T4 replacement therapy can be stopped temporarily in these children (trial off therapy) and thyroid function tests should be repeated after 4–6 weeks or earlier if the child is symptomatic. If TSH and FT4 are normal, he/she should be monitored every 3 months for a year and 6 monthly thereafter. If they are abnormal, L-thyroxine therapy should be restarted. Monitoring is required lifelong.

Local examination of the thyroid gland and regional lymph nodes should be done in each visit. Detailed anthropometry including weight, height, and body mass index is noted. Pubertal staging is noted in adolescents. Scholastic performances and psychological problems (if any) are assessed.

Central Hypothyroidism

These children are also treated with L-thyroxine. Lower doses are required compared to primary hypothyroidism. Coexisting pituitary hormone deficiencies should be treated especially glucocorticoid deficiency. Administration of T4 in a glucocorticoid-deficient child without proper glucocorticoid replacement may precipitate adrenal crisis.[60] These children should be periodically reviewed for improvement in clinical parameters. Thyroid stimulating hormone has no value in the follow up unlike in primary hypothyroidism. Free T4 should be measured and the dose of T4 is adjusted in such a way that FT4 level is in the upper limit of reference range.

Subclinical Hypothyroidism (Isolated Hyperthyrotropinemia)

In this situation, TSH levels are high but T4 (or FT4) levels are normal. In most cases, it is transient or a benign self-limiting process and only follow-up is required. However, children with positive antibody (autoimmune thyroiditis) may develop overt hypothyroidism; hence, require close monitoring. Children with Down syndrome have high incidence of subclinical hypothyroidism. Treatment, however, remains controversial.[61] A recent United States consensus statement recommends observation in patients with TSH levels below 10 µU/mL, regardless of the antibody titers.[62] When the signs and symptoms suggestive of hypothyroidism are present, they should be put on L-thyroxine.[61,63,64]

Isolated Hypothyroxinemia

This condition is common in premature children. Rarely does it occur in older children. Prader-Willi syndrome is an example and is believed to be due to hypothalamic dysfunction. Routine L-thyroxine administration is not recommended in this condition. In children on growth hormone replacement, a mild reduction of T4 (or FT4) is common. This is due to stimulation of deiodination by growth hormone.[65] Thyroxine replacement results in early skeletal maturation and epiphyseal fusion.

Juvenile Hypothyroidism

Nonthyroidal Illness

This condition is characterized by initial fall in serum T3 levels. When the primary disease is prolonged, fall in T4 and TSH occurs with thyroid function tests resembling that of central hypothyroidism. T4 replacement is not advocated in this condition, and the thyroid hormone levels become normal on recovery from the primary illness. Similar abnormal thyroid function results are seen in adolescents with anorexia nervosa.

Surgical Treatment

Surgical removal of the thyroid gland is indicated in case of thyroid malignancy or if the gland shows some compressive symptoms like dysphagia, chocking spells, dyspnea, or hoarseness of voice.

CASE SCENARIOS

CASE 1

A 9-year-old girl was brought with history of attaining menarche 2 weeks back. She was noticed to have progressive weight gain for the past 3 years along with significant breast enlargement at the same time; but this was not given much importance by parents.

Examinations

Examination revealed a short girl with puffy eyelids and a dull facial expression. Her weight was 32 kg (around 75th centile) with height 112 cm (<3rd centile) and body mass index (BMI) 25.6 kg/m² (90th centile). The heart rate was 74/min and blood pressure 90/60 mmHg. She had a thyroid swelling which was diffuse, firm and nontender with smooth surface (Fig. 3). The breast development corresponded to stage 4. Pubic and axillary hairs were absent (Tanner stages P1 and A1, respectively). Abdominal examination revealed vague masses of size 4 × 5 cm on both lumbar regions, which were nontender, nonfluctuating, and mobile.

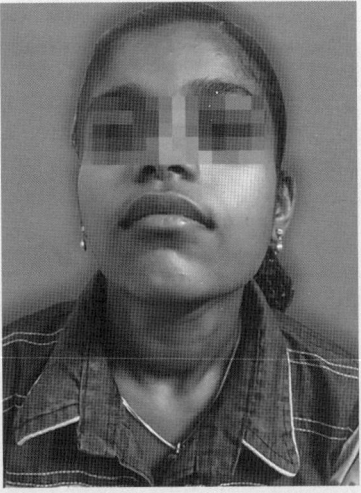

FIG. 3: Girl with short stature and thelarche. Goiter and ovarian masses: Van Wyk Grumbach syndrome

Investigations

Investigations showed normocytic normochromic blood picture with hemoglobin 9 g/dL. Bone age was delayed and was corresponding to 5 years. Thyroid function tests revealed low serum T4 (4.1 µg/dL) and elevated serum TSH (>100 µU/mL). The anti-TPO antibody levels were high (280 IU/mL) with luteinizing hormone (LH) levels 0.09 IU/L, follicle-stimulating hormone (FSH) 5.8 IU/L and estradiol 71 pg/mL. Ultrasound of abdomen showed bilateral enlarged ovaries (left measuring 16 × 12.5 × 8 cm and right 17 × 10 × 9.5 cm) with multiple cysts, each of which had size of 2–3 cm (Fig. 4). Uterus was enlarged (7.8× 4 cm) with endometrial thickness of 11 mm.

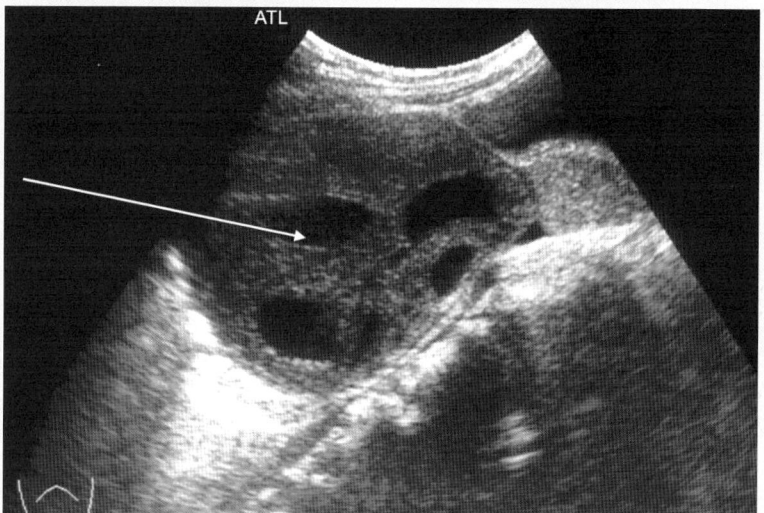

FIG. 4: Ultrasound of the abdomen showing ovarian enlargement with multiple cysts

She was started on L-thyroxine in a dose of 25 µg/day. Dose was gradually increased every 3–4 weeks. Currently, she is on L-thyroxine 100 µg/day. Her height showed a good increment; present height after 1 year is at 10th centile. Her weight showed gradual reduction initially, but stabilized at 28 kg (at 50th centile). She did not report any more menstrual bleeds. Her scholastic performance has improved now. Uterus and ovarian follicles showed reduction in size in a repeat ultrasound taken 6 months after initiation of treatment.

Discussion

Primary hypothyroidism is characterized by delayed linear growth and puberty. Rarely, this condition is associated with pseudoprecocious puberty. This condition was described in detail by Van Wyk and Grumbach in 1960 and hence known as Van Wyk and Grumbach syndrome.[66] The constellation of symptoms includes hypothyroidism with delayed linear growth and bone age with precocious puberty (thelarche and menarche, but delayed pubarche). Bilateral ovarian masses or cysts are often palpable.[67] These symptoms regress once the patient is treated with L-thyroxine. There are many postulations about the cause of this condition; the most accepted is that TSH acts on FSH receptor since it shares a common β subunit with FSH, LH, and human chorionic gonadotropin. Early clinical suspicion and prompt management prevent unnecessary surgical interventions in many girls.

CASE 2

A 10-year-old girl was brought for evaluation of short stature. She was the second child of nonconsanguineously wed couple with a birth weight of 2,800 g. Her milestones were delayed with head control attained at 6 months, sitting at 8 months, standing at 1 year and walking at 1½ years. Language development was also delayed and her academic performance was poor. She was shown to a pediatrician when she was 1 year of age with history of constipation and developmental delay; but unfortunately thyroid function tests done at that time were reported as normal with total T4 7 µg/dL and TSH 5.5 µU/mL (probably a lab error). She was not evaluated for thyroid dysfunction later even though she was a frequent visitor in the pediatric clinic.

Examinations

Examination revealed dysmorphic facial features (Fig. 5A). She had puffy eyelids and an expressionless facies. On anthropometry, her height was 108 cm (<3rd centile), weight 30 kg (between 50 centiles and 75 centiles) and BMI at 90th centile. Upper segment/lower segment ratio slightly higher (1.1:1) compared to chronological age. There was no visible thyroid swelling. Tanner staging was prepubertal.

Investigations

Investigation revealed normocytic normochromic anemia with hemoglobin 9.2 g/dL. Bone age was markedly delayed (3 years). Other routine investigations were unremarkable. Her thyroid functions showed an elevated serum TSH (150 µU/mL) and low total T4 (4.6 µg/dL). Ultrasound evaluation did not demonstrate thyroid tissue in the neck. Radioisotope study revealed a sublingual thyroid (Fig. 6). She was put on L-thyroxine at a small dose (25 µg/day) and was titrated up. She is on 125 µg of T4 now and showed good acceleration of height velocity. Her facial appearance also showed marked improvement (Fig. 5B). But she continues to be poor at her studies, especially in mathematics.

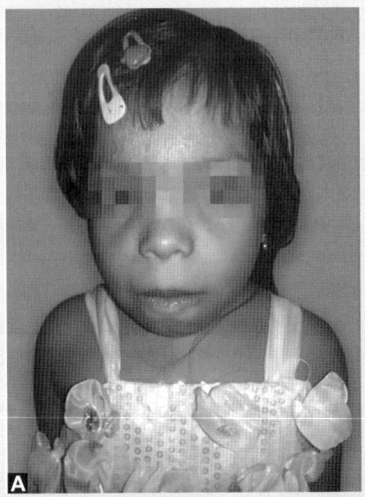 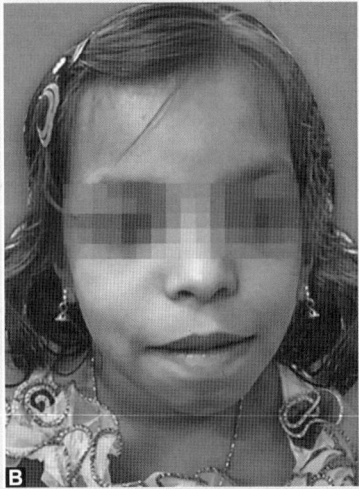

FIG. 5: A, A clinical photograph of a 10-year-old girl with congenital hypothyroidism due to ectopic thyroid. Note the dysmorphic facial features, depressed nose, puffy eyelids and edematous facial appearance; **B,** The same girl 1 year after treatment with L-thyroxine. Note the disappearance of facial edema and the puffiness around the eyelids.

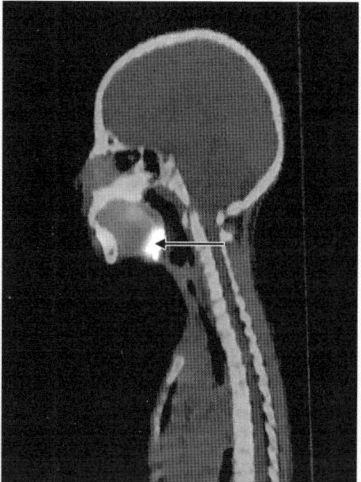

FIG. 6: Single-photon emission computed tomography image (after administration of technitium) showing a focal nodular area in the posteroinferior aspect of the tongue with intense uptake of tracer (arrow) *(For color version, see Plate 7)*

Discussion

Since India lacks a universal thyroid screening program, many cases of congenital hypothyroidism are missed in the newborn period and present late with developmental delay, mental retardation, poor scholastic performance, or short stature. These include cases of partial agenesis and ectopic thyroid glands. Nonreliable laboratory testing in peripheral centers add to the problem. We recommend that thyroid function test should be done (more than once) in any case of developmental delay, poor scholastic performances and short stature where there is a high index for the suspicion of hypothyroidism.

CONCLUSION

Thyroid dysfunction is a common endocrine problem in children. Clinical features of hypothyroidism are often subtle and nonspecific; hence, many cases will be missed or diagnosed late. Autoimmune thyroiditis constitutes the commonest autoimmune disorder affecting children and is the most common cause of thyroid swelling in this age group. Unfortunately, many cases are diagnosed as "puberty goiter" and left alone. Thus, a high index of clinical suspicion is essential for early diagnosis and proper management. All cases need lifelong follow up and titration of the drug dose based on thyroid hormone levels.

REFERENCES

1. Brent GA, Weetman AP. Hypothyroidism and Thyroiditis. In: Melmed S, Polonsky KS, Larsen R, Kronenberg HM (Eds). Williams Textbook of Endocrinology, 13th edition. Philadelphia: Elsevier Saunders; 2016. pp. 416-47.
2. Fagge CH. On Sporadic Cretinism, occurring in England. Br Med J. 1871;1:279.
3. Murray GR. Note on the treatment of myxoedema by hypodermic injection of an extract of the thyroid gland of a sheep. Br Med J. 1891;2:796-7.
4. Haynes RC Jr. Thyroid and antithyroid drugs. In: Gilman AG, Rall TW, Nies AS, Taylor P (Eds). Goodman and Gilman's: The Pharmacological Basis of Therapeutics, 8th edition. New York: Pergamon Press; 1990. pp. 1361-522.

5. Hashimoto H. Zur Kenntniss der lymphomatosen Veranderung der Schilddruse (struma lymphomatosa). Arch Klin Chir. 1912;97:219-248.
6. Kendall EC. The isolation in crystalline form of the compound containing iodine which occurs in the thyroid: its chemical nature and physiological activity. Trans Assoc Am Physicians. 1915;30:420-9.
7. Braverman LE, Ingbar SH, Sterling K. Conversion of thyroxine (T4) to triiodothyronine (T3) in athyreotic human subjects. J Clin Invest. 1970;49:855-64.
8. Parmentier M, Libert F, Maenhaut C, Lefort A, Gérard C, Perret J, et al. Molecular cloning of the thyrotropin receptor. Science. 1989;246:1620-2.
9. Fisher DA. Hypothyroidism. Pediatr Rev. 1994;15:227-32.
10. Virmani A, Menon PS, Karmarkar MG, Gopinath PG, Padhy AK. Profile of thyroid disorders in a referral centre in north India. Indian Pediatr. 1989;26:265-9.
11. Shankar SM, Menon PSN, Karmarkar MG, Gopinath PG. Dysgenesis of thyroid is the common type of childhood hypothyroidism in environmentally iodine deficient areas of north India. Acta Paediatr. 1984;83:1047-51.
12. Desai M, Colaco MP, Samuel AM, Vas FE. Etiology of childhood hypothyroidism. Indian Pediatr. 1989;26:212-22.
13. Desai MP. Disorders of thyroid gland in India. Indian J Pediatr. 1997;64:11-20.
14. Zak T, Noczyńska A, Wasikowa R, Zaleska-Dorobisz U, Golenko A. Chronic autoimmune thyroid disease in children and adolescents in the years 1999-2004 in Lower Silesia, Poland. Hormones (Athens). 2005;4:45-8.
15. Rivkees SA. Thyroid diseases in children and adolescents. In: Sperling MA (Ed). Pediatric Endocrinology, 4th edition. Philadelphia: Elsevier Saunders; 2014. pp. 444-70.
16. Cappa M, Bizzarri C, Crea F. Autoimmune diseases in children. J Thyroid Res. 2011;2011:675703.
17. Wasniewska M, Salerno M, Cassio A, Corrias A, Aversa T, Zirilli G, et al. Prospective evaluation of the natural course of idiopathic subclinical hypothyroidism in childhood and adolescence. Eur J Endocrinol. 2009;160:417-21.
18. De Luca F, Santucci S, Corica D, Pitrolo E, Romeo M, Aversa T. Hashimoto's thyroiditis in childhood: presentation modes and evolution over time. Ital J Pediatr. 2013;39:8.
19. Brown RS. Autoimmune thyroiditis in childhood. J Clin Res Pediatr Endocrinol. 2013;5(Suppl 1):45-9.
20. Zaletel K, Gaberšček S. Hashimoto's thyroiditis: From genes to the disease. Curr Genomics. 2011;12:576-88.
21. La Franchi SH, Huang SA. Hypothyroidism Thyroiditis. In: Kliegmann RM, Stanton BF, Geme III JW, Schor NF (Eds). Nelson Textbook of Pediatrics, 1st South Asia edition. New Delhi: Elsevier; 2016. pp. 2665-76.
22. De Vries L, Bulvik S, Phillip M. Chronic autoimmune thyroiditis in children and adolescents: at presentation and during long-term follow-up. Arch Dis Child. 2009;94:33-7.
23. Gopalakrishnan S, Chugh PK, Chhillar M, Ambardar VK, Sahoo M, Sankar R. Goitrous autoimmune thyroiditis in a pediatric population: a longitudinal study. Pediatrics. 2008;122:e670-4.
24. Demirbilek H, Kandemir N, Gonc EN, Ozon A, Alikasifoglu A. Assessment of thyroid function during the long course of Hashimoto's thyroiditis in children and adolescents. Clin Endocrinol. 2009;71:451-4.
25. Rallison ML, Dobyns BM, Keating FR, Rall JE, Tyler FH. Occurrence and natural history of chronic lymphocytic thyroiditis in childhood. J Pediatr. 1975;86:675-82.
26. Aust G, Krohn K, Morgenthaler NG, Schröder S, Edelmann J, Brylla E. Graves' disease and Hashimoto's thyroiditis in monozygotic twins: case study as well as transcriptomic and immunohistological analysis of thyroid tissues. Eur J Endocrinol. 2006;154:13-20.
27. Desai MP, Karandikar S. Autoimmune thyroid disease in childhood: a study of children and their families. Indian Pediatr. 1999;36:659-68.
28. Gopalakrishnan S, Marwaha RK. Juvenile autoimmune thyroiditis. J Pediatr Endocrinol Metab. 2007;20:961-70.
29. Radetti G, Gottardi E, Bona G, Corrias A, Salardi S, Loche S. The natural history of euthyroid Hashimoto's thyroiditis in children. J Pediatr. 2006;149:827-32.
30. Jaruratanasirikul S, Leethanaporn K, Khuntigij P, Sriplung H. The clinical course of Hashimoto's thyroiditis in children and adolescents: 6 years longitudinal follow-up. J Pediatr Endocrinol Metab. 2001;14:177-84.
31. Thomas I. Thyroid diseases. In: Jain V, Menon RK (Eds). Case Based Reviews in Pediatric Endocrinology, 1st edtion. New Delhi: Jaypee Brothers Medical Publishers Pvt Ltd.; 2015. pp. 49-56.
32. Simon A, Zacharin M. Thyroid Disorders. In: Zacharin M (Ed). Practical Pediatric Endocrinology in a Limited Resource Setting, 2nd edition. San Diego, USA: Elsevier; 2013. pp. 69-95.
33. Lim M, Hacohen Y, Vincent A. Autoimmune encephalopathies. Pediatr Clin North Am. 2015;62:667-85.
34. King K, O'Gorman C, Gallagher S. Thyroid dysfunction in children with Down syndrome: a literature review. Ir J Med Sci. 2014;183:1-6.

35. Graber E, Chacko E, Regelmann MO, Costin G, Rapaport R. Down syndrome and thyroid function. Endocrinol Metab Clin North Am. 2012;41:735-45.
36. Aversa T, Lombardo F, Valenzise M, Messina MF, Sferlazzas C, Salzano G, et al. Peculiarities of autoimmune thyroid diseases in children with Turner or Down syndrome: an overview. Ital J Pediatr. 2015;41:39.
37. Menon PS, Vaidyanathan B, Kaur M. Autoimmune thyroid disease in Indian children with type 1 diabetes mellitus. J Pediatr Endocrinol Metab. 2001;14:279-86.
38. Korzeniowska K, Ramotowska A, Szypowska A, Szadkowska A, Fendler W, Kalina-Faska B, et al. How does autoimmune thyroiditis in children with type 1 diabetes mellitus influence glycemic control, lipid profile and thyroid volume? J Pediatr Endocrinol Metab. 2015;28:275-8.
39. Vijayakumar M. Adrenal insufficiency and polyglandular failure. In: Gupta P, Menon PSN, Ramji S, Lodha R (Eds). PG Textbook of Pediatrics, 1st edition. New Delhi: Jaypee Brothers Publishers; 2015. pp. 2345-51.
40. Melse-Boonstra A, Jaiswal N. Iodine deficiency in pregnancy, infancy and childhood and its consequences for brain development. Best Pract Res Clin Endocrinol Metab. 2010;24:29-38.
41. Andersson M, de Benoist B, Rogers L. Epidemiology of iodine deficiency: Salt iodisation and iodine status. Best Pract Res Clin Endocrinol Metab. 2010;24:1-11.
42. Schomburgh L, Köhrle J. On the importance of selenium and iodine metabolism for thyroid hormone biosynthesis and human health. Mol Nutr Food Res. 2008;52:1235-46.
43. Zimmermann MB, Köhrle J. The impact of iron and selenium deficiencies on iodine and thyroid metabolism: biochemistry and relevance to public health. Thyroid. 2002;12:867-78.
44. Laurberg P, Nohr SB, Pedersen KM, Fuglsang E. Iodine nutrition in breast-fed infants is impaired by maternal smoking. J Clin Endocrinol Metab. 2004;89:181-7.
45. den Brinker M, Joosten KF, Visser TJ, Hop WC, de Rijke YB, Hazelzet JA, et al. Euthyroid sick syndrome in meningococcal sepsis: the impact of peripheral thyroid hormone metabolism and binding proteins. J Clin Endocrinol Metab. 2005;90:5613-20.
46. Mebis L, Van den Berghe G. Thyroid axis function and dysfunction in critical illness. Best Pract Res Clin Endocrinol Metab. 2011;25:745-57.
47. Yamada M, Mori M. Mechanisms related to the pathophysiology and management of central hypothyroidism. Nat Clin Pract Endocrinol Metab. 2008;4:683-94.
48. Smyczynska J, Hilczer M, Stawerska R, Lewinski A. Thyroid function in children with growth hormone (GH) deficiency during the initial phase of GH replacement therapy - clinical implications. Thyroid Res. 2010;3:2.
49. Van Wyk JJ, Grumbach MM. Syndrome of precocious menstruation and galactorrhea in juvenile hypothyroidism. An example of hormonal overlap in pituitary feedback. J Pediatr. 1960;57:416-35.
50. Erdogan M, Kosenii A, Ganidagli S, Kulaksizoglu M. Characteristics of anemia in subclinical and overt hypothyroid patients. Endocr J. 2012;59:213-20.
51. Laurberg P. Iodine intake as a determinant of thyroid disorders in populations. Best Pract Res Clin Endocrinol Metab. 2010;24:13-27.
52. Raghupathy P. Hypothyroidism and thyroiditis. In: Gupta P, Menon PSN, Ramji S, Lodha R (Eds). PG Textbook of Pediatrics. 1st edition. New Delhi: Jaypee Publishers; 2015. pp. 2313-7.
53. Van Vliet G, Deladoëy J. Interpreting minor variations in thyroid function or echostructure. Pediatr Clin North Am. 2015;62:929-42.
54. Setian NS. Hypothyroidism in children: diagnosis and treatment. J Pediatr (Rio J). 2007;83(5 Suppl):S209-16.
55. Foley TP Jr. Mediators of thyroid diseases in children. J Pediatr. 1998;132:569-70.
56. Brenta G, Fretes O. Dyslipidemias and hypothyroidism. Pediatr Endocrinol Rev. 2014;11:390-9.
57. Hong HS, Lee EH, Jeong SH, Park J, Lee H. Ultrasonography of various thyroid diseases in children and adolescents. a pictorial essay. Korean J Radiol. 2015;16:419-29.
58. Tonacchera M, Pinchera A, Vitti P. Assessment of nodular goiter. Best Pract Res Clin Endocrinol Metab. 2010;24:51-61.
59. Leger J, Olivieri A, Donaldson M, Torresani T, Krude H, van Vliet C, et al. European Society for Paediatric Endocrinology consensus guidelines on screening, diagnosis, and management of congenital hypothyroidism. J Clin Endocrinol Metab. 2014;99:363-84.
60. Davis J, Sheppard M. Acute adrenal crisis precipitated by thyroxine. Br Med J (Clin Res Ed). 1986;292:1595.
61. Biondi B. Natural history, diagnosis and management of subclinical thyroid dysfunction. Best Pract Res Clin Endocrinol Metab. 2012;26:431-46.

62. Gharib H, Tuttle RM, Baskin HJ, Fish LH, Singer PA, McDermott MT. Consensus statement: subclinical thyroid dysfunction: a joint statement on management from the American Association of Clinical Endocrinologists, the American Thyroid Association, and the Endocrine Society. J Clin Endocrinol Metab. 2005;90:581-5.
63. Monzani A, Prodam F, Rapa A, Moia S, Agarla V, Bellone S, et al. Natural history of subclinical hypothyroidism in children and adolescents and potential effects of replacement therapy: a review. Eur J Endocrinol. 2012;168:R1-11.
64. Bona G, Prodam F, Monzani A. Subclinical hypothyroidism in children: natural history and when to treat. J Clin Res Pediatr Endocrinol. 2013;5(Suppl 1):23-8.
65. Portes ES, Oliveira JH, MacCagnan P, Abucham J. Changes in serum thyroid hormones levels and their mechanisms during long-term growth hormone (GH) replacement therapy in GH deficient children. Clin Endocrinol (Oxf). 2000;53:183-9.
66. Durbin KL, Diaz-Montes T, Loveless MB. Van Wyk and Grumbach Syndrome: an unusual case and review of the literature. J Pediatr Adolesc Gynecol. 2011;24:e93-6.
67. Sharma Y, Bajpai A, Mittal S, Kabra M, Menon PS. Ovarian cysts in young girls with hypothyroidism: follow-up and effect of treatment. J Pediatr Endocrinol Metab. 2006;19:895-900.

CHAPTER 15

Neonatal Hypothyroidism

Anjana Hulse

INTRODUCTION

Neonatal hypothyroidism is a common and preventable cause of intellectual disability. In the past 5 decades, there has been a revolution in the process of diagnosis and management of newborns with congenital hypothyroidism (CH). Neonates affected with CH may be symptom free during the first few weeks making early diagnosis impossible even for the experts in this field.[1,2] Biochemical evidence of CH appears much before clinical signs appear. Newborn screening (NBS) which is a routine in developed world has contributed not only for early detection of neonatal hypothyroidism, but also for significant reduction in disease burden associated with CH. Unfortunately in many developing countries, NBS is still not a part of preventive health screening programs leading to delayed presentation of CH as illustrated in the following case scenario.

CASE 1

An 8-week-old male infant was presented with history of poor feeding, constipation, dry skin, and hoarse cry. He was born in a district general hospital at term following a normal vaginal delivery. He weighed 2,800 g at birth and did not require resuscitation. His APGAR (Appearance, Pulse, Grimace, Activity, and Respiration) score was 8 and 10 at 1 and 5 minutes, respectively. There were no complications during pregnancy. There was no history of thyroid illnesses in the family.

Examination

On examination, the infant was failing to thrive. He weighed 2,900 g and his length was 48 cm. He had a hypothyroid facies with large protruding tongue and coarse facial features. The skin was dry. There was generalized hypotonia and an umbilical hernia. Anterior fontanel was wide open and posterior fontanel had not closed. There was hoarse cry. The baby did not fix and follow.

Investigations

Since this was a typical clinical presentation of hypothyroidism, venous samples were sent for serum thyroid stimulating hormone (TSH) and serum free T4 analysis. Serum TSH was found to be more than 100 mIU/L and serum freeT4 0.2 ng/dL. An ultrasonogram of the neck showed an absence of thyroid gland. Therefore, an isotope scan using technetium 99 was performed which showed no tracer uptake confirming thyroid agenesis.

Treatment

The infant was started on thyroxine 37.5 µg (12.9 µg/kg/day) and was followed up closely. The dose of thyroxine was titrated based on clinical features and serial monitoring of serum TSH and free T4. During the follow-up, serum free T4 was maintained in the upper normal range and serum TSH in the normal rage. Now, at the age of 1 year, the baby is able to stand with support, has a pincer grasp, makes single syllable sounds and can understand simple commands.

Discussion

This is a classic case of CH who presented late at the age of 2 months. Neonatal screening for hypothyroidism was not done in this case. Hence, the infant presented with typical clinical features of hypothyroidism. It is known that, in case of CH, if the treatment is started within the first 2 weeks, and serum free T4 maintained in the upper normal range, patients do well irrespective of the severity of the hypothyroidism.[3] In this scenario, even though the motor development at 1 year of age appears to be normal, since there was delay in starting treatment with thyroxine, the infant needs further follow-up and assessment to evaluate speech and language and intellectual abilities.

THYROID SYSTEM IN FETUS

Development of thyroid gland starts during the first trimester of gestation. The thyroid gland arises at the base of the tongue (foramen cecum). It develops from a median anlage derived from the primitive pharyngeal floor and lateral anlagen from the pharyngobranchial pouch. By 7 weeks, the median and lateral anlagen would fuse and the thyroid gland migrates to anterior neck from foramen cecum where it was formed originally. Several transcription factors (TTF1, TTF2, PROP1, PIT1, and PAX8) are involved in morphogenesis, differentiation, and migration of thyroid system. The fetal thyroid starts concentrating iodide by as early as 10 weeks. Fetal thyroid hormone synthesis requires adequate quantities of iodide. By 12 weeks, thyroxine production starts and it increase steadily. Fetal TSH increases from a low level at 12 weeks to normal level (7–10 mIU/L) by term. Following delivery, there is TSH surge in response to stress of parturition and changes in the environmental temperature. At 30 minutes postdelivery, TSH may be as high as 70 mIU/L. This TSH surge initiates increased thyroxine production during 24–48 hours following delivery. Serum TSH normalizes by 3–5 days.

Maternal placenta is impermeable to TSH. Therefore, fetal thyroid develops autonomously, independent of maternal thyroid system. However, significant amount of maternal T4 is passed to fetus throughout the pregnancy. This is evident from the fact that maternal hypothyroxinemia during the first trimester is associated with low intelligence quotient (IQ) in the child.[4]

EPIDEMIOLOGY

Incidence of CH in neonates has been reported as ranging from 1 in 2,000 to 1 in 4,000 live births. A number of epidemiological studies have reported an increase in the incidence of CH since past few decades.[5] In the United States, CH has been increasing at a rate of 3% per year.[5] In Asia, an increase of up to 10% per year has been reported.[6] Studies from United States have reported that there is difference in prevalence of CH in different ethnic groups.[6] In New Zealand, although the incidence of CH has increased, it is reported that, this is due to changes in the country's ethnic composition.[7] Increased detection rates of even milder forms of CH as well as transient CH, as a result of newborn screening programs adopted by most of the developed countries could be the reason for the increase in incidence of CH. Male to female ratio in CH is 1:2.

Box 1: Etiological classification of congenital hypothyroidism	

Primary hypothyroidism
• Dysgenesis
   ○ Aplasia
   ○ Hypoplasia
   ○ Ectopia
• Dyshormonogenesis
   ○ Defective iodide transport
   ○ Defective organification
   ○ Thyroglobulin synthesis abnormalities
   ○ Defects in deiodination
   ○ Resistance to thyroid stimulating hormone
   ○ Defect in thyroid hormone transport
• Thyroid hormone resistance
• Maternal antibodies (thyroid stimulating hormone receptor blocking antibodies)
• Maternal drugs (iodide, amiodarone, propylthiouracil, methimazole)
• Iodine deficiency
	Hypothalamic pituitary hypothyroidism (central hypothyroidism)
	• Isolated thyroid stimulating hormone deficiency, thyrotropin releasing hormone deficiency, panhypopituitarism, genetic defects (e.g., PIT1, PROP1)

ETIOLOGY

Hypothyroidism in neonates can be primary (thyroidal), secondary (pituitary), or tertiary (hypothalamus) and permanent or transient. Permanent primary CH is the commonest cause of hypothyroidism in neonates. Hence, this chapter focuses mainly on permanent primary CH in neonates. Etiological classification of CH is listed in box 1.

DYSGENESIS

Common forms of permanent primary CH include dysgenesis (80–90%) and dyshormonogenesis (10–15%). Thyroid dysgenesis represents developmental defects of thyroid gland such as absence (agenesis) or arrested migration of embryonic thyroid (ectopic) or hypoplastic thyroid gland. Ectopic thyroid can be sublingual, suprahyoid, subhyoid, suprasterna, or in the anterior mediastinum, based on the location of the thyroid tissue. Thyroid dysgenesis is usually sporadic. However, 2–3% of these cases are familial and associated with mutations in homeobox genes such as TTF1 and 2 or PAX8.[8-10] In trisomy 21, prevalence of dysgenesis is higher than in the general population. Agenesis of thyroid can be confirmed on thyroid scintigraphy or by measuring thyroglobulin levels. However, one should be aware of apparent athyreosis in cases where there is transfer of maternal TSH receptor blocking antibodies to the newborn which leads to neonatal hypothyroidism. In such cases, thyroid gland can be seen in its place on ultrasound scan.

It has been stated that first degree relatives of children with thyroid dysgenesis have increased prevalence of thyroid gland abnormalities such as thyroglossal cysts, thyroid hemiagenesis, and ectopic thyroid.[11-13] This supports the hypothesis that in some cases of thyroid dysgenesis, there could be a common genetic component with variable phenotypes.

DYSHORMONOGENESIS

Thyroid dyshormonogenesis comprises 10–15% of newborns with CH. Dyshormonogenesis results because of defects involved at various steps of thyroid hormone biosynthesis. These include defective iodide transport, defective organification, thyroglobulin synthesis abnormalities, defects in deiodination, resistance to TSH, and defect in thyroid hormone transport. Often, these defects are a result of autosomal recessive mode of inheritance.

Defect of Iodide Transport

The transport of iodide across the thyroid follicular cell membrane is the first step in thyroid hormone biosynthesis. Defect of iodide transport involves mutations in the sodium-iodide symporter. High incidence has been reported from Japan. Neonates may present with goiter, limited or absent radioiodine and pertechnate uptake, and elevated serum TSH. This condition may respond to Lugol's iodine, but treatment with L-thyroxine is preferable.

Organification Defects (Peroxidase System Defects)

Thyroid peroxidise coupling and organification defects are commonest of thyroid hormone biosynthetic defects. In thyroid follicular cells, iodide which is trapped gets rapidly oxidized and bound in organic form. Organification of iodide involves oxidation and iodination of thyroglobulin bound tyrosine to form monoiodotyrosine (MIT) and diiodotyrosine (DIT). Two DIT combine to form T4. Monoiodotyrosine and DIT one each combine to form T3. The process is catalyzed by thyroid peroxidise enzyme system. Defect in any component of this system (quantitative or qualitative defect of thyroid peroxidase or defect in generation of hydrogen peroxide) may lead to dyshormonogenesis. The defect can be diagnosed by perchlorate discharge test.

Pendred Syndrome

Pendred syndrome is an autosomal recessive condition presenting with congenital deafness and goiter. Prevalence of Pendred syndrome is unknown. It is one of the commonest causes of congenital deafness. Patients with Pendred syndrome present with goiter and euthyroidism or mild hypothyroidism during childhood. This condition may not be diagnosed in neonates unless they are in an iodine deficient environment. A mutation in the chloride iodide transport protein known as Pendrin, common to the thyroid gland and cochlea, is responsible for this condition.

Defects of Thyroglobulin Synthesis

Thyroglobulin is essential for organification. The thyroglobulin gene is located on chromosome 8. Newborns with this condition may present with goiter, increased serum TSH, low T4 levels, and absent or low levels of thyroglobulin levels.

Defects in Deiodinataion

Deficiency of the iodotyrosine deiodinase can lead to severe wastage of iodine because the nondeiodinated MIT and DIT leak out of the thyroid gland and are excreted in urine. These enzymes are present within the thyroid cells as well as peripheral tissues, and the defect may be confined to thyroid cells or peripheral tissue or both. Radioiodine uptake in this condition may be rapid and radioiodine discharge is also rapid. Genetic defects involving specific genes have been reported.

Defects in Thyroid Hormone Transport

Defects in plasma membrane transporters which facilitate passage of thyroid hormone into the cells have been reported in multiple patients. Mutations in *MCT8* gene located on X chromosome leading to CH with neurological manifestations are characteristics of this disorder (Allan-Herndon-Dudley syndrome). Clinical features include severe developmental delay, hypotonia, involuntary athetoid movements, dystonia, hyper-reflexia, and nystagmus. Biochemically this condition is characterized by elevated serum T3, low serum free T4, and mildly elevated or normal serum TSH.

RESISTANCE TO THYROID STIMULATING HORMONE

This is an autosomal dominant disorder characterized by increased serum T3 and T4 with normal or increased serum TSH. Phenotypically, these disorders can be classified as generalized resistance to thyroid hormone, pituitary resistance to thyroid hormone, and peripheral resistance to thyroid hormone. Many affected patients may be clinically euthyroid. Older children may present with some features of hypothyroidism or even thyrotoxicosis. Syndrome of attention deficit hyperactivity has been reported in a significant number of these cases. This condition may be detected in newborns on neonatal screening if their TSH is raised. No treatment is required unless growth is affected.

HYPOTHALAMIC: PITUITARY HYPOTHYROIDISM

Prevalence of central hypothyroidism in neonates is far less common than primary hypothyroidism. Prevalence is thought to be in the range of 1 in 20–30,000 newborns.[14] These newborns are not detected on neonatal screening programs which screen for increased TSH. The majority of these newborns have multiple pituitary hormone deficiencies and present with persistent jaundice, hypoglycemia, and midline defects.

Congenital TSH deficiency can occur in *PIT1*, *PROP1*, and *HESX1* mutations. *HESX1* mutation may be associated with septo-optic dysplasia. Isolated deficiency of TSH also has been reported in some familial cases.[8] Several families with autosomal recessive inheritance have been reported from Japan. Mutations in the TRH receptor gene also have been reported.

Neonates with central hypothyroidism have low serum free T4 with low or normal TSH level. When TSH deficiency is suspected, other pituitary hormones such as growth hormone and cortisol should be assessed to rule out multiple pituitary hormone deficiency. Magnetic resonance imaging of the brain with focus on pituitary and hypothalamus may through light on structural defects.

THYROID DYSFUNCTION IN PREMATURE NEONATES

Premature infants have relatively immature hypothalamo-pituitary-thyroid systems. When compared to term infants, preterm and low birth weight infants have lower TSH surge on D1 and low T4 during the first 1 week of life. Moreover, the complications of prematurity such as respiratory distress syndrome, sepsis, necrotizing enterocolitis, hypoxia, and cardiac dysfunction may affect functioning of their hypothalamic-pituitary-thyroid axis. They are prone to develop transient primary hypothyroidism and transient hypothyroxinemia of prematurity. It is important to keep in mind the possibility of transient hypothyroidism in preterm neonates who are exposed to iodide containing disinfectants for cleaning their skin in the neonatal intensive care unit. Extremely preterm infants (<28 weeks of gestation) may have very low thyroxine and may need thyroid hormone replacement for a short period of time.[8]

TRANSIENT CONGENITAL HYPOTHYROIDISM

Transient CH has been reported in about 2% neonates diagnosed by newborn screening.[15] Higher incidence is reported in some studies. The most common causes are use of lower TSH cutoffs for diagnosing CH, iodine deficiency, maternal drugs, maternal TSH receptor blocking antibodies, and excess iodine exposure. If the condition is related to maternal antibodies, it may take up to 6 months to resolve. If CH persists beyond 2 weeks of age, these neonates should be started on treatment. Here is an example of a case of transient CH.

CASE 2

A 3-week-old male infant was referred to pediatric endocrine clinic for high serum TSH (44 mIU/L) on newborn screening. He was already started on thyroxine 25 μg/day by his pediatrician without performing an etiological workup. He was born at term by normal vaginal delivery without any complications, weighing 3,100 g. He was feeding well and was gaining weight. The mother was a 26-year-old primigravida. She was on thyroxine 100 μg/day during pregnancy as she was a known case of hypothyroidism since the age of 18 years. Maternal thyroid function remained normal during pregnancy but, thyroid antibody status was not known.

Examination
On examination, the infant was well, weighed 3,500 g. Systemic examination was normal.

Investigation
Since the baby was already on thyroxine for a week, serum TSH and free T4 were repeated. Serum TSH was 25 mIU/L and serum free T4 0.6 ng/dL. Since the mother was on thyroxine, thyroid peroxidise, thyroglobulin, and thyroid receptor blocking antibody (TRAb) levels were also measured. Thyroid receptor blocking antibody levels were high. An ultrasonogram confirmed the presence of thyroid tissue in the normal anatomical position in the neck. Thyroid isotope scan was not done as the baby was already on thyroxine. Maternal antibodies were also checked. Maternal thyroid peroxidise and TRAb antibody levels were high. Furthermore, the infant was followed up closely with serial thyroid function tests (serum TSH and free T4).

Treatment
The baby was initially on thyroxine 25 μg/day. By 4 months of age, serum TSH decreased to 0.8 mIU/L and free T4 was 1.9 ng/dL. Thyroxine dose was reduced to 12.5 μg/day. Presence of TRAb and reduction in thyroxine requirement with maternal hypothyroidism confirmed the diagnosis of transient hypothyroidism in this infant. At the age of 5 months, thyroxine was stopped. The infant remained euthyroid during the follow-up over the next few months.

Discussion
Transient CH caused because of maternal blocking antibodies is rare. This diagnosis should be considered for infants with CH whose mother is hypothyroid. Maternal antibodies disappear from infant's circulation by about 4–6 months of age. Therefore, thyroid hormone replacement should be continued till the age of 4–6 months.

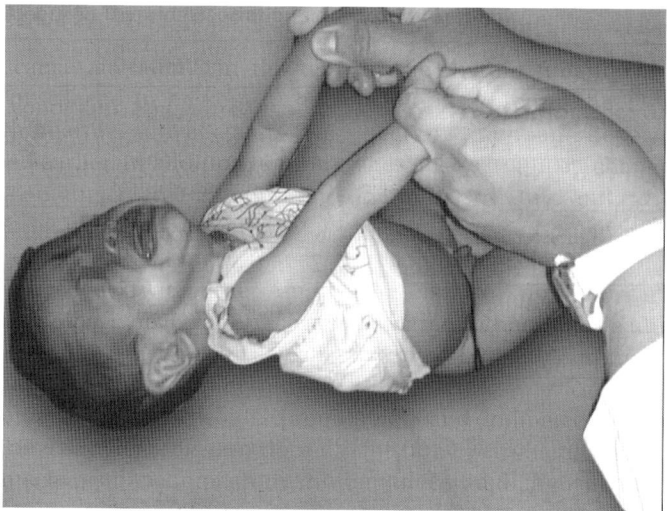

FIG. 1. Global developmental delay (note: head lag) in a 9-month-old baby with untreated congenital hypothyroidism

CLINICAL FEATURES OF CONGENITAL HYPOTHYROIDISM

Newborns with CH are often asymptomatic at birth. This may be related to transplacental passage of maternal T4 which may provide partial protection for the newborns. During early neonatal period, even for most experienced medical professionals, recognizing the subtle clinical features of CH can be difficult and challenging. Therefore, clinicians depend on newborn screening for the early diagnosis of CH. The symptoms and signs of CH in infants include failure to thrive, developmental delay, poor feeding, hoarse crying, constipation, umbilical hernia, wide fontanels, hypotonia, prolonged jaundice, and dry skin. About 10% of newborns with CH may have associated abnormalities such as cardiac anomalies, genitourinary anomalies, and hearing problems.

If CH is not diagnosed during the first 2-3 weeks or untreated, it may lead to irreversible consequences on developing brain. Untreated infant will develop severe stunting of growth and typical hypothyroid face with coarse facial features, depressed nasal bridge, swollen eyelids, large protruding tongue, and coarse brittle hair. Skin may be dry and scaly. Global developmental delay becomes more and more evident later in infancy (Fig. 1).

INVESTIGATIONS

Neonatal Screening

Newborn screening has now become universal in most of the developed countries. The fact that, CH is difficult to diagnose clinically in a newborn and if untreated can lead to irreparable damage, makes it an ideal condition for screening in preventive health screening programs. Newborn screening started in United States in 1960s, initially for phenylketonuria and later for CH and many other disorders. Pilot screening program for CH was started in Quebec (Canada) and Pittsburgh (Pennsylvania) in 1974. Later on, NBS was adopted by various countries.[16]

Newborn screening is a simple method wherein few drops of blood are collected from newborns by heel prick method on a filter paper (Guthri card) and analyzed. The best time to collect the blood sample in neonates is at 3–5 days of age. Samples obtained too early (on day 1 or 2) may give a false positive results because of postnatal physiological TSH surge. However, these days, since the families are opting for early discharge of mother and newborn (in the absence of any medical complication), cord blood sample could be used to measure TSH. The TSH cutoff to diagnose CH may vary from center to center, depending on timing of the sample and the assay used. Generally, in most screening programs, when the sample is obtained between day 3 and 5, threshold value of serum TSH for diagnosing CH is 20–25 mU/L.[8] For TSH measured on day 1, higher threshold value should be used.

Most NBS programs measure serum TSH. These programs may miss the diagnosis of central hypothyroidism. Therefore some centers, such as Northwest Regional Newborn Screening Program, Oregon, use T4 measurement as primary assay in their program.[17] It has been reported that about 5% of the newborns with CH are missed in NBS programs. This is often related to technical errors at various levels in the program. However, occasionally it may be related to delayed TSH response because of immaturity of hypothalamic-pituitary-thyroid axis. To overcome this, some NBS programs include both TSH and T4 measurements. This has shown to increase the detection rates of central hypothyroidism. Repeat testing at 2–6 weeks of age also has been shown to increase the detection rates.

Further Evaluation of the Newborn with Congenital Hypothyroidism

Neonates with positive screening test should be recalled as soon as possible and thoroughly evaluated. A detailed history including maternal history of autoimmunity should be obtained. Thorough examination should be performed together with further investigations. A venous sample from the newborn should be obtained. The diagnosis of CH is confirmed by measuring serum TSH and free T4 and/or total T4. In the neonatal period (2–6 weeks), serum T4 less than 6.4 µg/dl, serum free T4 less than 0.8 ng/dL, and serum TSH more than 10 mIU/L suggest CH.[8]

Infants diagnosed with CH should have the etiological workup. Commonly used modalities include ultrasound and thyroid scintigraphy. If there is no provision to get the scan done, treatment with thyroxine should not be delayed. In such situations etiological workup can be done after the age of 3 years when it is safe to stop thyroxine. Since availability of radioiodine 123 is often limited, technetium is frequently used for radioisotope scan. Technetium is trapped in the follicular cells but it is not organified. Presence of tracer uptake in an abnormal site is used to diagnose ectopic thyroid. Absence of tracer uptake suggests thyroid agenesis, but some neonates may have absent/poor uptake of radioisotope due to TSH receptor defect, iodide trapping defect, or because of maternal antibodies blocking TSH receptor. In such cases, thyroid ultrasound scan is useful to detect the presence of thyroid gland. Thyroid stimulating hormone receptor blocking antibodies also could be measured in the mother and newborn.

Measurement of thyroglobulin levels may be useful in some situations. A very low or absent thyroglobulin with absent uptake on nuclear scan suggests agenesis of thyroid gland. A low thyroglobulin level and normal radioisotope scan suggests a defect in thyroglobulin synthesis. Infants with thyroid dysgenesis have elevated thyroglobulin level.

TREATMENT

Treatment for CH should begin as soon as possible after the confirmation of diagnosis. The preferred thyroid hormone preparation to treat CH is L-thyroxine. The dose of thyroxine should normalize serum T4 as quickly as possible so that there is no irreversible damage to the developing brain. It is desirable to maintain free or total T4 in the upper normal range. To achieve this, initial thyroxine dose of 10–15 µg/kg/day is recommended. In some infants with CH, despite high normal T4, serum TSH may remain elevated for few months. Therefore, it is important to measure both serum TSH and free T4. After the first few weeks of treatment, TSH is a very reliable marker for titration of thyroxine dose.

Infants with transient CH may need to be treated if their T4 continues to be low with high TSH, beyond 2 weeks of age. Therapy could be discontinued after 8–12 weeks if thyroid function normalizes. Transient CH because of maternal TSH receptor blocking antibody also need to be treated if serum T4 levels are low. This condition resolves by 6 months as the antibodies undergo degradation by then.

Neonates with CH initially should have their biochemical thyroid profile repeated 2–4 weeks after starting treatment, every 1–2 months during the first 6 mounts of life, every 3–4 months between 6 months and 3 years of age, every 6–12 months thereafter until growth is complete.[18] Thyroid profiles should be repeated after 4 weeks when there is change in dose of thyroxine.

PROGNOSIS

Neonates with CH who are started on adequate treatment within the first 2 weeks of age tend to do well in term of IQ. Physical growth normalizes in most of the infants with CH. Intelligence quotient deficit has been reported in cases where there has been delay or inadequacy of treatment. Studies on outcome report up to 10% of patients with residual problems regarding neorodevelopmental delay despite early diagnosis.[19] It has been shown that patients with CH who are treated within 2 weeks of age with adequate thyroxine (>9.5 µg/kg/day) and maintain their free T4 in the upper normal range throughout infancy can achieve normal psychomotor development, irrespective of the severity of the disease.[3]

CONCLUSION

Congenital hypothyroidism is one of the commonest endocrine problems seen in newborns. Prompt diagnosis and initiation of treatment within 2 weeks of age generally leads to normal neurodevelopmental outcome. Even though NBS is universal in industrialized nations, developing countries are yet to adopt NBS as a routine. Scientists and medical professionals should work towards creating awareness about universal NBS for diagnosis of CH in newborns all over the world.

REFERENCES

1. Buyukgebiz A. Congenital hypothyroidism clinical aspects and late consequences. Pediatr Endocrinol Rev. 2003:1:185-90.
2. Jacobsen BB, Brandt NJ. Congenital hypothyroidism in Denmark: incidence, type of thyroid disorders, and age at onset of therapy in children. Arch Dis Child. 1981:56:134-6.

3. Bongers-Schokking, JJ, Koot, HM, Wiersma, D. Influence of timing and dose of thyroid hormone replacement on the development in infants with congenital ypothyroidism. J Pediatr. 2000;136:292-7.
4. Mitchell ML, Klein RZ. The sequelae of untreated maternal hypothyroidism. Eur J Endocrinol. 2004;151(Suppl 3):U45-8.
5. Hinton CF, Harris KB, Borgfeld L, Drummond-Borg M, Eaton R, Lorey F, et al. Trends in incidence rates of congenital hypothyroidism related to select demographic factors: data from the United States, California, Massachusetts, New York, and Texas. Pediatrics. 2010;125 Suppl (2):S37-47.
6. Chen CY, Lee KT, Lee CT, Lai WT, Huang YB. Epidemiology and Clinical Characteristics of Congenital Hypothyroidism in an Asian Population: A Nationwide Population-Based Study. J Epidemiol. 2013;23(2):85-94.
7. Albert BB, Cutfield WS, Webster D, Carll J, Derraik JG, Jefferies C, et al. Etiology of increasing incidence of congenital hypothyroidism in New Zealand from 1993–2010. J Clin Endocrinol Metab. 2012;97(9):3155-60.
8. Sperling M. Pediatric endocrinology. Elsevier Health Sciences; 2008.
9. DeFelice M, DiLauro R. Thyroid development and its disorders: Genetic and molecular mechanisms. Endocrine Rev. 2004;25:722.
10. Topaloglu AK. Athyreosis, dysgenesis, and dyshormonogenesis in congenital hypothyroidism.Pediatr Endocrinol Rev. 2006;3 Suppl 3:498-502.
11. Léger J, Marinovic D, Garel C, Bonaïti-Pellié C, Polak M, Czernichow P. Thyroid developmental anomalies in first degree relatives of children with congenital hypothyroidism. J Clin Endocrinol Metab. 2002;87(2):575-80.
12. Kumorowicz-Czoch M, Tylek-Lemanskaz D, Wyrobek L, Grodzicka T, Starzyk J. Thyroid developmental anomalies among first-degree relatives of children with thyroid dysgenesis and congenital hypothyroidism. J Pediatr Endocrinol Metab. 2012;25(5-6):413-8.
13. Sindhuja L, Dayal D, Sodhi KS, Sachdeva N, Bhattacharya A. Thyroid dysfunction and developmental anomalies in first degree relatives of children with thyroid dysgenesis. World J Pediatr. 2016;12(2):215-8.
14. van Tijn DA, de Vijlder JJ, Verbeeten Jr B, Verkerk PH, Vulsma T. Neonatal detection of congenital hypothyroidism of central origin. J Clin Endocrinol Metab. 2005;90(6):3350-9.
15. Brown RS, Bellisario RL, Botero D, Fournier L, Abrams CA, Cowger ML, et al. Incidence of transient congenital hypothyroidism due to maternal thyrotropin receptor-blocking antibodies in over one million babies. J Clin Endocrinol Metab. 1996;81(3):1147-51.
16. Working Group on Neonatal Screening of the European Society for Paediatric Endocrinology. Revised guidelines for neonatal screening programmes for primary congenital hypothyroidism. Horm Res. 1999;52:49-52.
17. Hunter MK, Mandel SH, Sesser DE, Miyahira RS, Rien L, Skeels MR, et al. Follow-up of newborns with low thyroxine and nonelevated thyroid-stimulating hormone–screening concentrations: Results of the 20-year experience in the Northwest Regional Newborn Screening Program. J Pediatr. 1998;132(1):70-4.
18. American Academy of Pediatrics; Rose SR; Section on Endocrinology and Committee on Genetics, American Thyroid Association; Brown RS; Public Health Committee, Lawson Wilkins Pediatric Endocrine Society; Foley T, Kaplowitz PB, Kaye CI, Sundararajan S, Varma SK 2006 Update of newborn screening and therapy for congenital hypothyroidism. Update of newborn screening and therapy for congenital hypothyroidism. Pediatrics. 2006;117(6):2290-303.
19. Ng SM, Anand D, Weindling AM. High versus low dose of initial thyroid hormone replacement for congenital hypothyroidism. Cochrane Database Syst Rev. 2009;(1):CD006972.

CHAPTER 16

Sick Euthyroid Syndrome

Bipin K Sethi, Jayant V Kelwade, Harsh Y Parekh, Vaibhav V Dukle

INTRODUCTION

Increasing possibilities of measuring thyroid hormone with little or no clinical finding has created two distinct syndromes in thyroidology. In the ambulatory patients, subclinical hypothyroidism or thyrotoxicosis, and in critically ill, the nonthyroidal illness syndrome (NTIS). Critically ill patients have one or more features that can simulate overt thyroid dysfunction or the tests are ordered in an attempt to uncover significant contributor in a critically ill patient who is not well or not responding to treatment. Limited knowledge about exact pathophysiological mechanism, correlation with outcome, and no clear guidelines regarding treatment further obscure the condition. The authors reviewed the literature about pathophysiology of nonthyroidal illness, its correlation with morbidity and mortality, and the need for and treatment outcome.

CASE 1

A 42-year-old lady, recently diagnosed with type 2 diabetic on oral antidiabetic drugs, visited our clinic with the history of fever, weight loss (4 kg in 20 days), and palpitations.
Examination
- Febrile (102°F), pulse rate 120/min
- Grade 1 goiter present
- Tremors absent.

Investigation
- Fasting blood sugar: 370 mg/dL, post lunch blood sugar: 450 mg/dL
- Glycosylated hemoglobin: 9.8%
- Urine examination: plenty of pus cells
- Thyroid-stimulating hormone (TSH): 0.1 IU/mL (0.3– 5IU/mL)
- Thyroxine (T4): 6.3 g/dL (5–12g/dL)
- Triiodothyronine (T3) 0.33 ng/mL (0.6–2.1 ng/mL)
- Impression: Sick euthyroid syndrome or non-thyroidal illness
- Management: Observation with repeat thyroid profile after 8 weeks

Discussion
This lady presented with acute illness and had symptoms similar to hyperthyroidism of weight loss and palpitation. On evaluation, though her TSH was low, the T4 was normal while T3 was low which indicated sick euthyroid syndrome. Weight loss and palpitations were due to uncontrolled diabetes and presence of infection, respectively. She was managed with antibiotics and insulin with which she improved and her repeat thyroid profile was normal after 8 weeks. TSH: 0.76 IU/mL, T4: 10.3 g/dL, T3: 0.87 ng/mL

> **CASE 2**
> A 50-year-old postmenopausal female was admitted in intensive care unit (ICU) with lower respiratory tract infection with sepsis and shock. She was on dopamine. She was febrile with temperature of 101°F. Her pulse rate was 120/min and blood pressure was 100/70 mmHg. On routine evaluation she had:
> - TSH: 0.1 IU/mL (0.3–5IU/mL)
> - Total T3: 0.5 ng/mL (0.6–2.1 ng/mL)
> - Total T4: 3.0 g/dL (5–12g/dL)
> - Endocrinologist was called upon to rule out secondary (central) hypothyroidism
> - Random cortisol, follicle-stimulating hormone (FSH), and electrolytes were ordered and reported as:
>   - Random cortisol: 22.41 g/dL
>   - FSH: 78 IU/mL
>   - Na: 137 mEq/L
>   - K: 3.9 mEq/L
> - Impression: Sick euthyroid syndrome
>
> **Discussion**
> This 50-year-old lady had low T3, T4, and TSH level with normal cortisol suggesting secondary hypothyroidism but high FSH level (as is expected in menopause and appropriately high cortisol ruled out that possibility). Hence, diagnosis of sick euthyroid syndrome was made. She has fulminant course and succumbed to her illness with multiple organ failure. The low T4 in this instance was a marker of this outcome.

DEFINITION

Nonthyroidal illness refers to changes in the thyroid homeostasis during acute illness (Table 1). While the abnormalities of reverse T3, T4, and regulatory hormone TSH are varied, the common finding is a low T3 level; hence, it is also called as low T3 syndrome. Other name given to this condition is the sick euthyroid syndrome.[1]

TABLE 1: Thyroid hormonal changes during acute illness

Parameter	Observed changes	Possible causes
TRH	↓TRH	↓ Leptin ↑ Type 2 deiodinase
TSH	↓	↓ TRH Inhibition by cytokines
T3	Low	↓ Type 1 deiodinase, ↓ thyroxine-binding globuline Inhibitors of protein binding ↓ TRH, TSH
rT3	Acute illness: High Late illness: Normal/low	↑ Type 3 deiodinase ↓ T4, TSH
T4	Acute illness: Normal/increased Chronic illness: Decreased	↑ Type 1 deiodinase, binding inhibitors ↓ TRH, TSH
Thyroid receptors	Acute illness: Low Chronic illness: High	–
Tissue uptake	Low	–

T4, thyroxine; T3, triiodothyronine; rT3, reverse triiodothyronine; TSH, thyroid-stimulating hormone; TRH, thyrotropin-releasing hormone.

EPIDEMIOLOGY

Although very few and small sample size studies are there, low T3 is a consistent finding in all of them. Low T3 and, in particular, low T4 consistently is also associated with poor outcome. Different studies have showed prevalence of NTIS between 32 and 84%.[2-4]

In a study by Katharina Plikat et al.[2] involving patients in ICUs, 44.1% had low free T3 (FT3) levels indicating an NTIS, either with normal (23.6%) or reduced (20.5%) serum thyrotropin levels. Free T4 (FT4) was also reduced in 23.3%. The combination of low FT3 and FT4 correlated well with high Acute Physiology and Chronic Health II scores, mortality, length of hospital stay, and the need for mechanical ventilation.

Gomez et al.[3] evaluated NTIS in five groups of patients with acute severe bacterial infection (16 patients), acute myocardial infarction (22 patients), diabetic ketoacidosis (24 patients), nonketotic hyperosmolar decompensation (8 patients) and protein-calorie undernutrition (12 patients). They found similar results with low T3 in 57.3%, and low T4, FT4 and the FT4 index in 26.8, 20.7, and 10.9%, respectively. The level of reverse T3 (rT3) was increased in 39% of cases. The TSH level was normal in majority with few showing marginal suppression but none had TSH elevation.

In another small study on 100 critically ill patients, Loh et al.[4] observed altered thyroid function in 84% of the patients. The low T3 and the low T3 plus T4 accounted for 55 and 29% of the NTIS cases, respectively. They also observed significantly higher mortality in patients with NTIS as compared to the patients without NTIS (40% vs. 6%).

Zargar et al.[5] studied thyroid hormonal changes in acutely ill patient and followed them up to 24 weeks. Low T3 was most common finding (32.6% cases with acute illness and 20.6% cases of chronic illness). Interestingly, nearly 7% of patient showed increase in T4 levels. Although small variations in TSH were observed, average TSH level was normal.

PATHOPHYSIOLOGY

The exact mechanisms behind nonthyroidal illness are unclear and it is still controversial whether these changes are protectively designed to conserve energy or have a maladaptive response to the illness. Changes are observed at all levels of hypothalamic-pituitary-thyroid axis (HPT axis). The alterations in thyroid functions in early part of acute illness are mainly because of peripheral mechanisms while central mechanisms are operative later.

Hypothalamic-pituitary-thyroid Axis

Since TSH levels in most cases are normal, an inappropriate TSH response in face of low thyroid hormones has been taken as pointer toward suppressed HPT axis. While different mechanisms have been put forth, increased activity of type 2 deiodinase in brain appears to be most appealing.[6] Type 2 deiodinase is involved in synthesis of T3 in brain and its increased expression in acute stress can cause local increase in T3 at hypothalamic level with resultant decrease in thyrotropin-releasing hormone (TRH). This would lead to decrease expression of *TRH* gene and TRH messenger RNA at paraventricular nucleus documented in post mortem hypothalamic tissue of patients with sick euthyroid syndrome, lending credence to the role of TRH in NTIS.[7,8]

Increased cytokines [interleukin (IL)-1, IL-6, tumor necrosis factor-α] and drugs like dopamine and corticosteroid along with depressed level of leptin in acute illness, all have negative influence on TRH expression and can impair TRH and therefore TSH secretion.[9-12]

Thyroid-stimulating hormone levels vary with the stage of the illness. While it is usually normal in early part of disease, the level goes down during prolonged illness. In recovery phase, TSH level may go up temporarily due to reactivation of HPT axis due to the yet low T4 level and picture may appear as that of primary hypothyroidism.[13,14]

Triiodothyronine

As indicated earlier, low T3 is the most consistent finding in NTIS and this is on account of decreased conversion of T4 to T3 due to inhibition of the type 1 deiodinase.[15] Though it is not clear why type 1 deiodinase is specifically inhibited while there is increase activity of other deiodinases, it may be the adaptive response of chronically starved body to cut down the metabolism by decreasing T3 level to conserve energy. This may be because of circulating inhibitors of deiodinase activity like free fatty acids, cytokines such as tumor necrosis factor, interferon-α, NF-κ-B, and IL-6, and drugs (amiodarone, propranolol, glucocorticoids).[16] Selenium is required for activity of type 1 deiodinase and its deficiency may also be contributory.[17]

Isolated mild decrease in T3 level is usually observed in very mild NTIS and usually does not have any prognostic importance. With suppression of HPT axis and decrease in thyroxine-binding globulin (TBG), T3 levels decrease further along with decrease in T4 level which strongly point toward poor outcome.[18]

While low T3 is due to decreased neogenesis, decrease in T4 and T3 may also be due to displacement of T4 from its binding protein, so that it is rapidly metabolized.[19]

Thyroxine

The level of T4 varies and depends on the severity of acute illness. While it may be normal or more rarely increased in earlier part of disease, with increasing severity and duration of illness, the T4 levels fall.[20,21] This is mainly because of decrease in TBG in early part of disease and suppressed secretion of TRH or TSH later.[20] Under normal circumstance less than 0.05% of the hormone circulates unbound (free) in plasma, while rest is attached to globulin, albumin, and transthyretin. In NTIS, thyroid hormone-binding protein levels decease as a result of decreased synthesis, increased breakdown and movement of protein from plasma, contributing to the decrease in the thyroid hormone level.[22,23] Rapid metabolism of T4 displaced from the binding proteins may also contribute to the lower T4 levels (vide supra).

Free Thyroxine

The levels of FT4 depends upon the type of assay and analytical methods used, and values differ in different methods.[24,25] Although majority shows depressed level, it may be elevated or normal in early part of disease. With downregulation of HPT axis, FT4 eventually becomes low.[26]

Reverse Triiodothyronine

Changes in rT3 in NTIS are nonspecific and the level is governed by the ambient T4 level. While its level increases in early part of disease due to increased activity of type 3 deiodinase, they fall later in parallel with the decrease in the T4 level and rT3 level also reduces.[22]

Thyroid Hormone Receptors and Metabolism

Thyroid hormone act by binding to thyroid receptors. There are three types of thyroid hormone receptors (THRs)—THRa1, THRb1, and THRb2—all bind to T3 with similar affinity and has equal transactional activity. In NTIS, with decrease in T3 level, THR gets downregulated as evident in recent studies on mice treated with lipopolysaccharide or cytokines and patients with septic shock.[27,28] In another study on the rabbit model with prolonged (7 days) burn injury by Mebis et al.,[29] THRs were found unchanged. Thus, in early stage of acute illness, THR gets down regulated while in prolonged illness, it may be normal or increased.

Role of Cytokines

Various cytokines including IL-1β, soluble IL-2 receptor (sIL-2R), IL-6 and tumor necrosis factor-α, and hypoxia-induced changes in metabolites can cause decrease in thyroid hormonal levels. This is due to central inhibition of TRH secretion with direct suppression of TSH as well.[30] However, infusion of antagonists against these cytokines failed to increase the depressed T3, T4, and TSH in an experiment by van der Poll et al. questioning their role in NTIS.[31]

Correlation with Morbidity and Mortality

Different studies have indicated that low T3 and T4 strongly correlate with poor outcomes and mortality. The possibility of death was found to be about 50% with T4 less than 4 µg/dL and it increased further to 80% with lower T4 (<2 µg/dL).[32]

Giorgio Iervasi et al.[33] studied 573 consecutive cardiac patients admitted to hospital and followed them for over 1 year. Those with low T3 level had significantly higher mortality compared to their counterparts with normal T3 level. Low FT3 was most important risk factor for cumulative death. Similar findings were reported by Pingitore[34] on 281 patients with ischemic and nonischemic dilated cardiomyopathy; low FT3 was found to be an independent risk factor for increased mortality and heart failure.

Michael[18] studied 86 patients hospitalized in an ICU. They observed decreased thyroid hormone levels with normal TSH in 22% of the patients. They observed increased mortality correlating with T4 levels; mortality being 84, 50, and 15% in patients with T4 levels less than 3 µg/dL, 3–5 µg/dL and more than 5 µg/dL, respectively.

Other randomized clinical trials involving patients with multiple trauma,[35] bone marrow transplantation,[36] elderly (undergoing surgery),[37] and children (with meningococcal septicemia treated with dopamine)[38] have drawn similar conclusions.

Should Nonthyroidal Illness be Treated?

Significant association between low T3 and T4 level and poor clinical outcome have led to attempts of correcting these thyroid hormonal abnormalities with the hope of improving the clinical outcomes.

In this context, Brent and Hershman[39] supplemented patients having T4 less than 5 µg/dL admitted in ICU with thyroxin intravenously for 2 weeks. Thyroxine and FT4 levels increased significantly on day 3 of treatment and were normalized by day 5. Surprisingly, T3 recovered earlier in untreated patients (7 days vs. 10 days). No significant mortality benefit was observed with this intervention. In another study by Acker et al.,[40] who supplemented patients of acute renal failure with thyroxine, T4 and TSH got normalized promptly but mortality increased in treated group (43% vs. 13%) and this correlated with the decrease in TSH level.

Since the lack of benefit with T4 supplement could be attributed to the persistently low level of T3; attempts have been made to directly supplement T3. Klemperer et al.[21] studied the effect of T3 supplementation in coronary artery bypass patients with low T3 level. While T3 supplementation normalized T3 levels in these patients and also augmented cardiac output reducing the need for pressor support, again there was no mortality benefit. Effect of thyroid replacement on cardiac function in a patient of heart failure, cardiac transplant, and coronary artery bypass were studied in many small trials and have been reviewed by Farwell.[41]

Becker et al.[42] tried T3 in burn patients but failed to show any mortality benefits. Acker et al.[43] in their follow-up study supplement their postrenal transplant acute tubular necrosis patient with T3 in hope of fasten recovery but did not show the results.

A novel approach is giving continuous infusion of intravenous TRH that increases TSH as well as T4 and T3 levels. Van den Berghe et al.[44] studied the effect of continuous infusion of TRH in critically ill patient over two nights and observed increase in TSH (twofold), T4 (40-54%) and in T3 (52-116%) while rT3 level remains same. It may be more physiological method of treatment rather than supplementing individual hormones. However, TRH has been withdrawn and is not available for clinical use.

Although low T3 and T4 in NTIS significantly correlates with poor clinical outcomes, and there are various options for correcting these, interventions which supplement thyroid hormone do not show any significant benefit in terms of clinical outcome, except in cardiac patients where it showed some improvement in heart failure. On the contrary, some may have detrimental effect on final outcome.

INVESTIGATIONS AND DIAGNOSIS

In view of the foregoing, thyroid function test should not be done as a routine in all critically ill patients until there is a high suspicion for hypo- or hyperthyroidism. Thyroid stimulating hormone along with T3 and T4 should be ordered as only TSH may not provide correct information. While high TSH level points toward probable permanent hypothyroidism, low TSH with increased T4 and T3 level would indicate hyperthyroidism. Decrease in T4 and T3 and increase in rT3 level with low TSH make the diagnosis of NTIS.

Appropriate cortisol rise and elevated gonadotropins in postmenopausal patient would suggest against central hypothyroidism. Detailed drug history including those of dopamine, corticosteroid, dilatin, and aspirin should be asked as they may cause decrease in thyroid hormone levels.

Whom to Treat and How to Treat?

This is a controversial topic, and experts differ in their opinions. In general, treatment should be restricted to those with very low T4 level (<4 μg/dL) and should possibly include both T4 and T3 supplementation. Triiodothyronine should be given in replacement dose of 50 μg/day and increased up to 75 μg/day in early part of the disease for rapid normalization of hormonal levels. Thyroxine and T3 levels should be kept at lower normal range and frequently monitored (every 48 h). Once it normalizes, doses can be tapered gradually.[45]

Since cardiac patient with decrease in left ventricular ejection fraction below 45% have been shown to derive benefit with supplementation of thyroid hormone, they should also be supplemented likewise.

LONG-TERM FOLLOW-UP

With recovery from illness, serum TSH and thyroid hormone concentrations eventually return to normal. In initial part of recovery, TSH level may go up and usually represents recovery of HPT axis and should not be treated with thyroid hormone supplement. In general, T3 and T4 take longer time than TSH to recover, suggesting that recovery of HPT axis is essential for the normalization of thyroid hormones.

Hamblin et al.[46] followed 60 patients of burns, septicemia, and acute renal failure. Thyroxine got normalized in all patients who survived and usually preceded by rise in TSH level. Similarly, findings are observed by Zargar et al.[5] who followed patient with sick euthyroid syndrome over 24 weeks. In their study, TSH rose temporarily above normal during early recovery while T3 and T4 took longer time to recover. Triiodothyronine and T4 continued to be low at 3 weeks even when clinical recovery had taken place; T3 continued to be low even at 6 months.

CONCLUSION

Abnormalities in thyroid axis are common in acute illness. These abnormalities are varied and depend on degree, type of stress, and timing of the sample, although low T3 is the most consistent finding. While low T3 and T4 have prognostic implications, they are of little therapeutic value, and it is not advisable to perform thyroid function tests routinely in sick patients until there is compelling indication to do them. Evidence for benefit by intervention is small and restricted to a small subset of patients. Finally, while the contributions of NTIS to patient care and outcome is questionable, it has inadvertently added to our understanding of thyroid homeostasis.

REFERENCES

1. Wartofsky L, Burman KD. Alterations in thyroid function in patients with systemic illness: the "Euthyroid sick syndrome". Endocr Review 1982;3:164-217.
2. Plikat K, Langgartner J, Buettner R, Bollheimer LC, Woenckhaus U, Schölmerich J, et al. Frequency and outcome of patients with nonthyroidal illness syndrome in a medical intensive care unit. Metabolism. 2007;56:239-44.
3. Gomez JM, Virgili N, Navarrom A, Roca M, Moutana E, Soler J. Study of thyroid function parameters and thyrotropin in general nonthyroid disease. Med Clin (Barc). 1989;91:5-9.
4. Loh KC, Eng PC. Prevalence and prognostic relevance of sick euthyroid syndrome in a medical intensive care unit. Ann Acad Med Singapore. 1995;24:802-6.
5. Zargar AH, Ganie MA, Masoodi SR, Laway BA, Bashir MI, Wani AI, et al. Prevalence and pattern of sick euthyroid syndrome in acute and chronic non-thyroidal illness—its relationship with severity and outcome of the disorder. J Assoc Physicians India. 2004;52:27-31.
6. Coppola A, Liu ZW, Andrews ZB, Paradis E, Roy MC, Friedman JM, et al. A central thermogenic-like mechanism in feeding regulation: an interplay between arcuate nucleus T3 and UCP2. Cell Metab. 2007;5:21-33.
7. Fliers E, Guldenaar SE, Wiersinga WM, Swaab DF. Decreased hypothalamic thyrotropin-releasing hormone gene expression in patients with nonthyroidal illness. J Clin Endocrinol Metab. 1997;82:4032-6.
8. Fliers E, Alkemade A, Wiersinga WM, Swaab DF. Hypothalamic thyroid hormone feedback in health and disease. Prog Brain Res. 2006;153:189-207.
9. Hermus RM, Sweep CG, van der Meer MJ, Ross HA, Smals AG, Benraad TJ, et al. Continuous infusion of interleukin-1 beta induces a non-thyroidal illness syndrome in the rat. Endocrinology. 1992;131:2139-46.

10. Spencer C, Eigen A, Shen D, Duda M, Qualls S, Weiss S, et al. Specificity of sensitive assays of thyrotropin (TSH) used to screen for thyroid disease in hospitalized patients. Clin Chem. 1987;33:1391-6.
11. Brabant G, Brabant A, Ranft U, Ocran K, Köhrle J, Hesch RD, et al. Circadian and pulsatile thyrotropin secretion in euthyroid man under the influence of thyroid hormone and glucocorticoid administration. J Clin Endocrinol Metab. 1987;65:83-8.
12. Blake NG, Eckland DJ, Foster OJ, Lightman SL. Inhibition of hypothalamic thyrotropin-releasing hormone messenger ribonucleic acid during food deprivation. Endocrinology. 1991;129:2714-8.
13. Spencer CA. Clinical utility and cost-effectiveness of sensitive thyrotropin assays in ambulatory and hospitalized patients. Mayo Clin Proc. 1988;63:1214-22.
14. Stockigt JR. Guidelines for diagnosis and monitoring of thyroid disease: nonthyroidal illness. Clin Chem. 1996;42:188-192.
15. Kaplan MM. Subcellular alterations causing reduced hepatic thyroxine-53-monodeiodinase activity in fasted rats. Endocrinology. 1979;104:58-64.
16. Jakobs TC, Mentrup B, Schmutzler C, Dreher I, Kohrle J. Proinflammatory cytokines inhibit the expression and function of human type I 5'-deiodinase in HepG2 hepatocarcinoma cells. Eur J Endocrinol. 2002;146:559-66.
17. Berger MM, Reymond MJ, Shenkin A, Rey F, Wardle C, Cayeux C, et al. Influence of selenium supplements on the post-traumatic alterations of the thyroid axis: a placebo-controlled trial. Intensive Care Med. 2001;27:91-100.
18. Slag MF, Morley JE, Elson MK, Crowson TW, Nettle FQ, Shafer RB. Hyperthyroxinemia in critically ill patients as a predictor of high mortality. JAMA. 1981;245:43-5.
19. Mendel CM, Laufhton CW, McMahon FA, Cavalieri RR. Inability to detect an inhibitor of thyroxine-serum protein binding in sera from patients with nonthyroidal illness. Metabolism. 1991;40:491-502.
20. Warner MH, Beckett GJ. Mechanisms behind the non-thyroidal illness syndrome: an update. J Endocrinol. 2010;205:1-13.
21. Klemperer JD, Klein I, Gomez M, Helm RE, Ojamaa K, Thomas SJ, et al. Thyroid hormone treatment after coronary-artery bypass surgery. N Engl J Med. 1995;333:1522-7.
22. Afandi B, Schussler GC, Arafeh AH, Boutros A, Yap MG, Finkelstein A. Selective consumption of thyroxine-binding globulin during cardiac bypass surgery. Metabolism. 2000;49:270-4.
23. Peeters RP, Wouters PJ, Kaptein E, van Toor H, Visser TJ, Van den Berghe G. Reduced activation and increased inactivation of thyroid hormone in tissues of critically ill patients. J Clin Endocrinol Metab. 2003;88:3202-11.
24. Kaptein EM, MacIntyre SS, Weiner JM, Spencer CA, Nicoloff JT. Free thyroxine estimates in nonthyroidal illness: comparison of eight methods. J Clin Endocrinol Metab. 1981;52:1073-7.
25. Nelson JC, Weiss RM. The effect of serum dilution on free thyroxine concentration in the low T4 syndrome of nonthyroidal illness. J Clin Endocrinol Metab. 1985;61:239-46.
26. Beckett GJ. Thyroid function and thyroid function tests in non-thyroidal illness. CPD Bulletin: Clin Biochem. 2006;7:107-16.
27. Beigneux AP, Moser AH, Shigenaga JK, Grunfeld C, Feingold KR. Sick euthyroid syndrome is associated with decreased TR expression and DNA binding in mouse liver. Am J Physiol Endocrinol Metab. 2003;284:E228-36.
28. Rodriguez-Perez A, Palos-Paz F, Kaptein E, Visser TJ, Dominguez-Gerpe L, Alvarez-Escudero J, et al. Identification of molecular mechanisms related to nonthyroidal illness syndrome in skeletal muscle and adipose tissue from patients with septic shock. Clin Endocrinol (Oxf). 2008;68:821-7.
29. Mebis L, Debaveye Y, Ellger B, Derde S, Ververs EJ, Langouche L, et al. Changes in the centralcomponent of the hypothalamus-pituitary-thyroid axis in a rabbit model of prolonged critical illness. Crit Care. 2009;13:R147.
30. Cannon JG, Tompkins RG, Gelfand JA, Michie HR, Stanford GG, van der Meer JW, et al. Circulating interleukin-1 and tumor necrosis factor in septic shock and experimental endotoxin fever. J Infect Dis. 1990;161:79-84.
31. van der Poll T, Van Zee KJ, Endert E, Coyle SM, Stiles DM, Pribble JP, et al. Interleukin-1 receptor blockade does not affect endotoxin-induced changes in plasma thyroid hormone and thyrotropin concentrations in man. J Clin Endocrinol Metab. 1995;80:1341-6.
32. Maldonado LS, Murata GH, Hershman JM, Braunstein GD. Do thyroid function tests independently predict survival in the critically ill? Thyroid. 1992;2:119-23.
33. Iervasi G, Molinaro S, Landi P, Taddei MC, Galli E, Mariani F, et al. Association between increased mortality and mild thyroid dysfunction in cardiac patients. Arch Intern Med. 2007;167:1526-32.
34. Pingitore A, Landi P, Taddei MC. Ripoli A, L'Abbate A, Iervasi G. Triiodothyronine levels for risk stratification of patients with chronic heart failure. Am J Med. 2005;118:132-6.
35. Schilling JU, Zimmermann T, Albrecht S, Zwipp H, Saeger HD. Low T3 syndrome in multiple trauma patients—a phenomenon or important pathogenetic factor? Med Klin (Munich). 1999;94 Suppl 3:66-9.
36. Schulte C, Reinhardt W, Beelen D, Mann K, Schaefer U. Low T3-syndrome and nutritional status as prognostic factors in patients undergoing bone marrow transplantation, Bone Marrow Transplant. 1998;22:1171-8.

37. Girvent M, Maestro S, Hernandez R, Carajol I, Monné J, Sancho JJ, et al. Euthyroid sick syndrome, associated endocrine abnormalities, and outcome in elderly patients undergoing emergency operation. Surgery. 1998;123:560-7.
38. den Brinker M, Joosten KF, Visser TJ, Hop WC, de Rijke YB, Hazelzet JA, et al. Euthyroid sick syndrome in meningococcal sepsis: the impact of peripheral thyroid hormone metabolism and binding proteins. J Clin Endocrinol Metab. 2005;90:5613-20.
39. Brent GA, Hershman JM. Thyroxine therapy in patients with severe nonthyroidal illnesses and lower serum thyroxine concentration, J Clin Endocrinol Metab. 1986;63:1-8.
40. Acker CG, Singh AR, Flick RP, Bernardini J, Greenberg A, Johnson JP. A trial of thyroxine in acute renal failure. Kidney Int. 2000;57:293-8.
41. Farwell AP. Thyroid hormone therapy is not indicated in the majority of patients with the sick euthyroid syndrome. Endocr Pract. 2008;14:1180-7.
42. Becker RA, Vaughan GM, Ziegler MG, Seraile LG, Goldfarb IW, Mansour EH, et al. Hyper-metabolic low triiodothyronine syndrome of burn injury. Crit Care Med. 1982;10:870-5.
43. Acker CG, Flick R, Shapiro R, Scantlebury VP, Jordan ML, Vivas C, et al. Thyroid hormone in the treatment of post-transplant acute tubular necrosis (ATN). Am J Transplant. 2002;2:57-61.
44. Van den Berghe G, de Zegher F, Baxter RC, Veldhuis JD, Wouters P, Schetz M, et al. Neuroendocrinology of prolonged critical illness: effects of exogenous thyrotropin releasing hormone and its combination with growth hormone secretagogues. J Clin Endocrinol Metab. 1998;83:309-19.
45. De Groot LJ. Non-thyroidal illness syndrome: A form of hypothyroidism. In: De Groot LJ, Jameson JL (Eds). Endocrinology Adult and Pediatric, 7th edition. Philadelphia: Elsevier; 2016. pp. 1557-69.
46. Hamblin PS, Dyer SA, Mohr VS, Le Grand BA, Lim CF, Tuxen DV, et al. Relationship between thyrotropin and thyroxine changes during recovery from severe hypothyroxinemia of critical illness. J Clin Endocrinol Metab. 1986;62:717-22.

INDEX

Page numbers followed by *f* refer to figure and *t* refer to table

A

Addison disease 151-153
Adenocarcinoma 28
Adenoma 27
  follicular 107
  toxic 12, 72, 74, 94
Adenovirus 53
Agranulocytosis 14
Alanine transaminase 54
Allan-Herndon-Dudley syndrome 125, 176
Alopecia 1, 83, 151, 152
Alzheimer's disease 66
Amenorrhea 1
American Thyroid Association's risk scoring system 34*t*
Aminoglutethimide 148
Amiodarone 148, 155, 174
Anemia 157
  aplastic 14
  hemolytic 148
  pernicious 83, 151, 152
Ankle jerks 1
Antibodies
  anti-insulin 14
  anti-thyroglobulin 106
  maternal 174
Antithyroid
  agents 23
  antibodies 67, 79, 80, 82, 104, 108, 149, 152
  peroxidase 106
  drugs 6, 13, 16, 23, 126, 148
APGAR score 172
Aplasia 174
Arthralgias 54
Aspartate transaminase 54
Atrial fibrillation 73
Autoimmune encephalitis 151
Autoimmune polyglandular syndromes 148, 151, 152
Azathioprine 142

B

Bacterial infection 51
Ballet sign 137
Benzodiazepines 155
Bethesda scoring system 35, 35*t*
Biopsy 162
Body mass index 5, 15
Bone 116
  metastasis 46
  mineral density 71
Borrelia burgdorferi 150
Boston's sign 137
Bradycardia 158
Breast imaging reporting and data system 33, 90

C

Calcitonin 106
Carbimazole 13, 14
Carcinoma
  follicular 39, 102, 107
  medullary 28
  mucoepithelial 28
  papillary 37
Cardiac dysrhythmia 83*b*
Carotid 87
  artery, internal 88*f*
Carpenter syndrome 152
Celiac disease 151, 152
Cell membrane thyroid hormone transport defects 120
Central nervous system 4, 65, 73, 116
Cerebrospinal fluid 151
Cervical lymph node 91*f*
Chemosis 140
Chromosomal syndromes 148
Cold nodule 96*f*
Collier's sign 137
Congestive heart failure 83
Cowden's syndrome 29

Coxsackievirus 150
Craniopharyngioma 148
C-reactive protein 55
Cyclophosphamide 142
Cyclosporine 142
Cystinosis 148
Cysts
    ovarian 3
    thyroglossal 109
Cytokines, role of 186
Cytomegalovirus 53
Cytotoxic T-cell activation 143

D

Dalrymple's sign 137
De Quervain's thyroiditis 51, 52, 57
Dementia 83
Depression 65
Diabetes 4, 83, 131
    mellitus 148, 151, 152
Diiodotyrosine 153, 175
Dopamine 155
Down syndrome 148, 151, 152, 164
Drug-induced hypersensitivity syndrome 53
Dysgenesis 148, 174
Dyshormonogenesis 148, 156, 174, 175
Dyslipidemia 81
Dysphagia 165
Dyspnea 165
Dysthyroid optic neuropathy 134, 137

E

Ectodermal dysplasia 152
Ectopia 174
Ectopic thyroid 148, 162*f*, 167*f*
    tissue 95
Edematous facial appearance 167*f*
Epiphyseal dysgenesis 161
Epstein-Barr virus 53
Erythrocyte sedimentation rate 52, 55
Euthyroid ophthalmopathy 134, 136
Euthyroid sick syndrome 148
External beam radiation therapy 43

F

Familial adenomatous polyposis 29
Farnsworth-Munsll panel detects 137
Fatigue 54, 66
Fetal growth retardation 24
Fibrosarcoma 28

Fine needle aspiration cytology 27, 34, 56, 87, 91, 92*f*, 93, 104, 106, 107
Fluorodeoxyglucose positron emission tomography 32, 98*f*, 99*f*, 101
Follicle stimulating hormone 46
Foramen cecum 173
Free thyroxine 6, 126, 129, 163, 185
Free triiodothyronine 6, 126
Furosemide 155

G

Galactorrhea 3, 157
Giant cell 53
    multinuclear 56
    thyroiditis 51
Gifford's sign 137
Glasgow Coma Scale 2
Glucocorticoids 130, 155
Glycosaminoglycan 135
Glycosylated hemoglobin 4, 182
Goiter 51, 118, 150, 154, 158, 165*f*
    chronic lymphocytic 148
    endemic 148, 153
    euthyroid 148
    fetal 24
    multinodular 94, 94*f*, 104, 105, 120
    staging of 159
    toxic 108
Goitrogens 154
Gonadotropins 5
Graves' disease 10-17, 23, 24, 29, 32, 54, 56, 74, 96*f*, 102, 120, 128, 130, 134, 136, 150
Graves' hyperthyroidism 24
Graves' ophthalmopathy 15, 16, 134
Graves' orbitopathy 143
Graves' thyrotoxicosis 10, 17, 102

H

Hashimoto's encephalopathy 151
Hashimoto's thyroiditis 2, 27, 51, 147, 150, 156, 157, 162
Hashitoxicosis 150
Head trauma 148
Helicobacter pylori 150
Helper T-cell proliferation 143
Hemithyroidectomy 109
Hepatic injury 14
Hepatitis
    cholestatic 14
    toxic 14
Hirschberg principle 140

Histiocytosis 148
Human chorionic gonadotropin 12, 20, 53, 72
Human herpes viruses 53
Human immunodeficiency virus 53, 150
Human leukocyte antigen 51, 135, 149
Hurthle cell 37
    neoplasm 37
Hydrops fetalis 24
Hyperemesis gravidarum 22
Hyperglycemia 143
Hyperplasia, glandular 27
Hyperprolactinemia 5, 157
Hyperreflexia 11
Hypertension 11, 131, 143
Hyperthyroidism 11, 12, 17, 22, 24, 59, 150
    endogenous subclincal 75
    euthyroid 24
    exogenous subclinical 75
    fetal 24
    gestational 24
    primary 12
    secondary 12
    subclinical 71, 72t, 73, 76t
    treatment of 83
Hyperthyrotropinemia 164
Hyperthyroxinemia, familial dysalbuminemic 126
Hypertrophy, pseudomuscular 3
Hypoglycemia 14, 158
Hypoosmolar euvolemic hyponatremia 3
Hypoplasia 148, 174
Hypoprothrombinemia 14
Hypothalamic disorders 148
Hypothalamic pituitary
    gonadal axis 5
    hypothyroidism 174
    region, inflammatory disorders of 3
    thyroid axis 151, 116, 184
Hypothyroidism 1, 3-6, 8, 59, 65, 66, 68, 72, 147-150, 154, 161, 174
    acquired 148, 157, 158t
    autoimmune 118, 150
    central 74, 148, 156, 158, 164, 174, 176
    congenital 148, 153, 157, 158t, 162, 167f, 172, 174, 178, 178f, 179
    diagnosis 5
    drug-induced 148
    etiology 3
    juvenile 147, 148, 156, 163
    management of 21
    neonatal 65, 172
    overt 3, 20, 80
    pituitary 176
    presentation 3
    prevalence of 19
    primary 1f, 3, 6, 158, 166, 158t, 174
    secondary 2f, 3, 6t, 149, 156
    subclinical 3, 6, 21, 66, 67, 77-80, 80t, 83, 84t, 85, 150, 151, 164
    symptoms of 158
    tertiary 149
    treatment 6
Hypothyroxinemia 164

I

Infections 148
Infertility 3
Inflammatory disorders 148
Influenza virus A, B 53
Iodide transport, defect of 174, 175
Iodine
    deficiency 3, 148, 153, 154, 174
    diseases, spectrum of 154t
    disorder 158, 159
    excess 154
Iodotyrosine deiodinase, deficiency of 175

J

Jendrassik's sign 137
Joffroy's sign 137
Juvenile hypothyroidism 148, 156
    causes of 148b

K

Kinase inhibitor therapy 47
Klinefelter syndrome 148, 151
Knies' sign 137
Kocher's sign 137
Kocher-Debre-Semelaigne syndrome 3, 157

L

Leukemia 148
Levator muscle 136
Levothyroxine 5, 21, 119
Levotriiodothyronine suppression test 120
Lithium 148
Lobectomy plus isthmectomy 109
Longus coli muscles 87
Lugol's iodine 109
Lugol's solution 109
Lymphoma 28

M

Madarosis 1
Malaise 54
Marcus Gunn pupil 137
McCune-Albright syndrome 12
Memory loss 66
Meningioma 148
Meningoencephalitis 148
Mental retardation 1, 158
Metastatic disease, management of 45
Methimazole 13, 148, 174
Methotrexate 142
Minimally invasive, video-assisted thyroidectomy 110
Mobius sign 137
Modified American Thyroid Association 2009 risk stratification 41*t*
Monoiodotyrosine 153, 175
Muller's muscle 136
Muscles
  sternocleidomastoid 87
  weakness 11
Muscular hypertrophy 157
Myalgias 54
Myxedematous syndrome 159

N

Neck pain 55
Necrotizing enterocolitis 176
Neoplasm, follicular 35, 37
Newborn screening 172, 178
Nocardia asteroides 58
Nodular thyroid disease 54
Nodules 93
  autonomous 97*f*
  functional status of 94
  multiple 94*f*
  rapid growth of 31
Nonsteroidal anti-inflammatory drugs 56
Nonthyroidal illness syndrome 148, 156, 182
Noonan syndrome 151

O

Obesity 5
Ophthalmopathy, thyroid associated 139*t*, 140*t*
Opiates 155
Orbital radiotherapy 144
Orbitopathy, thyroid associated 134, 135, 137*t*, 140-142, 144
Ovarian masses 165*f*, 166

P

Pancreatitis 14
Panhypopituitarism 174
Papillary thyroid
  cancer 28, 40, 41
  microcarcinoma 40, 41
Papilledema 137
Paranoid schizophrenia 65
Pendred syndrome 175
  prevalence of 175
Peroxidase system defects 175
Phenobarbitone 148, 155
Phenytoin 148
Pituitary hormone deficiencies 158
Polyendocrinopathy, autoimmune 152
Polyserositis 3
Polyuria 158
Povidone iodine 155*t*
Pregnancy 22, 25, 128
Propranolol 130, 155
Propylthiouracil 13, 130, 148, 174
Pseudogiant cell 51
Psychiatric disorders 83
Psychosis, steroid-induced 143

R

Radiation 28
  safety precautions 99
  thyroiditis 59
Radioactive iodine 28, 41, 104
  refractory 46
  therapy 42
Radioiodine 17, 148
  ablation 14
Recurrent laryngeal nerve 105, 158
Regional lymph nodes 158, 164
Retroviruses 150
Riedel's thyroiditis 51, 60

S

Sarcoidosis 148
Schizophrenia 66
Schmidt syndrome 152
Sheehan's syndrome 2, 2*f*
Sistrunk's operation 109
Snellen-Rieseman's sign 137
Sodium iodide symporter 30, 149
Solitary nodule 96*f*, 97*f*, 107
Spongiform nodules 35
Squamous cell epidermoid carcinoma 28

Index

Stellwag's sign 137
Stereotactic body radiotherapy 45
Steroid therapy 56
Strabismus 140
Strain tissue elastography image 92*f*
Stromal cells 116
Struma granulomatosa 51
Struma ovarii 12
Suker's sign 137
Sulfonamides 155
Superior laryngeal nerve 105
Surgery 16, 38, 104

T

Tachycardia 11, 24
Tanner stage 1
Thalassemia 148
Thalidomide 148
Thelarche 165*f*
Thionamides 19, 23
Thrombocytopenia 14
Thyroglobulin 55, 163
   serum 106
   synthesis
      abnormalities 174
      defect of 175
Thyroid 87, 155
   abscess 54
   antibodies 19
   autoantibodies 5, 160
   biopsy of 162
   cancer 28, 32, 38, 40, 44, 46, 47, 89, 108
      follicular 29, 33, 40, 41
         staging of 96
   carcinoma 28, 29, 40*t*, 158*t*
   destruction, causes of 12
   disease 10, 88, 106
      autoimmune 3, 20, 24, 61, 83, 148, 149, 151, 152, 164, 168
   disorder 19, 25, 104, 124, 152
   dysfunction 82, 126, 155, 168, 176
      subclinical 83
   dysgenesis 161
   dyshormonogenesis 175
   enlargement 158
   function test 3, 6*t*, 20, 106, 108, 124, 126*f*
   gland 12, 27, 33, 51, 72, 90, 95*f*, 100, 100*f*, 101f, 155, 158, 159, 164, 165
      agenesis of 162*f*
      fetal 82
   normal 88*f*
   palpation of 157
   radioiodine ablation of 3
   hormone 3, 4, 12, 22, 65, 67, 115, 116, 118, 119, 121, 124, 127, 147, 159, 186
      cell membrane transport defects 121
      levels 164
      maternal 19
      metabolism defect 120, 121
      receptor 116, 116*t*, 117, 117*f*, 125, 186
      replacement 112
      resistance 115, 120, 174
      response element 116, 117
      transport 174, 176
   illness 80, 124
   infection, chronic 59
   lesions, benign 90*f*
   neoplasms 29
   nodule 25, 27, 28, 31, 32*t*, 34, 57, 161
      classification of 28*t*
   peroxidase 51, 77, 83
      antibodies 53, 55
   receptor 183
      antibodies 23
      blocking antibody 177
   removal of 148
   scintigraphy 91
   solitary nodule of 27
   status, fetal 24
   stimulating hormone 6, 10, 12, 19-21, 24, 30, 32, 55, 74, 77, 78, 80, 82, 82*f*, 83, 97, 106, 115, 126, 147, 159, 160, 163, 174, 176, 182, 183
      deficiency 174
      measurement 129
      receptor 19, 28, 174
      secreting pituitary tumor 119
   suppression 36
   surgery 83, 111, 148
   surgical problems of 109
   swellings, management of 113
   tissue 94, 98*f*
   ultrasonography of 161
Thyroidectomy 16, 38
   complications of 111
   subtotal 109
   total 105, 109
Thyroiditis 6, 12, 51, 52, 59, 72, 92, 95*f*, 151
   acute infectious 58
   atrophic 150
   autoimmune 153, 156*f*, 158*t*

causes of 59
chronic
   autoimmune 59
   lymphocytic 53
infectious 51, 58
lymphocytic 51
nonsuppurative 51
painful 52
   subacute 51, 52
painless 51, 59
postpartum 24, 54, 55, 60, 61
recurrence of 57
secondary 51
subacute 12, 51, 53, 57, 72
suppurative 51
trauma induced 59
Thyroperoxidase 149, 163
Thyrotoxicosis 11, 12, 17, 72
   causes of 12
   gestational 12
   signs of 11
   symptoms of 55
Thyrotropin releasing hormone 3, 19, 119, 163, 183
   deficiency 148, 174
   stimulation test 120, 160
Thyroxine 6, 19, 55, 69, 83, 159, 163, 182, 183, 185
   binding globulin 20, 185
   therapy 44, 84
TNM staging system 39
Topolanski's sign 137
Toxic multinodular goiter 12, 71, 72, 74
Toxoplasmosis 148
Trachea 87, 88
Tracheostomy 105
Triiodothyronine 19, 55, 83, 117, 124, 159, 163, 182, 183, 185
   measurement 129
   toxicosis 14
Tubercles of Zuckerkandl 105
Tuberculosis 148
Tumors 148
   metastatic 28
   suppressor genes 31
Turner syndrome 148, 151, 152
Tyrosine kinase inhibitors 126

V

Valproate 148
Van Wyk Grumbach syndrome 3, 157, 165f, 166
Vasculitis 14
Video-assisted thyroidectomy 110
Vigouroux sign 137
Vitamin
   A deficiency 154
   D supplement 112
Vitiligo 151
von Graefe's sign 137

W

Wilder's sign 137
Williams syndrome 148
Wolff-Chaikoff effect 154

Y

Yersinia *enterocolitica* 150

Z

Zinc deficiency 154